ADULT AND FAMILY NURSE PRACTITIONER CERTIFICATION EXAMINATION:
Review Questions and Strategies

THIRD EDITION

Jill E. Winland-Brown, EdD, MSN, APRN, BC
Professor and Family Nurse Practitioner
Christine E. Lynn College of Nursing
Florida Atlantic University
Boca Raton, Florida

Lynne M. Dunphy, PhD, APRN, BC
Professor and Routhier Chair of Practice
Family Nurse Practitioner
College of Nursing
University of Rhode Island
Kingston, Rhode Island

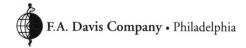
F.A. Davis Company • Philadelphia

F. A. Davis Company
1915 Arch Street
Philadelphia, PA 19103
www.fadavis.com

Printed in the United States of America

Last digit indicates print number: 10 9 8 7 6 5 4 3

Publisher, Nursing: Joanne P. DaCunha, RN, MSN
Developmental Editor: Barbara Tchabovsky
Director of Content Development: Darlene Pedersen, RN, MSN
Project Editor: Kristin L. Kern
Art & Design Manager: Carolyn O'Brien

ISBN 10: 0-8036-1819-0
ISBN 13: 978-0-8036-1819-0

As new scientific information becomes available through basic and clinical research, recommended treatments and drug therapies undergo changes. The author(s) and publisher have done everything possible to make this book accurate, up to date, and in accord with accepted standards at the time of publication. The author(s), editors, and publisher are not responsible for errors or omissions or for consequences from application of the book, and make no warranty, expressed or implied, in regard to the contents of the book. Any practice described in this book should be applied by the reader in accordance with professional standards of care used in regard to the unique circumstances that may apply in each situation. The reader is advised always to check product information (package inserts) for changes and new information regarding dose and contraindications before administering any drug. Caution is especially urged when using new or infrequently ordered drugs.

I would like to dedicate this book to my husband, Harvey, who is my "true north," and to my daughter, Cydney, who keeps putting up with me through multiple editions.

Jill E. Winland-Brown

To my dear husband, Jim, with thanks for his steadfastness, good humor, loyalty, and affection, and to Bradley James Arthur Hektor, the best teenager in the world!

Lynne M. Dunphy

Preface

When we originally began this process, review books were available for just physician assistants and physicians. As nurse educators who had been preparing undergraduates for the NCLEX exam for many years, we knew the importance of taking sample exams in the discipline that reflect the test content. Thus, the idea for this book was born. With the advent of the doctorate in nursing practice (DNP) as the entry into advanced-practice nursing, this book is more essential than ever for staking the parameters of discipline identity.

Research shows that answering numerous sample test questions is the best way to prepare for taking a multiple-choice exam such as the current certification exam. We saw a tremendous need for a book that contained a large number of sample test questions with rationales, as well as reinforcement in test-taking skills. In the second edition, we updated information using new standards and guidelines. We also increased the number of questions. In this third edition, relying heavily on evidenced-based practice, we updated content, added new medications, and utilized new practice guidelines. We increased the number of questions for each chapter, each practice examination in the back of the book, and the CD examination. Success on multiple-choice exams is a skill that can be learned like any other skill—for example, playing tennis—and the outcomes improve with practice.

We suggest reading Chapters 1 and 2 first to get a feel for both taking the exam and setting up an individualized study plan. Next, you might want to take one of the practice tests in the back of the book to assess your baseline score. These practice tests simulate the certification examination both in content and the number of questions. This will help you identify your weaknesses and design your individual study plan. We then suggest you go to the chapter containing test questions for the content area in which you feel you are weakest.

Because medicine is rapidly changing and is an art, as well as a science, there are many conflicting viewpoints and practices regarding treatment options. Every effort has been made to ensure that the content is current and relevant, and several sources were used for the rationales of each question. For further information regarding content, the references used for the questions appear at the end of each chapter. This book can be used as a companion to *Primary Care: The Art and Science of Advanced Practice Nursing*, which will elaborate further on each rationale.

After you pass the certification exam, this text can be used as a study guide to continually refresh your knowledge base. We suggest writing comments next to each question that will assist you in remembering and noting ideas to be researched further. We sincerely wish you success on certification and hope that this book contributed in a small way to that success. Best of luck.

—*Jill E. Winland-Brown*
—*Lynne M. Dunphy*

Acknowledgments

I would like to thank Bruce Wishnov, DO, for his mentorship and having never been too busy or too irritable for any questions!!! You are a caring physician and an all-around great guy.

LMD

We would both like to thank the entire F. A. Davis team, especially Joanne DaCunha, publisher, F. A. Davis, for her enthusiasm, support, and friendship, and Barbara Tchabovsky, developmental editor, for her firm hand and expertise.

JW-B & LMD

Contributors

Denise Coppa, PhD, APRN, BC
Family Nurse Practitioner
Associate Professor, Director of NP Program
College of Nursing
University of Rhode Island
Kingston, Rhode Island

Diane Gerzevitz, MSN, APRN, BC
Family Nurse Practitioner
Assistant Professor
College of Nursing
University of Rhode Island
Kingston, Rhode Island

Janice S. Hayes, PhD, RN
Associate Professor
School of Nursing
University of Northern Colorado
Greeley, Colorado

Allison M. Jedson, MSN, APRN, BC
Family Nurse Practitioner
Adjunct Faculty
College of Nursing
University of Rhode Island
Kingston, Rhode Island

Deborah A. Raines, PhD, RNC
Professor
Christine E. Lynn College of Nursing
Florida Atlantic University
Boca Raton, Florida

Lorraine M. Schwartz, MSN, APRN, BC
Gerontological Nurse Practitioner
Kingston, Rhode Island

Susan Elaine Sloan, MSN, APRN, BC
Cardiovascular Nurse Clinician
The Cardiology Center
Delray Beach, Florida

Douglas H. Sutton, EdD, APRN, BC
Adult Nurse Practitioner
Associate Professor
Christine E. Lynn College of Nursing
Florida Atlantic University
Boca Raton, Florida

Marcella R. Thompson, MSN, RN
PhD candidate
College of Nursing
University of Rhode Island
Kingston, Rhode Island

Sharon A. Thrush, MSN, APRN, BC
Family Nurse Practitioner
Palm Beach Family Physicians
West Palm Beach, Florida
Adjunct Faculty
Christine E. Lynn College of Nursing
Florida Atlantic University
Boca Raton, Florida

Contents

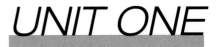

INTRODUCTION

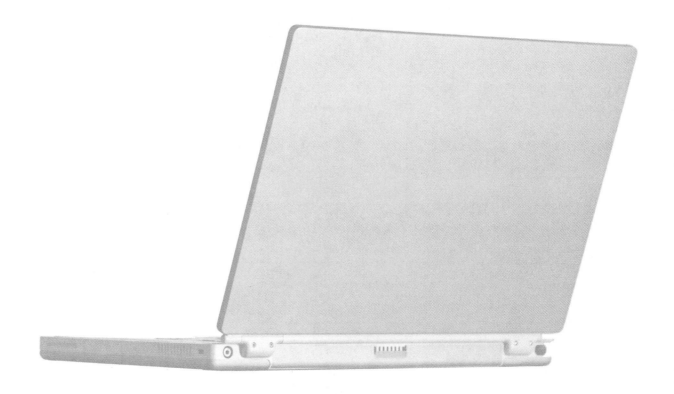

Chapter 1: *Achieving Success on a Certification Exam*

DOUGLAS H. SUTTON
LYNNE M. DUNPHY

Congratulations! With the purchase of this book, you have taken your first step along the road to becoming a certified advanced-practice nurse. The earlier in your educational process you begin preparing for the certification examination (we will be using the term *exam* from now on), the greater your chance of success. If you are a practitioner who has been "out there" for a number of years, this book will help you understand the certification process and the steps you need to take to be successful on the certification exam of your choice. Regardless of your situation, the important point is that you have begun! Remember, the longest journey begins with a single step.

Certification and Why It Is Important

There are basic differences between becoming licensed (something you achieved at the completion of your basic nursing program by sitting for the state boards or the National Council Licensure Examination for Registered Nurses [NCLEX-RN]) and becoming certified. A good understanding of these differences is important to your ultimate success on the certification exam. Becoming "test savvy" demands a thorough understanding of

the underlying premises and purposes of the exam for which you are sitting.

LICENSURE

Licensure is a legal requirement. You must be licensed by a state to practice nursing in that state. The purpose of licensure is to protect the public from unsafe practitioners. Legal regulation of nursing practice is the joint responsibility of the state legislature and the state board of nursing. Minimum competency is assessed on a licensure exam. This exam asks: Have you met the basic criteria for safe and effective nursing practice? The test questions on the licensure exam are from frequently updated job analyses of entry-level nursing practice. They reflect the concepts and functions that a registered nurse (RN) needs to know and perform for safe entry-level practice.

Currently, the licensure exam is prepared and administered by the National Council of State Boards of Nursing (NCSBN). Composed of representatives from every nursing board in the United States and five of its territories, this body is responsible for setting a national standard for safe and effective entry-level nursing practice and assessing it through administration of a national licensing exam, the NCLEX-RN. Every state now mandates passage of this exam as a prerequisite for state licensure as a registered nurse.

CERTIFICATION

Certification is the process by which a nongovernmental agency or association grants recognition to an individual who has met predetermined standards for specialty practice. The purpose of certification (Table 1-1) is quite different from that of licensure. Certification is a voluntary process, although currently most states require passage of the appropriate certification exam as a prerequisite to licensure to perform advanced-practice nursing functions.

Certification validates entry-level knowledge of an advanced nursing specialty; the process of recertification recognizes continued proficiency in that specialty. In 1974 the American Nurses Association (ANA) initiated a national voluntary certification process to recognize excellence in nursing practice. By 1978 the purpose had broadened to include the assurance of quality in advanced nursing practice. This was done partly to recognize professional achievement but also to identify nurses who were potentially eligible for third-party reimbursement.

By the 1990s, the regulation of advanced-practice nursing had become a topic of increasing concern within the nursing profession. Whether a secondary level of licensure, rather than certification, is the more appropriate regulatory mechanism has been debated for some time. This debate is ongoing, while at the same time certification requirements have continued to be implemented across the United States. Currently only New York and California do not require certification prior to obtaining licensure to practice as an advanced-practice registered nurse (APRN).

The current system for recognizing advanced-practice nursing through certification was established by, and has been operated by, various specialty nursing organizations since the 1970s. An umbrella board, the American Board of Nursing Specialties (ABNS), was

established in 1991. Modeled after the American Board of Medical Specialties, this board recognizes advanced-practice nursing certifying bodies by establishing that these bodies have met certain uniform standards, such as education.

In 2006 the National Council of State Boards of Nursing released a draft of a vision paper titled "The Future Regulation of Advanced Practice Nursing." This paper has further fueled the debate regarding the regulation of advanced nursing practice in the United States. However, continuation of voluntary certification administered through professional associations such as the ANA subsidiary, the American Nurses Credentialing Center (ANCC), and the American Academy of Nurse Practitioners (AANP) remains the only nationally recognized means available for validating advanced-practice nursing knowledge. Table 1-2 lists associations and organizations offering advanced-practice nursing certification.

National certification and specialty designation play an increasingly central role in state licensure at an advanced-practice level, as well as in reimbursement for advanced nursing services. They are also linked to prescriptive authority in certain states. Some forms of reimbursement are contingent on national certification. Since 1998, certification has been a prerequisite to Medicare reimbursement. The Veterans Affairs Medical Systems now mandate national certification for advanced-practice nurses. Likewise, certain managed care organizations, as well as hospitals, require national certification as a criterion for credentialing providers.

The purpose of certification is to assure the public that an individual has mastery of a body of knowledge and has acquired the skills necessary to function in a particular specialty. APRNs are expected to have expert competence, knowledge, and skills in the delivery of nursing and medical services to individuals, families, and groups. Consensus has increasingly emerged regarding what these competencies and skills are. In 2006 the National Organization of Nurse Practitioner Faculties (NONPF), a nongovernmental, noncertifying organization, released the domains and core competencies for advanced practice. These domains and core competencies continue to provide guidance for curriculum development across programs and are consistent with certifying agencies' (AANP and ANCC) examination content. The domains and core competencies include the following:

- Management of patient health/illness status
- Nurse practitioner–patient relationship

TABLE 1-1. PURPOSE OF CERTIFICATION

- Required for practice in most states.
- Indicates specialized and advance knowledge base.
- Provides greater career opportunities.
- Increasingly required for third-party reimbursement.

TABLE 1-2. ASSOCIATIONS AND ORGANIZATIONS OFFERING ADVANCED PRACTICE NURSING CERTIFICATION

ASSOCIATION OR ORGANIZATION	*ADVANCED-PRACTICE NURSING CERTIFICATION*
American Academy of Nurse Practitioners	**Nurse Practitioner** • Adult • Family
American Nurses Credentialing Center	**Nurse Practitioner** • Acute care • Adult • Family • Gerontological • Pediatric • Advanced diabetes management • Psychiatric, adult • Psychiatric, family **Clinical Nurse Specialist** • Public community health • Gerontological • Adult health • Psychiatric and mental health (adult) • Psychiatric and mental health (child and adolescent) • Advanced diabetes management • Pediatric
American Association of Nurse Anesthetists	**Certified Registered Nurse Anesthetist**
American College of Nurse-Midwives	**Certified Nurse Midwife**
Pediatric Nursing Certification Board	**Nurse Practitioner** • Pediatric
National Certification Corporation for the Obstetric, Gynecologic, and Neonatal Nursing Specialties	**Nurse Practitioner** • Neonatal • Women's health
Oncology Nursing Certification Corporation	**Advanced Oncology Nursing for Nurse Practitioners and Clinical Nurse Specialists**

• The teaching-coaching function
• Professional role
• Managing and negotiating health-care delivery systems
• Monitoring and ensuring the quality of health-care practice
• Providing culturally sensitive care

Although the specific language of each of NONPF's domains and core competencies may differ from that of the certifying agency, it is the greater concept of each of the domains and core competencies that is essential for the candidate sitting for a certification exam to understand. In summary, the candidate for certification as an APRN should recognize that certification is a formal process, conducted by nongovernmental organizations, to validate the knowledge, skills, and abilities of a candidate, based on predetermined standards.

YOUR ROLE

You are making an important, timely, and professionally astute decision by choosing to become certified. In 1998 Margretta Madden Styles, president of the ANCC, noted in *Credentialing News*, "As the global tide turns from governmental regulation and public protectionism toward competitive quality improvement of services and informed consumer choice, voluntary credentialing is a movement whose time has come." We concur.

Certification Exams

This book is geared toward the nurse who is seeking certification as an adult nurse practitioner (ANP) and/or family nurse practitioner (FNP). The ANP certification exam is designed to assess your abilities as an APRN in the delivery of primary care services to an adult population, defined as adolescence through old age. The FNP certification exam is designed to assess your abilities as an APRN in the delivery of primary care services, including prepartum and postpartum care and pediatrics, to a population covering the entire family life span. Table 1-3 lists the requirements for nurse practitioner certification by the ANCC and AANP.

AMERICAN NURSES CREDENTIALING CENTER

In 1973 the ANA established a certification program to recognize professional achievement in a defined clinical or functional area of nursing. This was in response to the proliferation of specialties in nursing, as well as to the increasing emphasis on clinical specialization in graduate nursing education.

The exams were first offered in 1974. Certification was a voluntary process, and 691 nurses were initially certified, including psychiatric mental health clinical nurse specialists, the first group of APRNs to promote certification and use it for reimbursement. A master's degree was required to sit for this advanced-practice certification. In 1978 10 generalist and specialty-level certification examinations were available. By 2008 the number of exams available had expanded to 32. More than 250,000 nurses have achieved certification at both the generalist or specialty and advanced-practice

levels since 1990, and more than 75,000 APRNs are currently certified with the ANCC. Exams are available in five broad categories—nurse practitioner (NP), clinical nurse specialist (CNS), advanced diabetes management, nursing administration, and specialty nursing. Of the 32 exams offered by the ANCC, eight are designed for nurse practitioner certification and seven are designed for the clinical nurse specialist.

In 1991 the ANCC was established as a separate subsidiary of the ANA. This is in compliance with nationally accepted standards for certification, which require that credentialing bodies be separate from their parent organizations to prevent conflicts of interest.

To qualify to take an examination and become certified at either the specialty or advanced level, a nurse must (1) meet requirements for clinical or functional practice in a specialized field and (2) show evidence of having pursued education beyond basic nursing preparation, and in the case of both the ANP and FNP exam, provide evidence of successful completion of an approved master's-level curriculum. In some specialties, nurses must also receive the endorsement of their peers. After meeting these criteria as they relate to a given specialty, the nurse must take and pass the relevant certification exam. Only then will the nurse be certified in that specialty.

Once you have sent in your application for the ANCC exam, you will receive a copy of the *Candidate's Handbook*, a valuable source of help in preparing for the exam. The ANCC Web site, as well as the *Handbook*, contains a test content outline (TCO) that describes the major categories and domains of practice, as well as related topics and subtopics that will be covered on the exam. The exam currently consists of 175 questions, 150 of which are scored and 25 pretest questions that are not scored. The nonscored questions cannot be distinguished from the scored items.

The TCO includes information about how the content is weighted—that is, how many or what percentage of the test questions are in each of the major domains. Table 1-4 lists the major categories or domains of practice for the FNP exam and includes an approximate number of questions and the overall percentage for each category. Table 1-5 provides similar information for the ANP exam.

The importance of reviewing the current TCO prior to sitting for the exam cannot be overstated. To facilitate understanding of each of the major domains, the ANCC also includes subcategories in a topical outline format. For example, the largest category or domain, clinical

TABLE 1-3. REQUIREMENTS FOR NURSE PRACTITIONER CERTIFICATION

AMERICAN NURSES CREDENTIALING CENTER (ANCC)	AMERICAN ACADEMY OF NURSE PRACTITIONERS (AANP)
Specialty Areas • Acute care nurse practitioner • Adult nurse practitioner • Family nurse practitioner • Gerontological nurse practitioner • Pediatric nurse practitioner • Advanced diabetes management nurse practitioner • Psychiatric nurse practitioner, child and adolescent • Psychiatric nurse practitioner, adult	• Adult nurse practitioner • Family nurse practitioner • Gerontological nurse practitioner
Requirements • Master's-level nurse practitioner program from an accredited institution of higher learning • Meet practice requirements specific to certification type	• Master's-level nurse practitioner program from an accredited institution of higher learning (nurse practitioners without this degree may petition the certification board for permission to sit for the examination)
Examinations • Check ANCC Web site. • Sylvan Technology Centers operates more than 300 centers. • Check Web site for current cost.	• Check AANP Web site. • Check Web site. • Check Web site for current cost.
Contact ANCC 600 Maryland Ave, SW Suite 100 West Washington, DC 20024-2571 800-284-2378 http://www.ana.org/ancc/index.htm	AANP Certification Program Capitol Station PO Box 12926 Austin, TX 78711 512-442-5202 http://www.aanpcertification.org email: certification@aanp.org

management (32%–34%), includes eight relevant subcategories. One subcategory under clinical management is standards of advanced practice. Within that subcategory the following clarifying statement is provided, "Standards are authoritative statements by which the nursing profession describes the responsibilities for which its practitioners are accountable."

For the candidate to adequately prepare for the certification exam, all elements of the TCO should be understood and studied. Table 1-6 lists the six major categories or domains of practice, as well as the related subcategories, that are currently being tested on both the ANP and FNP exam.

Additionally, all questions are classified according to life span and problem-focused content areas. The life span dimension for the ANP exam includes non–age-specific content, as well as specific content pertaining to the adolescent, the adult, and the

TABLE 1-4. ANCC FAMILY NURSE PRACTITIONER CERTIFICATION EXAMINATION CONTENT OUTLINE

DOMAINS OF PRACTICE	NUMBER OF QUESTIONS	PERCENT
Clinical management	53	34%
Professional role and policy	7	6%
Nurse practitioner and patient relationship	16	11%
Assessment of acute and chronic illness	39	26%
Research	4	2%
Health promotion and disease prevention	31	21%
TOTAL	**150**	**100%**

TABLE 1-5. ANCC ADULT NURSE PRACTITIONER CERTIFICATION EXAMINATION CONTENT OUTLINE

DOMAINS OF PRACTICE	NUMBER OF QUESTIONS	PERCENT
Clinical management	48	32%
Professional role and policy	13	9%
Nurse practitioner and patient relationship	18	12%
Assessment of acute and chronic illness	33	22%
Research	9	6%
Health promotion and disease prevention	29	19%
TOTAL	**150**	**100%**

aging adult. The FNP life span dimension includes the same content as the ANP exam, plus content relating to children, infants, and childbearing women.

The last dimension is related to problem areas and organizes question content by body system—for example, cardiovascular, endocrine, and respiratory.

What this means is that each test question is characterized across three dimensions. For example, a test question that asks about the treatment of a 70-year-old woman with a diagnosis of osteoporosis would be characterized as follows:

Dimension One—Clinical Management

Dimension Two—Life Span: Older Adult

Dimension Three—Problem Area: Musculoskeletal

Be aware that the TCO may change from exam to exam, so you need to review your handbook carefully for the most current content breakdown.

In 2006 the exam results were based on 150 *scored* questions for both the ANP and FNP exams. A total of 1115 people took the ANP exam and 889 (79.7%) passed. A total of 2423 people took the FNP exam and 2209 (91.2%) passed.

To assess each examinee's level of specialty knowledge independent of the group taking the exam, a *criterion-referenced standard* is used. In this approach, each examinee's score is compared with an absolute number determined by the content experts who develop the exam.

The test development committee determines the passing score after careful consideration of the content of the test questions. The passing score is always expressed in terms of the number of questions you must correctly answer on the total test, as well as statistical examinations of the reliability and validity of the "piloted" test questions. Additional statistical examination of the piloted questions is assessed for inclusion in the final graded pool of test questions on the next exam.

Your score report will provide you with detailed information regarding how many test questions you correctly answered in each of the major content domains. However, it is your performance on the total test that determines your success or failure. The report will be mailed to you 5 to 7 days after you take the test.

You will need to be recertified every 5 years. This may be accomplished by accumulating continuing education credits. Please check the ANCC Web site for the most current information because guidelines for recertification are subject to change.

TABLE 1-6. FNP/ANP EXAM: DOMAINS OF PRACTICE AND RELATED SUBCATEGORIES

MAJOR CATEGORY OR DOMAIN OF PRACTICE	SUBCATEGORIES
Clinical management	Standards of advanced practice
	Clinical guidelines
	Pharmacotherapeutics
	Clinical therapeutics
	Clinical decision making
	Documentation
	Safety
	Theory application
Professional role and policy	Health care/public policy
	Ethics
	Scope of practice
	Access to care
	Coordination of care
Nurse practitioner and patient relationship	Cultural competence
	Therapeutic communication
	Teaching/coaching
	Patient advocacy
Assessment of acute and chronic illness	Epidemiology/disease control
	Anatomy
	Physiology
	Pathophysiology
	Psychosocial
	Diagnostic reasoning
Research	Research process/utilization
	Continuous process improvement
	Outcome evaluation
Health promotion and disease prevention	Epidemiology/risk analysis
	Genetics
	Risk reduction and health behavior guidelines
	Growth and development across the life span
	Screening
	Wellness assessment

AMERICAN ACADEMY OF NURSE PRACTITIONERS

The AANP offers competency-based national certification examinations for the ANP, FNP, and the geriatric NP (GNP). Reflecting nurse practitioner knowledge and expertise, the content areas of these exams include health promotion, disease prevention, and diagnosis and management of acute and chronic diseases. The exams given by the AANP were developed in conjunction with the Professional Examination Service, a not-for-profit organization with more than 50 years of experience in developing and administering national licensing and certification exams in health-related fields.

Historically, examinees were required to be graduates of approved master's-level ANP, FNP, or GNP programs. As of this writing, non–master's-prepared practitioners may petition the certification board for permission to sit for the examinations. This certification program is fully accredited by the National Commission for Certifying Agencies (NCCA).

The Academy Certification Program, in conjunction with the Professional Examination Service, conducted a role delineation study to determine areas of clinical knowledge to be tested. Based on the study's results, the exam tests clinical knowledge in the following areas: assessment, diagnosis, formulation and implementation of treatment plans, evaluation, follow-up, and applicable professional issues. The ANP exam tests knowledge of late adolescence, adult, and geriatric primary care, while the FNP exam tests clinical knowledge of prenatal, pediatric, adolescent, adult, and geriatric primary care. Examinees must be able to integrate knowledge of pathophysiology, psychology, and sociology with the assessment, diagnosis, and treatment of patients in primary care. Knowledge of health promotion and disease prevention is tested, as well as management of acute/episodic and chronic illness in the primary care setting.

Unlike the ANCC, the AANP does not publish exam statistics on its Web page. However, the AANP Certification Program does publish a *NewsBriefs* document, which provides score report information. According to the most current *NewsBriefs* (April 2007), during the calendar year 2005 a total of 521 ANPs and 1762 FNPs were tested; approximately 84% passed the exam.

Certification is good for 5 years, after which you must recertify. This may be accomplished by (1) sitting for the exam again or (2) keeping your practice current by working 1000 hours in your clinical area *and* pursuing 75 contact hours of continuing education in your relevant area of specialization.

Achieving Success

Practitioner programs generally focus on assessment, management, and evaluation of *disease*. Indeed, this is the role most of you perform in your respective work settings. The ability to diagnose and treat disease is paramount to your safe and effective functioning as an APN, and certification exams increasingly reflect this reality. However, it is important never to lose sight of the fact that these exams are certifying your abilities as an APN, and as such have an underlying bias toward health, health promotion, and human responses to health and illness.

As a nurse, your reaction to the various manifestations of health and illness phenomena is instinctively different from that of other primary care providers. This is manifested in different ways on each exam, but it is an important distinction to keep in mind as you sit and ponder various distractors and wonder what answer is the best. Similarly, the test blueprints and type of questions asked reflect a continued commitment to concepts of health promotion and disease prevention, as well as the underlying principles of therapeutic communication skills that are so essential to the forging of meaningful nurse-client relationships. Nursing-based elements of growth and development, nutrition, and therapeutic communication, as well as questions about cultural differences and cross-cultural communication, will be integrated with content concerning specific aspects of diagnosis, pharmacology, and disease management.

Questions testing physical assessment and history-taking skills, as well as content from advanced physical assessment courses, remain prominent. Although a certain amount of basic pharmacological content is included, the latest drugs and pharmacological interventions may not always appear because the exam questions are prepared and tested well in advance. (Note: Questions about your knowledge of safe prescribing for the pregnant woman almost always appear on the FNP exams.)

If you have been in active practice for some time, you must exercise care as you take the exam. Distractors (see chapter 2) will not necessarily correlate with what you currently see and do. Remember, the exam reflects the *ideal* answer according to the certifying body; this ideal answer may not always mirror the realities of your practice. Test answers draw on national guidelines and standards of practice promulgated by a variety of bodies. Your practice is likely to be focused on a specialty and to reflect the practice patterns and priorities of your particular geographic region and site. The questions on the exam are looking for much more generalized responses and might well reflect phenomena that you very seldom experience. Allowing yourself to become frustrated with the distractors will not help you but rather will hinder your ability to succeed. This is why it is essential that you study large numbers of sample test items (see chapter 2).

Being test savvy and succeeding on a multiple-choice exam is a far different skill from the expert skills you bring to your practice. But these skills are not mutually exclusive. It is a matter of having the correct mind-set. This mind-set is predicated on an awareness of the *nursing base* of the certification exam coupled with an understanding of the *test blueprint*. Develop a determination not to select an anecdotal answer based on experience from your own practice but rather to select an answer based on nationally recognized, clinically based guidelines and rooted in clinical literature.

You have taken the first step toward certification by purchasing this book! Mentally review the important reasons to become nationally certified. Fix the end goal vividly in your mind. Imagine how you will feel opening the envelope telling you that you have succeeded, that you are a nationally certified APRN. It is a satisfying and worthwhile goal to achieve.

Take the next step on the road to success by turning to chapter 2. It will assist you in the development of important test-taking skills, as well as provide guidelines for your individualized study plan.

You can succeed!

Bibliography

American Academy of Nurse Practitioners: National competency-based certification examinations for adult and family nurse practitioners. American Academy of Nurse Practitioners, Austin, TX, 2007.

American Academy of Nurse Practitioners: Position statement on nurse practitioner curriculum. American Academy of Nurse Practitioners, Austin, TX, 2007.

American Academy of Nurse Practitioners: http://www.aanp.org/certification.htm, Certification examination program description, 2007, accessed July 20, 2007.

American Nurses Certification Corporation certification Web page: http://www.nursecredentialing.org, accessed August 3, 2007.

Miller, SK: *Adult Nurse Practitioner Review and Resource Manual*, ed 2. American Nurses Credentialing Center, Silver Springs, MD, 2005.

National Certification Board of Pediatric Nurse Practitioners and Nurses: Pediatric nurse practitioner certification and certification maintenance programs. National Certification Board of Pediatric Nurse Practitioners and Nurses, Cherry Hill, NJ, 2007.

National Council of State Boards of Nursing: https://www.ncsbn.org/Draft_APRN_Vision_Paper.pdf, Draft vision paper: The future regulation of advanced practice nursing, 2006, accessed July 23, 2007.

National Organization of Nurse Practitioner Faculties: http://www.nonpf.com/NONPF2005/CoreCompsFINAL06.pdf, Domains and core competencies of nurse practitioner practice, 2006, accessed July 28, 2007.

National Organization of Nurse Practitioner Faculties and American Association of Colleges of Nursing: Nurse practitioner primary care competencies in specialty areas. Division of Nursing, Department Health and Human Services, Rockville, MD, 2002.

Resources

American Academy of Nurse Practitioners (AANP)
Capitol Station
PO Box 12926
Austin, TX 78711
512-442-5202
http://www.aanpcertification.org

American Nurses Credentialing Center (ANCC)
600 Maryland Ave, SW
Suite 100 West
Washington, DC 20024-2571
800-284-2378
http://www.ana.org/ancc/index.htm

Chapter 2: *Test-Taking Skills and Designing Your Study Plan*

Study Habits: Know Yourself

What Test-Taking Type Are You?

What Is Your Preferred Learning Style?

Active versus Passive Studying

Getting Started

Tips for Studying

Nature of the Exams
Test-Taking Skills: An Acquired Art

Basic Tools

Specific Strategies

Designing Your Study Plan

Assess

Plan and Implement

Evaluate

Last-Minute Preparations: Relaxed and Ready

Bibliography

DOUGLAS H. SUTTON
LYNNE M. DUNPHY

This chapter has several parts. The first part actively assists you in assessing your study and testing style. It prepares you to develop an individualized study plan that will enable you to achieve your goal: becoming a nationally certified advanced-practice nurse. Another part briefly explains the nature of the adult nurse practitioner and family nurse practitioner certification examinations (we will use the term exam from this point on). The remaining parts deal with the specifics of answering multiple-choice test questions and the skills necessary to succeed on a multiple-choice exam. We will specifically discuss the American Nurses Credentialing Center (ANCC) adult and/or family nurse practitioner exam and the American Academy of Nurse Practitioners (AANP) exam. Evaluating test-taking skills and developing a formal study plan are also covered.

Study Habits: Know Yourself

There are several approaches to developing good study habits and effective test-taking skills. Among them are recognizing what test-taking type you are and what your preferred learning style is; realizing the importance of active versus passive studying; and following basic tips for getting started and developing test-taking skills.

WHAT TEST-TAKING TYPE ARE YOU?

This fun exercise will allow you to diagnose your own studying and test-taking style. Are you a tortoise or a hare? Are you a peacock? Or are you more like a deer?

Knowing your style can assist you in designing your study plan for the exam and answering test questions on exam day. For example, are you a tortoise, moving slowly and laboriously through each question, taking far too long, and then having to rush at the end, thereby increasing your chance of error? Or are you a hare, racing through the exam questions as fast as you can, often misreading information, and likely to make quick guesses rather than carefully thought-out responses?

Are you preoccupied with grades and personal achievement, viewing the certification exam as a threat? Do you procrastinate about studying rather than developing and sticking to a well-designed study plan, thus increasing your anxiety? Do you argue with some test questions, convinced that none of the options is right according to your practice? Then you may be a peacock. Remember, exam questions are *not* perfect, but still require that you choose the *best* available option. Do *not* waste time and energy arguing mentally with a test question. Select what you feel is the best option and *move on!*

Or are you a deer? Do you easily lose self-confidence and tend to run away, doubting your initial response? Are you often academically successful but experience anxiety when information is presented in an unfamiliar format?

Table 2-1 will assist you in identifying your test-taking personality.

WHAT IS YOUR PREFERRED LEARNING STYLE?

Awareness of your learning style will also guide you in selecting study strategies. Learning styles are related to the pathways or channels through which you prefer to absorb information. The three types of learners are commonly identified as *visual*, *auditory*, and *tactile* (sometimes called *kinesthetic*).

Visual Learners

Visual learners learn better from reading and writing than from hearing and talking about information. They usually find background noise, such as music and television, distracting rather than helpful. Following are strategies for visual learners:

- Read texts in a quiet place.
- Watch appropriate videos.
- Use visual study aids such as concept maps, flash cards, and charts.
- Use highlighting markers or colored paper to take notes.

Auditory Learners

Auditory learners grasp information most effectively by listening and talking. Combining information with music often works well for auditory learners. Following are strategies for auditory learners:

- Read texts aloud.
- Listen to audiotapes of course material.
- Make up a song about the content and sing it aloud (especially helpful for assimilating difficult content).
- Listen to background music or other noise.
- Talk about the content with a study partner.

Tactile or Kinesthetic Learners

Tactile or kinesthetic learners prefer to learn "hands on." They have difficulty sitting still for long periods. During study sessions, they should stand and move around or take frequent stretch breaks. Integrating physical activity with study works well for these learners. Following are strategies for tactile learners:

- Move around while studying.
- Read while exercising on a stationary bicycle.
- Listen to tapes of learning material while walking or biking.
- Rewrite or type notes.

Although almost everyone is capable of learning through all of their sensory pathways, most have a preferred channel. Think about which of the three learning styles discussed works best for you. Time is often at a premium for nurses studying for certification, and capitalizing on your preferred learning style will help you study in the most efficient way. Keep strategies for your preferred learning style in mind as you develop your study plan.

ACTIVE VERSUS PASSIVE STUDYING

Regardless of your personal learning style, the more actively you are engaged in the material, the better your ability to retain and comprehend content. For example, many of us have had the experience of reading an entire chapter, or listening to a review CD, only to find that our mind drifted away sometime earlier and we have difficulty recalling even the most basic information. Time is a precious commodity, so it

TABLE 2-1. IDENTIFYING YOUR TEST-TAKING TYPE

HARE	*TORTOISE*	*PEACOCK*	*DEER*
Study Style			
• Crams • Feels anxious during study sessions	• Obsessive • Focuses on details; misses the bigger picture	• Procrastinates • Puts off studying; does not think there is a need to study	• Diligent • Smart; has good study habits but lacks self-confidence
Test-Taking Style			
• Often first to finish • Rushes; does not thoroughly read questions and answers • Makes quick guesses • Feels anxious when answer is not readily apparent	• Often last to finish • Spends too much time examining details and rereading questions and answers • May have to rush at end to complete exam in allotted time	• Reads own ideas into questions • Changes initial responses often because expected answer is not present • Selects answer based on anecdotal experience	• Questions own knowledge • Changes initial responses • Feels anxious when faced with information that is presented differently from expected way • Voices self-doubt during testing
Test-Taking Strategies			
• Develop and stick to a study plan; avoid last-minute cramming. • Focus on decreasing test-taking speed. • Read questions as though speaking them aloud in your head to avoid scanning. • Read all options. • Time yourself in practice tests; allow no less than 1 minute per question. • Keep a watch in front of you while taking the test; determine the halfway point and mark it on the exam.	• Focus on concepts and not details during study periods. • Use concept maps. • Focus on increasing testing speed. • Do not linger too long over one question. • Time yourself in practice tests; allow 45–60 seconds for each question.	• Develop and stick to a study plan. • Practice with sample tests. • Maintain objectivity; avoid adding own interpretation. • Avoid changing answers.	• Continue usual study activities. • Work on self-confidence. • Develop a self-confidence mantra to recite if you find yourself doubting your knowledge. • Use practice tests to increase confidence. • Avoid changing answers.

Continued

TABLE 2-1. IDENTIFYING YOUR TEST-TAKING TYPE—cont'd

HARE	*TORTOISE*	*PEACOCK*	*DEER*
Relaxation Techniques • Breathe deeply. • Practice positive visualization. • Avoid caffeine. • Develop a test-taking mantra to recite if you find yourself losing focus.	• Breathe deeply. • Practice positive visualization. • Avoid caffeine.	• Breathe deeply. • Practice positive visualization. • Avoid caffeine.	• Breathe deeply. • Practice positive visualization. • Avoid caffeine.

Source: Adapted from Sides, MB, and Korchek, N: *Successful Test-Taking Strategies*, ed. 3, Lippincott Williams & Wilkins, Philadelphia, 1998, p. 77; and Dickenson-Hazard, N: Test-taking strategies and techniques. In Kopac, CA, and Millonig, VL (eds): *Gerontological Nursing Certification Review Guide*, revised ed. Health Leadership Associates, Potomac, MD, 1996, pp. 3–5.

is far more efficient to learn actively the first time than to reread or relisten to an entire chapter a second time. Tips used to improve active learning include taking notes while reading, pausing after each heading or subheading, and summarizing the content. Can you identify the main idea that the author was attempting to impart? Did you pass over new terms without taking the time to become familiar with them? As you read a summary, do you realize that you really need to go back to a more detailed reference because your knowledge is insufficient? Although active engagement may slow you down initially, it will save you time in the long run because now you are involved in active learning and not simply hoping that something will stick as you speed by.

GETTING STARTED

Studying, like regular exercise, is good for the brain. As a health-care professional, you will find that it will always be your job to keep abreast of the professional literature and spend some time studying. To recertify, you are mandated to keep your practice current through a combination of a number of clinical hours and continuing education options. The earlier you begin to plan for certification or recertification, the better.

The principles of effective study are simple but often ignored. There is one central law about study—the law of mass effect. Any worthwhile studying takes time. And in today's world, time is a precious commodity. Therefore, if you want to study, you need to set aside adequate time and plan accordingly. Be prepared to delay the start of new projects until this one is complete and you have successfully taken the exam. There is no way around the hours involved. There are no shortcuts. But you need to make it easy to begin.

TIPS FOR STUDYING

Just as a cold engine will run a little rough, settling down to study when one is out of the habit can be difficult. The following suggestions should make it easier to begin studying and to return to it on a regular and consistent basis.

- **Create a pleasurable personal environment.** This is a very basic but frequently overlooked requirement for successful study. Organize all your study materials in one area. Try to create a pleasant and regular work space for yourself. Perhaps it will be just part of a room, but make it an inviting part. Decorate it with flowers, pictures, or whatever makes the area appealing to you. For the kinesthetic learner, an open area that allows free movement may be better than a small office. Some literature suggests that playing classical music, especially from the baroque era, in the background increases concentration and retention. Decide whether background music is helpful for you or distracting. Background music may be helpful for an auditory learner, whereas a visual learner may find it a distraction.

- **Plan your activities in advance and be realistic.** Plan in advance what you are going to work on and do not be overly ambitious. Blocks of 1½ hours at most are recommended, with a 10-minute break every 45 minutes. List the tasks beforehand; otherwise, you might spend valuable time trying to decide what material to review. Set specific targets for the time available.

- **Keep focused on the goal: becoming certified!** Keep the benefits of studying clearly in mind—in this case, the joy of receiving your passing score in the mail, followed by your embossed certificate. Visualize and imagine what the envelope will look and feel like when it comes in the mail. Feel your relief and joy when you open the envelope and read your passing score! Picture the certificate framed, hanging in your office. Write down a list of all the things you stand to gain from passing the exam and reread it when you are ready to begin to study. Maybe the list includes a raise, an advanced level of licensure, a new job, or prescriptive privileges. Focus on these results and how they make you feel. Close your eyes and allow the feelings to flood through you!

- **Use your knowledge of yourself and of basic tips.** There are a number of ways you can make studying more fun. Make use of your best time of day. For some, this might mean rising early while the rest of the household sleeps and stealing time alone, undisturbed, with a hot cup of tea or coffee. For others, evening is preferable. Study for short periods with frequent breaks. Remember to integrate whatever learning modalities work best for you. For example, if you are an auditory learner, use audiotapes. Listening to tapes while you are walking is especially good for tactile learners.

  Think in terms of "bite-size" pieces and structure your study plan accordingly. Use the "salami" principle: Cut large tasks into smaller ones and digest them one at a time. This will keep you from becoming overwhelmed and defeated before you begin.

  Variety is also essential. For example, divide your time between test question review and content review, or break up the study period into a variety of different tasks. Take notes part of the time and read for part of the time. Do not keep at any one activity—even your

practice exams—for longer than 45 minutes. Try studying with a study group part of the time. Discussing the materials with others is an especially good strategy for auditory learners. Study with your purpose in mind—in this case, passing the certification exam. As stated earlier, research has shown that two-thirds of your study time will be most effectively spent taking sample test questions. Do not lose sight of this! Studying does not necessarily mean sitting and reading textbooks. Reading books in a linear fashion is often not the most effective way to master information. Always keep the end result in mind.

- **Leave the environment in readiness for your next session.** Leave your work environment inviting for the next time. Put your materials away so that they are easily accessible. Do not leave the area cluttered; instead, make it more pleasing. Spend the last few minutes of your study time tidying up so that your environment is all set for your next session. This is also an excellent time to plan what you will do the next time you sit down to study. Believe it or not, these small, concrete habits can make a big dent in your natural tendency to procrastinate.

- **Reward yourself.** Last but not least, reward yourself! Reward yourself for each study period. You might decide that if you spend 3 hours studying on Saturday, you will see a movie on Saturday evening, or go to the mall, or treat yourself to a long, leisurely bubble bath! Be good to yourself.

Now that you understand yourself better and know how to approach studying for the exam, we will move on to providing some specific information about the certification exams.

Nature of the Exams

The ANCC and AANP certification exams consist of 150 multiple-choice questions and may include up to 25 additional pilot questions. The exam is administered on computers. The questions are at a variety of difficulty levels, administered in an integrated format. The questions cover pathophysiological content organized by body system. The exams are not computer adaptive at this time. (Computer-adaptive testing is the technique used for the NCLEX licensure exam. With computer adaptive tests, each answer, correct or incorrect, determines the difficulty level of the next question a participant receives, and each participant may answer a different number of questions to meet a minimum passing level.

The tests are computer based, so you will be expected to identify key words or phrases on a computer screen, not on the traditional paper format. Many test takers feel constrained when they are unable to underline or highlight key words and phrases. A helpful tip: Use the scratch paper and pencil provided to you when taking a computer-based examination to write down the key phrases if that helps you focus on the topic and/or issue being presented in the question. A reminder: Remember that the scratch paper is collected by the testing center staff before you may leave the testing area; this is done to maintain test question security.

The benefit of giving the exams via computer testing centers is flexibility as to the locations where the test is offered (more than 300) and the number of days when testing is available. The AANP exam is also given as a paper-and-pencil exam twice a year at a limited number of locations.

Test-Taking Skills: An Acquired Art

The ability to select the best response to each question is what determines your success on the exam. Knowledge of the content is, unfortunately, not enough to guarantee success. If you are not able to communicate your knowledge through the medium of a multiple-choice exam, you will not succeed in becoming certified.

Achieving success on a multiple-choice test is a skill, and like any other skill, it can be improved. Remember how you improve your other skills, such as playing an instrument or a sport: **practice.** The same holds true for test-taking skills. The best way to succeed on the exam is through practice, practice, and more practice.

The more you practice answering sample test questions, the better you will become at it. That is why we have written this book for you. This book will provide you with 2000 sample test questions. Research has shown that two-thirds of study time should be spent taking sample tests, and one-third of the time should be spent reviewing content. A number of exam preparation books are available to you; however, very few contain nearly the number of test questions you need to develop and flex your test-taking muscles. This book provides enough questions to enable you to do that.

To begin strengthening your test-taking skills, we discuss two basic tools to use when taking the exam and some specific strategies.

BASIC TOOLS

Two basic tools that are used in nursing—and that you should employ when taking the certification exam—are the nursing process and Maslow's Hierarchy of Needs.

The Nursing Process

The nursing process is a great tool when taking your certification exam because it can guide you through problem solving. As you recall from your basic nursing education program, the steps of the nursing process include assessment, diagnosis, planning, implementation, and evaluation. When a question provides you with a choice between assessment and implementation, you should remember these basic tips. The purpose of assessment is to validate or confirm the problem. When considering an answer choice that is an assessment, you should ask yourself, "Is this an assessment that is appropriate to the topic of the question?" If it is, you should carefully consider this as a very likely answer choice. If, however, you believe the correct answer choice is an implementation, you should ask yourself, "Do I have enough information to implement what it is the answer choice is asking me to do?" Lastly, if the answer choice is asking you to evaluate a situation, you should ask yourself, "What would be the outcome if I chose this answer choice?" The criteria for reference is always your textbook and/or guidelines, and you should avoid answer choices that are too narrow or reflective of an individual practice preference.

Maslow's Hierarchy of Needs

Another important tool is Maslow's Hierarchy of Needs. It is particularly helpful in making priority decisions. According to Maslow, there are five levels of human needs: physiological needs, a need for safety and security, a need for love and a sense of belonging, a need for self-esteem, and a need for self-actualization. Because survival is grounded in basic physiological needs, these needs take priority over any other human needs. It comes down to practicality. If you do not have oxygen to breathe or food to eat, your focus is not really on the stability of your love life. When trying to determine the priority between a physiological need of a client versus a psychosocial need, remember the priority is to meet the physical needs of the client. This doesn't imply that the correct answer is never psychosocial; it simply means that survival of the species requires us to address physiological needs first, before we advance through the other stages of human needs.

SPECIFIC STRATEGIES

The following specific strategies should help in answering the multiple-choice questions on the certification exam.

Strategy #1: Understand and Analyze the Anatomy of a Test Question

A multiple-choice test question consists of three parts:

- An *introductory statement*, which sets up the clinical scenario
- A *stem*, which poses a question
- *Options*, from which you must select the correct answer

The first step in analyzing a multiple-choice test question is to separate what the question *tells* you from what it *asks* you. The **introductory statement,** which may vary considerably in length, provides information about a clinical scenario, a disease process, or a nursing response. The **stem** poses a specific question, which you must answer on the basis of your advanced-practice nursing knowledge. Stems are worded in different ways. Some stems are in the form of a question; others are in the form of an incomplete statement that you must complete. You must select the one **option** that best answers the question or completes the incomplete statement from a number, usually four, of potential options, sometimes referred to as distractors.

Knowing these components will assist you in analyzing the information presented and in focusing on the question's intent or issue. Let's look at an example that includes an introductory statement in the form of a clinical scenario. The stem, which, in this example, is in the form of an incomplete statement, is in bold print.

EXAMPLE 1 _____

A 32-year-old woman comes to your office for a routine examination. Her blood pressure is 120/80. **You should recommend that the client have her blood pressure checked again in**
A. 6 months.
B. 1 year.
C. 2 years.
D. 5 years.

The first and most important step is to identify what the question is asking. You cannot expect to answer the question correctly until you understand the **topic** of the question. The introductory statement of Example 1 gives you information about the clinical situation—a 32-year-old female client came to your office for a routine exam and has a normal blood pressure; these are the topics. The stem asks you for a clinical judgment—when should she have her blood pressure checked again? You must select the option that provides the most accurate response—in this case, option C. This question is an example of a **recall (memory-based) question.** You need to remember the guidelines concerning the frequency of blood pressure measurements under different circumstances.

Nursing, however, is a practice-based discipline. Nurses must apply knowledge to specific situations. This ability is assessed through the second type of question designed to assess nursing knowledge—namely, **comprehension (application-based) questions.** Application of nursing knowledge is essential to safe, competency-based practice. Application frequently implies **analysis** of information. The certification exam is a test of "minimum competency," and simply recalling facts would not provide the certification bodies with sufficient information to determine your abilities. As such, you can expect the majority of questions to be comprehension and analysis type questions. These require you to integrate knowledge with the facts that are presented in order to choose the single best answer for each question. Review the following example.

EXAMPLE 2 _____

Julie, age 18 months, is up to date with her immunizations and is due to receive her diphtheria, tetanus, and pertussis (DTP) and oral polio (OPV) vaccinations today. Her father is bedridden at home with AIDS. Which immunizations should Julie receive today?
A. DTP and OPV as scheduled
B. DTP and inactivated polio vaccine (IVP)
C. DTP; IPV; and measles, mumps, and rubella (MMR)
D. DTP, OPV, and MMR

You must synthesize several concepts regarding immunizations to select the correct answer (option B) for this question. You must integrate your recall knowledge regarding standard and current immunization schedules (e.g., that Julie should receive DTP and polio immunizations on this visit) with the specific clinical scenario, which, in this case, includes a family member—her father who has AIDS. This calls for you to modify the regular regimen for immunizations and to administer a dose of inactivated polio vaccine (IPV) rather than the standard OPV because of Julie's close proximity to her father, who may be susceptible to the live poliovirus found in the standard OPV.

A common error test takers make in a multiple-choice testing format is to analyze the questions and answer choices with their eyes. Analysis is, however, done with the brain. Be careful of "looks good" choices. The reference for each and every correct answer is grounded in textbook and/or guideline knowledge. A common trap that test question writers use is to include answer choices that appear on the surface to be correct, but are not.

You should also determine if the stem is requesting a **positive response** or a **negative response.** Positive-response stems request an answer that is true, appropriate, or accurate, whereas negative-response stems request an option that is incorrect, false, inaccurate, or inappropriate. Negative-response stems frequently contain words such as *except, not, false,* or *least.* Consider this example.

EXAMPLE 3

Risk factors for osteoporosis include all of the following ***except***
A. alcohol.
B. obesity.
C. age.
D. sedentary lifestyle.

Example 3 is a straight recall question testing your knowledge about osteoporosis and its risk factors. The key word in the stem—*except*—is a negative. In other words, to select the correct response for this question, you must select the answer that is wrong or is *not* a positively correlated risk factor for osteoporosis. In this question, the correct response is B.

Strategy #2: Identify the Question's Critical Elements and Key Words

The ability to identify the **critical elements** and **key words** in a test question is crucial to a correct interpretation of the question. Critical elements, such as the key concepts and conditions, tend to appear in the introductory statement whereas key words usually appear in the stem of the question. Regardless of the placement of these words, remember that everything you need to be able to answer this question correctly is provided for you.

Key words are important words or phrases that help focus your attention on what the question is specifically asking. For example, key words determine whether the stem is asking for a positive or negative response. Examples of key words include *most, first response, earliest, priority, on the first visit, on a subsequent visit, common, best, least, except, not, immediately,* and *initial.* Often, but not always, these words appear in bold or italicized print. Take a look at this example.

EXAMPLE 4

Which of the following is an example of a ***primary*** *preventive intervention?*
A. Tetanus prophylaxis
B. Screening sigmoidoscopy
C. Papanicolaou smear
D. Blood pressure screening

Example 4 is a recall question with a positive-response stem. Although all of the interventions are preventive, the key word is *primary,* allowing you to choose the correct answer, A.

After identifying the topic of the question, you must also identify the **issue** the question is asking about. For example, the question, as in Example 5, may be requesting information about a disorder.

EXAMPLE 5

Mr. Williams, age 76, is seen in the ambulatory care clinic. He is complaining about incontinence, suprapubic pain, urgency, and dysuria. A urinalysis reveals the presence of white blood cells (WBCs), red blood cells (RBCs), and bacteria. What is your assessment?
A. Prostatitis
B. Nephrotic syndrome
C. Benign prostatic hypertrophy (BPH)
D. Cystitis

By selecting the correct answer, D, you have demonstrated knowledge related to a disease process, the **issue** about which this question requested information. Other examples of issues include drugs—for example, antibiotics or immunizations; diagnostic tests, such as urinalysis or serum glucose; toxic effects of a drug, such as rash or vomiting; problems, such as knowledge deficit or substance abuse; procedures, such as bone marrow aspiration or cardiac catheterization; behaviors—for example, agitation or overeating; and, occasionally, a combination of these. Consider this example.

EXAMPLE 6 _____

Which drug is not used in the treatment of acute gout?
A. An NSAID
B. Colchicine
C. An antibiotic
D. An analgesic

This is a **recall** question with a negative-response stem. The **key word** is negative—*not*—and the **issue** is knowledge of drugs. The correct answer is C.

Strategy #3: Use Therapeutic Communication

In communication-type questions, you are always looking for a **therapeutic response,** the cornerstone of the nurse-client relationship. To communicate therapeutically, you need to use communication tools and avoid communication blocks. Remember your basic therapeutic nursing role. The nurse, whether at a generalist or advanced-practice level, is *always* therapeutic. Your role is *not* that of an authority figure. This may cause some confusion for practitioners from other cultures in which health-care providers are conceptualized as authority figures who give directions. Remember, this is a nursing-based exam. Your **initial response** is *always* the therapeutic response— the acknowledgment and validation of the client's feelings.

EXAMPLE 7 _____

Ms. Doe, age 55, is very fearful because of a breast lump you have just identified. She begins to cry and states, "I'm afraid of having a mammogram." Your initial response is
A. "You must have the mammogram."
B. "Don't worry; I'm sure it is nothing."
C. "Wonderful advances have been made in breast cancer research."
D. "You're feeling scared?"

The correct answer is D. Communication skills learned in Nursing 101 are important components of successful test-taking strategies. Table 2-2 reviews communication techniques that facilitate therapeutic communication and those that block therapeutic communication.

Another important component in selecting the correct answer to questions that address your ability to communicate therapeutically is prioritization of responses. More than one option may contain a therapeutic response. But which is the **first, best,** or **most therapeutic** response in that situation? Communication theory emphasizes that it is a priority to address the client's **feelings first.** Validate, validate, validate. "You seem to be very sad today, Mr. George." "I can see that you are upset." "You seem very anxious, Mrs. Smith." This should always be done *before* clarifying or presenting information. Is there a need to address the feelings? If so, this takes priority. Empathy, restatement, reflection, and being silent, as well as remaining with the client, are all excellent nursing strategies that can potentially validate clients' feelings. The only exception to this rule would be the presence of a pressing or interfering physical problem.

Strategy # 4: Identify the Person Who Is the Focus of the Question

Another critical element is your ability to identify the person who is the focus of the question. This person might be the client or the person with the health-care problem, or a family member or neighbor of the person with the health-care problem, or another member of the health-care team. Take a look at this example.

EXAMPLE 8 _____

Mr. Boyd, age 84, has dementia and is in a long-term care facility. His daughter and son-in-law are visiting. As they get ready to leave and begin to say good-bye, Mr. Boyd grabs his daughter's arm and begins to cry, saying "Don't leave me here. I will die in this place." As she leaves the room, his daughter is visibly upset and asks you if she should visit again soon because it has so upset her father. The best reply for you to make is
A. "You might try telephoning next time instead of visiting. Your father will know that you are thinking of him then."
B. "I will give you the number of the social worker. She will be able to arrange a team conference and family meeting."
C. "This is a very upsetting time for all of you. However, it is important that you continue to visit regularly. For now, I will go in and sit with your father for a little while."
D. "He needs time to adjust to this new setting. Perhaps it might be easier on you all if you just didn't visit for a few days."

In this question, the person who is the focus of the question is Mr. Boyd's daughter, not Mr. Boyd. The **key word** in the stem is **best** response. It is also helpful to identify the **issue** the question is asking about. The issue in this question is one of therapeutic communication, specifically, Mr. Boyd's daughter's feelings of concern about her father. C is the correct response because it validates the daughter's feelings first.

TABLE 2-2. COMMUNICATION TECHNIQUES

Techniques That Facilitate Therapeutic Communication

TECHNIQUES	EXAMPLES
Offering self	"I'll stay with you …"
Showing empathy	"I see you are upset."
Silence	Remaining present but silent
Giving information	"You need to take this drug two times a day."
Restatement	"You feel hurt?"
Clarification	"You are saying that …"
Reflection	"You seem to be anxious."

Techniques That Block Therapeutic Communication

False reassurance	"Everything will be OK."
Disapproval	"That was wrong."
Approval	"That was right."
Requesting an explanation	"Why did you do that?"
Giving advice	"I think you should …"
Deferring	"You need to talk with your doctor about that."
Defensiveness	"We are understaffed!"
Devaluing feelings	"That's silly; don't be upset!"

Strategy #5: Determine the Best Response

There may be more than one option in a test question that is correct. But which is the **best, first,** or **most therapeutically sound** response to the question posed? Application-based test questions often involve decision making, which is based on prioritization. Therapeutic communication skills teach the acknowledgment of feelings first. Teaching and learning theory reminds us that unless the client is motivated to learn, no client teaching will be successful. If the client is not motivated, this issue must be addressed first.

To assist you in the correct answer selection, follow a few tips:

- Assessment always comes before diagnosis and treatment.
- The key word *initial* usually implies the need to assess.
- Remember Maslow's Hierarchy of Needs.
- In communication-based questions, you must address the client's **feelings first.**
- In teaching and learning situations, learning is contingent upon **motivation.**

As stated earlier, according to Maslow, physiological needs always come first. In determining which physiological needs have priority, you might recall the ABCs for basic cardiopulmonary support—A for airway, B for breathing, and C for circulation. This is handy to remember for questions that present a sudden emergency situation or any situation that is potentially life threatening for the client. Once basic physiological needs are met, **safety** is the next priority, followed by **psychosocial** needs.

Strategy #6: Avoid Common Pitfalls

A very common cause of test-taking errors is misreading the test question. To avoid common pitfalls, follow these tips:

- Ask yourself, "What is this question *really* asking?"
- Look for the key words.
- Restate the question in your own words. Eliminate any options that require you to make assumptions about information that was not presented in the case scenario and any options that contain information not

presented in the scenario. *Do not read anything new into or overanalyze the test question!* Go with your first, most straightforward response. It is usually your best bet for answering the test question correctly.

- Carefully review the question using the systematic format and strategies suggested in this book.

- Make a decision about each option as you read it; this is an efficient approach to test taking. Do not go back to that option once you have eliminated it, do not overcomplicate the case scenario presented, and do not rely on anecdotal data from your own practice. These are national exams with testing content based on national standards of practice.

Strategy #7: Select the Best Answer When You Do Not Know the Answer

We now discuss some more specific strategies for selecting the best answer. Imagine that you are beginning your exam. You have answered a few questions easily, but now you have come to a test question to which you do not know the answer. You have identified the introductory statement and the stem, have determined whether it is a positive-response stem or a negative-response one, and have read through the options. You have identified the issue and the person who is the focus of the question. But you are still uncertain of the answer. If this happens, follow these tips:

- **Eliminate incorrect options.** This is very important. Frequently, you will be able to eliminate two choices easily, and remember that if even a small part of the answer choice is incorrect the whole answer choice is incorrect and you must eliminate it from further consideration. Eliminating incorrect answer choices improves your chances of choosing the correct response even when you are unsure of the exact answer choice. The key is to not panic. It is not realistic to expect to know everything that you will be tested on, but through careful preparation, use of test-taking tools and strategies, and analysis of the content presented in the question, you will improve your chances of successfully answering the question—and passing the certification exam on the first attempt—a noteworthy goal!

- **Select the most global response option.** The option that offers the most comprehensive or general statement is often a better answer than an option that is more specific and thus more limited.

- **Eliminate similar options.** If two options say essentially the same thing, neither can be correct. If three of the four options sound similar, the "odd" one should win out. In other words, look for patterns or relationships within the answer choices to help you select the best answer.

- **Eliminate options that contain words like *always* or *never*.** Absolute options containing the words *always* or *never* are seldom correct.

- **Look for words or phrases in the option that are similar to those in the introductory statement or stem.** Try this strategy if you need to guess.

- **Be alert to relevant information from earlier questions.**

- **Watch for grammatical inconsistencies between the stem and the options.**

- **Look for the longest option.** It is often the correct response.

Key test-taking tips are given in Table 2-3.

Designing Your Study Plan

In creating your individual study plan, review and apply the phases of the nursing process: assess, plan, implement, and evaluate.

ASSESS

Begin by taking some sample exams. You might try an integrated content exam first and score yourself. This will give you an idea of your baseline and how intensive your study plan needs to be. Reflect, as part of your assessment, on your test-taking type, preferred learning style, and personality. Remember, speed is not necessarily your best friend and overanalysis can lead you to an incorrect answer choice, but careful analysis of each question is a prerequisite to success on the exam. The union of knowledge and strategy is what is needed to achieve a successful outcome on the certification exam. One complements the other and both are imperative if you are to attain your goal of becoming a board-certified advanced-practice nurse.

TABLE 2-3. KEY TEST-TAKING TIPS

- Eliminate options you know are incorrect. If you can eliminate two options, even a guess has a 50% chance of being correct.
- Answer all questions as if the situations were ideal.
- Read the test question carefully.
- Separate what the question tells you from what it is asking.
- Identify all false-response stems.
- Select the most global response.
- Eliminate options that are incorrect or similar or that contain words such as *always* or *never*.
- Look for grammatical inconsistencies between the stem and the options, words in the options that have appeared in the stem, and the longest option.
- Be alert to information relevant to answering the question in the stem or in earlier questions.

Use the analysis of scoring in Table 2-4 to help you make an accurate assessment of why you missed the questions you did. Failure to analyze why you missed a specific question is a commonly missed opportunity to improve your skills. Simply comparing your answer choice to the correct answer choice is a passive learning process. However, analyzing why you missed a question (assessment) and actively creating a strategy to correct the knowledge or skills deficit (implementation) will help you achieve the outcome

TABLE 2-4. ANALYSIS OF SCORING

Test-Taking Error

Review the sample test questions that you answered incorrectly and keep track of WHAT caused you to select the incorrect answer. Look for a pattern.

- Missed key word
- Did not read all of the distractors carefully
- Read into the question
- Misread or misunderstood the question
- Changed the answer
- Content weakness
- Forgot or did not recognize or understand the content
- Applied wrong concept or rationale

you are seeking. For example, did you miss the correct answer because you did not know or remember the content? This is a knowledge deficit. Or did you miss a key word, read into the test question, or change the answer? If so, you need to continue to work on test-taking skills. You must become proficient at both—content knowledge and test-taking skills. Recognizing where you are vulnerable and then taking steps to improve in that specific area gives you a significant edge in preparing for your examination and building your confidence. These objectives are best achieved through ongoing self-testing with sample exam questions such as the ones provided for you in this book. Evaluate what percentage of questions you missed because of (1) content issues, (2) testing errors, or (3) confidence issues. Design your study plan accordingly. As you study, use the analysis of scoring to continue to track your progress.

Aim for an 85% grade on your practice exams to demonstrate a good level of mastery of each content area. Begin working on areas in which your knowledge may be lacking and progress to areas in which you are stronger. Opening a book and beginning on page one may not serve you well. However, recognizing that you may be weak in cardiovascular content and prioritizing your study time to concentrate on that content area to eliminate knowledge deficits will be very helpful.

Any test score below 80% indicates a need to initiate a more aggressive and intensive exam review. A score of 80% or above, however, does not mean that you shouldn't prepare. You should still aim to review approximately 2000 to 3000 sample test questions before sitting for the exam, as well as do some basic content review. An initial score below 80% means you should aim to review a minimum of 5000 sample test questions before the exam, as well as complete an intensive content review. Attending a certification review class is an additional way to shore up your knowledge base.

PLAN AND IMPLEMENT

The certification exam time line and study calendar (Table 2-5) provide a suggested 6-week time line, providing a countdown to exam time from the day you register for your exam. Use the salami technique. Study a little every day. Improve your self-image. Believe you are a good student and behave like one. Stick to your study plan. Set clear-cut goals and objectives.

Answer approximately 100 test questions in a specific content area. Assess your score. If it is between

85% and 95%, move on. Feel confident—but continue to review sample test questions. If your score is lower than 85%, use the diagnostic grid.

As noted in chapter 1, both the ANCC and AANP exams cover pathophysiological content organized by body system. This is how you should organize your study time: by body system, as well as by associated content areas. We suggest following the table of contents of this book, which is modeled on the practice domains spelled out by both certifying bodies. After assessing your baseline knowledge through use of the integrated exams provided in this book, move on to the content areas in which you scored the lowest. This will allow you to customize your study plan and make the best use of your time. Remember, for some people, this might be the neurological content; for others, it might be the endocrine or psychiatric content, and so on.

To review disorders and help you prioritize, use the following tips:

- Organize content by body system.
- Begin with the system you find the most difficult.
- Review the pathophysiology of that system, if necessary.
- List pertinent disorders of that system.
- Review incidence and contributing factors.
- Review early and late disease manifestations.
- Review the sequelae, prognoses, and life-threatening complications.
- Determine treatment; adjust for age.
- Review associated teaching and learning needs.
- Review coping techniques, prevention, and health promotion.
- Remember that the certification exam focuses on common diseases and disorders; use this information as a tool for success and avoid studying topics that are rarely seen in a primary care setting.

Using content maps is another approach to mastering content. Figure 2-1 is an example of a content map approach to reviewing disease processes. A content map is a picture or pattern of information. It also shows relationships between pieces of information. Developing content maps can help you to find content areas in which you are weak and avoid studying content you already know. People are drawn to study what they already know. They feel comfortable with that information, whereas new information can produce anxiety. In the long run, however, this is not a good strategy. Few people can read a book and visualize the exact page, word for word, in their minds. A content map helps you find the information in your memory, where it is usually stored in patterns related to other memories. Using this structure, you can find out what areas you may not completely understand. Content maps start with general information and move to specifics. They can be helpful for people who spend so much time studying the details that they miss the bigger picture.

EVALUATE

To help you evaluate your progress, consider these tips:

- Take a sample test and use the test-taking analysis of scoring. Review one of your sample content area tests. Why did you answer the questions that you got wrong incorrectly? Remember, active learning improves retention.
- If content is forgotten, use a content review. Did you not recognize or remember the content? This would indicate a need to review content using a book of condensed information or an outline-review text, or attending a certification review. It does not mean that you should return to your textbook or class notes.
- If a rationale is misunderstood, go back to textbooks. Did you not comprehend the content? For example, perhaps your basic understanding of the cardiac cycle was not thorough enough to include the severity and implications of various murmurs (i.e., which ones are relatively normal physiological events and which ones are indicative of more severe pathology). This would indicate a need to go back to one of your textbooks, or perhaps obtain audiotapes and/or videotapes with more detailed content, and review basic pathophysiological processes.
- If the error is in test taking or you need to build confidence, continue to take the sample exams. Did you answer a question incorrectly because you missed a key word? Did you not read all the options carefully enough? Did you read something into the question? Did you change an answer? Did you choose the correct answer but bubble in an incorrect response? All of these are indications of test-taking errors and

TABLE 2-5. CERTIFICATION EXAM TIME LINE AND STUDY CALENDAR

SUNDAY	MONDAY	TUESDAY	WEDNESDAY	THURSDAY	FRIDAY	SATURDAY
Commitment						
	• Register for the exam. • Evaluate your test-taking type and preferred learning style. • Take assessment exam. • Evaluate exam with analysis of scoring. • Develop study plan and gather study materials. • Fill out study calendar and begin. • Make arrangements for going to the exam.					
(Dates)						
WEEK 1	Content: Score:	Content: Score:	Content: Score:	Content: Score:	Content: Score:	Content: Score:
(Dates)						
WEEK 2	Content: Score:	Content: Score:	Content: Score:	Content: Score:	Content: Score:	Content: Score:
Perseverance						
	• Continue studying. • Take a week off from studying.					
(Dates)						
WEEK 3	Content: Score:	Content: Score:	Content: Score:	Content: Score:	Content: Score:	Content: Score:
(Dates)						
WEEK 4	Content: Score:	Content: Score:	Content: Score:	Content: Score:	Content: Score:	Content: Score:
Focus and Reward						
	• Focus on content areas in which you scored less than 80% on sample questions. • Make final arrangements for going to the exam.					
(Dates)						
WEEK 5	Content: Score:	Content: Score:	Content: Score:	Content: Score:	Content: Score:	Content: Score:
(Dates)						
WEEK 6	Content: Score:	Content: Score:	Content: Score:	Content: Score:	Content: Score:	Content: Score:

* Source: Adapted from Hoefler, P: *Successful Problem-Solving and Test-Taking for Beginning Nursing Students,* ed 3. MEDS, Silver Spring, MD, 1997, p. 111.

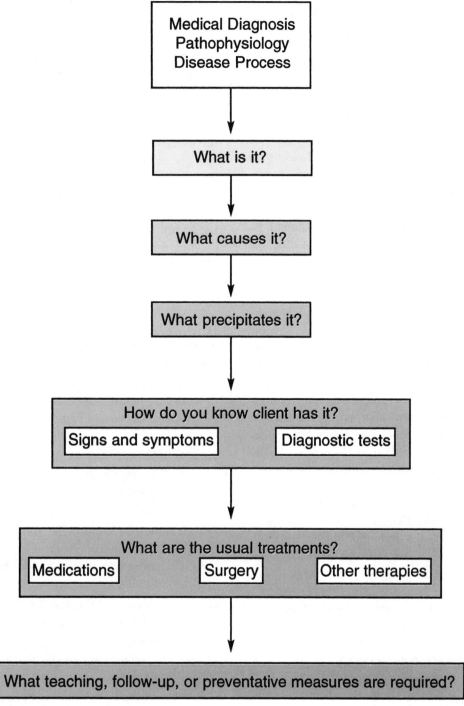

Fig. 2-1 Content map.

indicate an ongoing need for you to continue practicing your skills using sample exams. If you are consistently scoring well on practice exams, it will make you feel more confident and comfortable with testing.

- Practice, practice, practice sample test questions. Using the analysis of scoring as you

grade yourself on an integrated exam, followed by exams for specific body-system content, will enable you to design and update an individualized study plan that has specificity and relevance for you. For example, you may need to spend a week on neurological content but only a day on cardiac content. You *can* succeed in becoming certified!

Last-Minute Preparations: Relaxed and Ready

Well, you are finally there! The day of the exam has arrived. Several tried-and-true techniques can help you get through this day with success and confidence.

The night before the exam, get a good night's sleep. Last-minute all-night study sessions are *not* recommended. Since your examination will focus on comprehension and analysis, cramming the night before is not a test-taking strategy, and it often results in increased anxiety and lower test scores. However, taking time to review a few notes is acceptable. It might be better to do something relaxing and enjoyable like going to a movie.

Locate the exam site before the day of the actual exam and plan for possible traffic delays and bad weather on the day of the exam. Becoming lost or finding yourself stuck in traffic will only increase your anxiety. Know where to park and how long it will take you to get there.

The morning of the exam, do a few exercises to get your blood pumping to your brain. Eat lightly, but *do* have breakfast. Bring identification, your registration for the exam, at least two sharpened pencils if you are taking a paper-and-pencil exam, and a watch. Dress in layers. Avoid stimulants and depressants. Go light on the caffeine. Find the restroom, and use it before beginning the exam.

Pay careful attention to the instructions and tutorial for computer testing. Do deep breathing and positive relaxation exercises to calm yourself. In a testing center, others will be taking different exams and will have started at different times, so do not panic if people come and go while you are testing. Stay focused!

Pace yourself—do not spend too long on any one test question—and it is usually best if you go with your first choice. You should understand that the certification exams are *not* computer adaptive, meaning that you will be able to mark a question and return to it later if time permits. (In computer-adaptive exams, like the NCLEX-RN, after submitting your answer choice you are not permitted to return to a question and change your response.)

Use test-taking strategies when you do not know the answer. Identify distractions, such as backache or neck ache, noise, reading the same questions over and over, feeling tired, or thinking of your vacation. If these occur, *stop*, take a few deep breaths, refocus, then get back on track. Mental fatigue can certainly play a factor when you are taking a lengthy exam. We recommend that you pace yourself accordingly. For example,

prepare ahead of time to rest between each set of 25 questions or so. Allow yourself to disengage even for 1 minute; then you will be better able to refocus and continue answering questions. Stretch as needed. Practice positive visualization if your mind begins to drift and you find it difficult to concentrate, thus reducing your ability to identify key words and topics and increasing the likelihood of your answering a question incorrectly. Do not overcomplicate or overanalyze the test questions—everything you need to know to answer the question correctly is included in the question stem or answer choices. Move on! Think positively about your success. Stay focused on your goal: becoming a nationally certified advanced-practice nurse.

Begin now by using this book as suggested. After all, the longest journey begins with a single step. Take that step now. Turn the page and begin.

Bibliography

American Academy of Nurse Practitioners: National competency-based certification examinations for adult and family nurse practitioners. American Academy of Nurse Practitioners, Austin, TX, 2007.

American Nurses Certification Corporation certification Web page: http://www.nursecredentialing.org, accessed August 3, 2007.

Dickenson-Hazard, N: Test-taking strategies and techniques. In Kopac, CA, and Millonig, VL (eds): *Gerontological Nursing Certification Review Guide,* revised ed. Health Leadership Associates, Potomac, MD, 1996.

Hoefler, P: *Successful Problem-Solving and Test-Taking for Beginning Nursing Students,* ed 3. MEDS, Silver Spring, MD, 1997.

Miller, SK: *Adult Nurse Practitioner Review and Resource Manual,* ed 2. American Nurses Credentialing Center, Silver Springs, MD, 2005.

Sides, MB, and Korchek, N: *Successful Test-Taking,* ed 3. Lippincott Williams & Wilkins, Philadelphia, 1998.

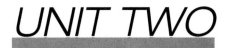

EVALUATION AND PROMOTION OF CLIENT WELLNESS

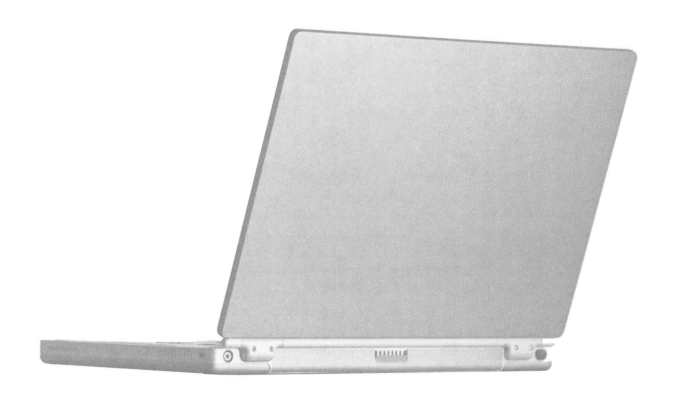

Chapter 3: *Health Promotion*

JILL E. WINLAND-BROWN
SHARON A. THRUSH

Questions

3-1 The American Cancer Society (ACS) recommends that mammography, as a method of screening for breast cancer, should be performed

A. every year after age 40.

B. only after a woman finds a lump when performing monthly breast self-examinations.

C. every 2 years from ages 40–80.

D. every 2 years from ages 40–50 and then annually until age 65, then every 2 years until age 80.

3-2 Which tumor marker is specifically elevated in prostate cancer?

A. Prostate cancer tumor marker (PCTM)

B. Cancer antigen (CA) 125

C. Carcinoembryonic antigen (CEA)

D. Prostate-specific antigen (PSA)

3-3 Sam, age 30, has a normal cholesterol level of 186 mg/dL. How often should he be screened for hypercholesterolemia?

A. Every 5 years

B. Every 2 years

C. Every year

D. Whenever blood work is done

3-4 Herbert, a 69-year-old man, comes to your office complaining of nocturia. On questioning Herbert, you find that for the past 3 months he has been getting up at least five times a night to void. He came in to seek help today because of his wife's insistence that he be checked out. When you perform the digital rectal exam, you find that his prostate protrudes 3–4 cm into the rectum. What grade would you assign to Herbert's prostate enlargement?

A. Grade 1

B. Grade 2

C. Grade 3

D. Grade 4

3-5 You are working with Iris, age 62, who has hypertension. Both of you are considering factors that contributed to her condition and will contribute to her probability of taking the appropriate plan of action. According to this information, you are formulating your plan using which of the following?

A. Social learning theory

B. Precede-proceed model

C. Health belief model

D. Nursing process model

3-6 What are the two leading causes of death in the United States for all ages?

A. Cancer and stroke

B. Heart disease and cancer

C. AIDS and heart disease

D. Accidents and heart disease

3-7 Sally, age 25, is of normal weight. She follows a diet of 70% carbohydrates, 10% fat, and 20% proteins. How do you respond when she asks you if this is a good diet?

A. "Yes, this is a good diet."

B. "No, you should eat more proteins."

C. "You should be eating only about 55% carbohydrates."

D. "Make sure your fats are divided among saturated, polyunsaturated, and monounsaturated fats."

3-8 The major public health and safety focus in the United States has shifted to

A. cardiovascular risk reduction.

B. domestic abuse and violence.

C. unintended pregnancies.

D. the threat of bioterrorism.

3-9 A conservative, preventive health approach for healthy adults is to recommend limiting salt intake to how many grams per day?

A. 2 g

B. 4 g

C. 6 g

D. 8 g

3-10 *Alcohol, especially when used with tobacco, is a dietary factor in which type of cancer?*

A. Liver

B. Esophagus

C. Bladder

D. Breast

3-11 *Josephine, a 60-year-old woman, presents to your office with a history of elevated total cholesterol, triglycerides, and low-density lipoprotein (LDL) cholesterol. She was started on a statin medication 4 weeks ago and is concerned about some muscle pains she has been experiencing. On questioning Josephine, you discover that she has had pain in both her thighs for the past 2 weeks. What possible complication of statin therapy are you concerned that Josephine might be experiencing?*

A. Liver failure

B. Renal failure

C. Rhabdomyolysis

D. Rheumatoid arthritis

3-12 *Jan's mother has Alzheimer's disease. She tells you that her mother's recent memory is poor and that she is easily disoriented, incorrectly identifies people, and is lethargic. Jan asks you, "Is this as bad as it gets?" You tell her that her mother is in which stage of the disease?*

A. Stage 1

B. Stage 2

C. Stage 3

D. Stage 4

3-13 *Which of the following criteria is not diagnostic for a child with attention deficit-hyperactivity disorder (ADHD)?*

A. The child frequently blurts out the answer to a question before the question is finished.

B. The child has difficulty following directions.

C. The child talks very little but is very restless.

D. The child often engages in physically dangerous activities.

3-14 *Carol, a nursing student, is at your office for her nursing school admittance physical exam and immunizations. On reviewing Carol's allergies, you find that she is allergic to baker's yeast. What would you tell Carol regarding the hepatitis B vaccine?*

A. You recommend that she receive the first hepatitis B vaccine today.

B. You advise her to wait until she is starting her clinical rotations to get the first hepatitis B injection.

C. You advise her that she cannot receive the hepatitis B vaccine because of her allergy to baker's yeast.

D. You instruct her to receive the first hepatitis B vaccine today, the second injection in 6 months, and the third injection in 1 year.

3-15 *Which statement is true regarding testicular cancer?*

A. White men are at a higher risk.

B. All races are equally susceptible.

C. Although testicular self-examination (TSE) alerts the person to the presence of a tumor, it has not been shown to decrease mortality.

D. TSE should be taught to all middle-aged men.

3-16 *An indicator of body fat measured by dividing weight in kilograms by height in meters is the*

A. weight/height chart.

B. body mass index.

C. body fat measurement.

D. anthropometric measurement.

3-17 *A lab value that is commonly decreased in older adults is*

A. creatinine clearance.

B. serum cholesterol.

C. serum triglyceride.

D. blood urea nitrogen.

3-18 *Anorexia nervosa is a steady, intentional loss of weight with maintenance of that weight at an extremely unhealthy low level. Which statement is true regarding anorexia nervosa?*

A. The poor eating habits result in diarrhea.

B. It may cause tachycardia.

C. It may occur from prepubescence into the early 30s.

D. It may cause excessive bleeding during menses.

3-19 *Mary, a 70-year-old woman with diabetes, is at your office for her 3-month diabetic checkup. Mary's list of medications includes Glucophage XR 1000 mg daily, an angiotensin-converting enzyme (ACE) inhibitor daily, and one baby aspirin (ASA) daily. Mary's blood work showed a fasting blood sugar of 112 and glycosylated hemoglobin (HgbA$_{1c}$) of 6.5. You tell Mary that her blood work shows*

A. that her diabetes is under good control and she should remain on the same medications.

B. that her diabetes is controlled and she needs to have her medications decreased.

C. that her diabetes is not controlled and her medications need to be increased.

D. that her diabetes has resolved and she no longer needs any medication.

3-20 *What is the term used to describe a disorder characterized by excessive sleep?*

A. Insomnia

B. Narcolepsy

C. Nocturnal myoclonus

D. Cataplexy

3-21 *The best defense against colds, flu, and respiratory syncytial virus is*

A. the flu shot.

B. prevention.

C. increased dosage of vitamin C.

D. rimantadine HCl (Flumadine).

3-22 *Susie, age 5, comes to the clinic for a well-child visit. She has not been in since she was 2. Her immunizations are up to date. What immunizations would you give her today?*

A. None; wait until she is 6 years old to give her booster shots

B. Diphtheria, tetanus, and pertussis (DTaP); *Haemophilus influenzae* type B (Hib); and measles, mumps, and rubella (MMR)

C. DTaP and IPV

D. DTaP, IPV, and MMR

3-23 *Which of the following is a true contraindication to immunizations?*

A. Mild-to-moderate local reaction to a previous immunization

B. Mild acute illness with a low-grade fever

C. Moderate or severe illness with or without a fever

D. Recent exposure to an infectious disease

3-24 *Which immunization may prevent meningitis?*

A. Hepatitis B

B. *Haemophilus influenzae* type B (Hib)

C. Measles, mumps, and rubella (MMR)

D. Varicella

3-25 *Gerald, a 67-year-old male retired maintenance worker, comes to your office for a physical. On reviewing Gerald's history, you discover that he has had pneumonia twice in the past 5 years. When you question Gerald about his immunization history, he reveals that his last tetanus and diphtheria (Td) immunization was 6 years ago, and his last flu shot was 8 months ago during the last flu season. He denies ever having had a pneumonia vaccination. Which immunizations should you offer to Gerald today?*

A. Td

B. Pneumococcal vaccine

C. Influenza

D. Td and pneumococcal vaccine

3-26 *How much higher are health-care costs for smokers than for nonsmokers?*

A. 20%

B. 40%

C. 60%

D. 80%

3-27 *The U.S. government report,* Healthy People 2010, National Health Promotion and Disease Prevention Objectives, *lists which of the following as leading health indicators?*

A. Obesity, substance abuse, and immunizations

B. Obesity, responsible sexual behavior, and driver education

C. Obesity, substance abuse, and driver education

D. Obesity, immunizations, and driver education

3-28 *Screening is considered a form of*

A. health counseling.

B. primary prevention.

C. secondary prevention.

D. tertiary intervention.

3-29   *The broad-based initiative led by the U.S. Public Health Service (PHS) to improve the health of all Americans through emphasis on prevention, rather than just treatment, of health problems throughout the next decade is*

A. the National Health Objectives Report.

B. *Healthy People 2010.*

C. the Surgeon General's Report.

D. the PHS Initiative.

3-30   *Performing range-of-motion exercises on a client who has had a cerebrovascular accident (CVA) is an example of which level of prevention?*

A. Primary prevention

B. Secondary prevention

C. Complications prevention

D. Rehabilitation prevention

3-31   *Emily, a healthy 26-year-old woman, asks you how she can prevent bone loss as she ages. She is concerned because both her maternal grandmother and now her mother have severe osteoporosis. What guidance would you give to Emily?*

A. Drink all the soda you like—it has no effect on your bone density.

B. It has not been proved that smoking affects bone loss.

C. Replace estrogen when you reach menopause.

D. Perform aerobic exercise at least three times a week.

3-32   *Which class of drugs causes the most adverse reactions?*

A. Chemotherapeutic agents

B. Anticonvulsants

C. Antibiotics

D. Antidepressants

3-33   *One of the major criteria for diagnosing chronic fatigue syndrome is*

A. generalized headaches.

B. unexplained, generalized muscle weakness.

C. sleep disturbance.

D. fatigue for more than 6 months.

3-34   *One of the most common causes of involuntary weight loss is*

A. malignancy.

B. pulmonary disease.

C. endocrine disturbances.

D. substance abuse.

3-35   *Which industry is responsible for the most injuries?*

A. Mining

B. Construction

C. Transportation and utilities

D. Manufacturing

3-36   *What is the most common type of occupational illness in the United States?*

A. Poisoning

B. Respiratory conditions caused by toxic agents

C. Disorders caused by physical agents

D. Skin disorders

3-37   *A 68-year-old woman presents to your office for screening for osteoporosis. Sandy states that her grandmother and mother both lost inches in their old age. Sandy has been postmenopausal for the past 15 years and never took any hormone replacement medications. She is Caucasian, weighs 108 lb, and is 5 ft 1 in. tall on today's measurement. When do postmenopausal women lose the greatest amount of bone density?*

A. The first 7 years after menopause

B. The first year of menopause

C. The first 10 years after menopause

D. Bone loss occurs continuously at the same rate from menopause to death.

3-38   *Margo, age 50, is perimenopausal. She tells you she is taking dehydroepiandrosterone (DHEA) and wants to start on hormone replacement therapy (HRT). When she asks for your opinion, you tell her that*

A. taking both DHEA and HRT is not recommended because it is like "double dosing."

B. DHEA is safe and will not affect prescribed medications.

C. she will be safe as long as she takes the minimum dose of both therapies.

D. DHEA has the same pharmacotherapeutic effects as HRT.

3-39   *In women with HIV infection, there is a high prevalence of additional infection from*

A. *chlamydia.*

B. syphilis.

C. human papillomavirus (HPV).

D. *candida.*

3-40   *Most anal cancers are potentially preventable. Which of the following is a cause of anal cancer?*

A. Sexually transmitted diseases (STDs)

B. A low-fiber diet

C. Hemorrhoids

D. Foreign bodies used as sexual stimulants

3-41   *When performing a sports physical exam on Kevin, a 16-year-old healthy boy, which question in the history is important to ask Kevin or his guardian?*

A. Did anyone in your family ever have sudden cardiac death?

B. Does anyone in your family have elevated cholesterol levels?

C. Did you ever have any injury requiring stitches?

D. Does anyone in your family have a history of asthma?

3-42   *What is an example of an active strategy of health promotion?*

A. Maintaining clean water

B. Introducing fluoride into the water

C. Enacting a stress management program

D. Maintaining a sanitary sewage system

3-43   *The best strategy to promote personal health is to*

A. instill a sense of responsibility in persons for their own health.

B. provide complete health information in many languages.

C. encourage health-promoting habits.

D. teach clients about appropriate risk factors.

3-44   *Women tend to outlive men by an average of*

A. 3–4 years.

B. 5–6 years.

C. 6–7 years.

D. 7 or more years.

3-45   *What is the goal of a sports physical?*

A. To clear all athletes for full participation in their sport activity

B. To limit the number of athletes participating in a sport activity

C. To identify health risks that may be minimized or cured in order to allow participation

D. To identify students at risk for health problems and limit their sports participation

3-46   *Harriet, a 76-year-old woman, comes to your office every 3 months for follow-up on her hypertension. Harriet's medications include one baby aspirin daily, lisinopril 5 mg daily, and calcium 1500 mg daily. On to-day's visit, Harriet's blood pressure is 168/88. According to the Joint National Committee (JNC) VII guides, what should you do next to control Harriet's blood pressure?*

A. Increase her dose of lisinopril to 20 mg daily.

B. Add a thiazide diuretic to the lisinopril 5 mg daily.

C. Discontinue the lisinopril and start a combination of ACE inhibitor and calcium channel blocker.

D. Discontinue the lisinopril and start a diuretic.

3-47   *Marvin is a gay man who is ready to "come out." What is the last step in the process of coming out?*

A. Testing and exploration

B. Identity acceptance

C. Identity integration and self-disclosure

D. Awareness of homosexual feelings

3-48   *Ethnocentrism is*

A. being concerned about the health needs of all Americans.

B. putting the group being studied at the center of dialogue.

C. thinking that ethnic groups other than one's own are inferior.

D. keeping a central focus on commonalities, not differences.

3-49 *The first step in alleviating the problem of homelessness is to*

A. increase available housing for low-income individuals.

B. make public assistance more readily available.

C. correct the public's perception of homeless persons.

D. provide community support for deinstitutionalized persons.

3-50 *Which health-care system delivers comprehensive health maintenance and treatment services to members of an enrolled group who pay a prenegotiated and fixed payment?*

A. Health maintenance organizations (HMOs)

B. Preferred provider organizations (PPOs)

C. Fee-for-service (FFS) independent practices

D. Exclusive provider organizations (EPOs)

3-51 *Marie, a Russian Jew, married Endo, a Filipino, and is adapting to his culture. This is referred to as*

A. acculturation.

B. biculturalism.

C. cultural relativity.

D. enculturation.

3-52 *Joseph, a 55-year-old man with diabetes, is at your office for his diabetes follow-up. On examining his feet with monofilament, you discover that he has developed decreased sensation in both feet. There are no open areas or signs of infection on his feet. What health teaching should Joseph receive today regarding the care of his feet?*

A. Wash your feet with cold water only.

B. See a podiatrist every 2 years, inspect your own feet monthly, and apply lotion to your feet daily.

C. Go to a spa and have a pedicure monthly.

D. See a podiatrist yearly; wash your feet daily with warm, soapy water and towel dry between the toes; inspect your feet daily for any lesions; and apply lotion to any dry areas.

3-53 *Sandra, a 27-year-old nurse, states that she does not want to get the hepatitis B virus vaccine because of its*

adverse effects. You tell her that the most common adverse effect is

A. fatigue.

B. headache.

C. pain at the injection site.

D. elevated temperature.

3-54 *In discussing sexuality with the mother of a 4-year-old, you should be concerned if the mother gives a yes answer to which of the following questions?*

A. Has your child asked questions about anatomical differences between sexes?

B. Does your child touch his or her own genitals?

C. Does your child play "doctor" with children of the opposite sex?

D. A yes answer to any of these questions is of no concern.

3-55 *Mimi, age 52, asks why she should perform a monthly breast self-examination (BSE) when she has an annual exam by the physician, as well as a yearly mammogram. You respond,*

A. "If you are faithful about your annual exams and mammograms, that is enough."

B. "More breast abnormalities are picked up by mammograms than by clinical exams or BSE."

C. "More than 90% of all breast abnormalities are first detected by self-examination."

D. "Self-examinations need to be performed only every other month."

3-56 *When does the National Cholesterol Education Program recommend cholesterol screening for persons with no family history of coronary heart disease before age 55?*

A. Starting at age 20 and then at least every 5 years if the cholesterol level remains normal

B. Whenever any other blood test is ordered

C. At the annual routine physical

D. Starting at age 20 and then annually

3-57 *A heart-healthy diet should be recommended to clients*

A. with a low-density lipoprotein (LDL) cholesterol level greater than 160 mg/dL.

B. with a total cholesterol level greater than 200 mg/dL.

C. with a high-density lipoprotein (HDL) cholesterol level below 35 mg/dL.

D. regardless of age or risk.

3-58   *Harvey, age 55, comes to the office with a blood pressure of 144/96 mm Hg. He states that he did not know if it was ever elevated before. When you retake his blood pressure at the end of the examination, it remains at 144/96. What should your next action be?*

A. Start him on an ACE inhibitor.

B. Start him on a diuretic.

C. Have him monitor his blood pressure at home.

D. Try nonpharmacological methods and have him monitor his blood pressure at home.

3-59   *Martha, age 82, has an asymptomatic carotid bruit on the left side. What do you recommend?*

A. ASA therapy

B. Coumadin therapy

C. Surgery

D. No treatment at this time

3-60   *According to the JNC VII guidelines for hypertension, Jesse, who has stage 1 hypertension, should be placed on which treatment plan for control of his hypertension?*

A. Thiazide diuretic

B. Diet and exercise

C. One drug from one of the following classes: ACE inhibitor, calcium channel blocker, or angiotensin receptor blocker (ARB)

D. Thiazide diuretic and either ACE inhibitor, calcium channel blocker, or an ARB

3-61   *Marian's husband, Stu, age 72, has temporal arteritis. She tells you that his physician wants to perform a biopsy of the temporal artery. She asks if there is a less invasive diagnostic test. What test do you tell her is less invasive?*

A. Computed tomography (CT) scan

B. Magnetic resonance imaging (MRI)

C. Electroencephalogram (EEG)

D. Color duplex ultrasonography

3-62   *Dennis, age 62, has benign prostatic hyperplasia (BPH). He tells you that he voids at least four times per night and that he has read about a preventive drug called terazosin hydrochloride (Hytrin) that might help him. What do you tell him?*

A. "It's not a preventive drug, but it relaxes smooth muscle in the prostate and bladder neck."

B. "It changes the pH of the urine and prevents infections caused by urinary stasis."

C. "It relaxes the urethra."

D. "It shrinks the prostate tissue."

3-63   *Molly, age 48, is healthy except for her well-controlled asthma. She asks if she should get an annual flu vaccination. You tell her that she should*

A. get it only after she reaches age 65.

B. get it only during the fall season when her asthma is bothering her.

C. get it on an annual basis.

D. not get it because she has a respiratory problem (asthma).

3-64   *How do you respond when Mattie, who is taking levothyroxine (Levothroid, Synthroid), says she has read that she should not eat brussels sprouts?*

A. "Brussels sprouts contain a high amount of iodine, and therefore you should not eat them."

B. "Brussels sprouts interfere with the absorption of the medication."

C. "There is no reason why you should not eat brussels sprouts."

D. "It is safe if you take the medication in the morning and don't eat brussels sprouts until the evening."

3-65   *A child's head circumference should be measured until the child reaches what age?*

A. 6 months

B. 12 months

C. 18 months

D. 24 months

3-66 *When should children have their first visual acuity testing?*

A. When they are able to read

B. When they enter kindergarten

C. At age 2

D. At age 3

3-67 *When should children be screened for lead poisoning?*

A. Only if they are in high-risk groups

B. At age 12 months

C. At age 3 years

D. Only if they live in or regularly visit a house built before 1960

3-68 *How do you respond when Jill, age 42, asks you what constitutes a good cardiovascular workout?*

A. Exercising for at least 30 minutes every day

B. Exercising a total of 2 hours per week

C. Exercising for at least 20 minutes, 3 or more days per week

D. Exercising for at least 30 minutes, 5 days per week

3-69 *Bone density studies to screen for osteoporosis should be performed on which of the following?*

A. Perimenopausal women who used to smoke but no longer do

B. All women after menopause

C. All women who have had hysterectomies

D. Women with drinking problems

3-70 *When can Pap smears be safely discontinued?*

A. At age 80

B. At age 65 if the previous three Pap smears have been normal

C. Never; they should be continued throughout life

D. After menopause or hysterectomy

3-71 *Utilization review refers to a system*

A. of reviewing access to and utilization of health-care services.

B. that uses retrospective review of client records to reveal problems that may be addressed in the future.

C. to monitor diagnosis, treatment, and billing practices to assist in lowering costs.

D. that has clients use an identification card to be able to use health-care services.

3-72 *Which federal insurance program went into effect in 1966 to provide funds for medical costs for persons age 65 and older, as well as disabled persons of any age?*

A. Medicare

B. Title XIX of the Social Security Act

C. Medicaid

D. Omnibus Reconciliation Act

3-73 *Which part of Medicare is basic hospital insurance?*

A. Medicare Part A

B. Medicare Part B

C. Medicare Part C

D. Medicare Part D

3-74 *A diagram that depicts each member of a family, shows connections between the generations, and includes genetically related diseases is referred to as a*

A. family assessment diagram.

B. family generation illustration.

C. generations diagram.

D. genogram.

3-75 *Lewin's change theory involves fundamental shifts in persons' behaviors to evoke and successfully implement change. The final phase is referred to as*

A. implementation.

B. refreezing.

C. finalizing.

D. change.

3-76 *The primary objective of screening is to*

A. prevent a disease.

B. detect a disease.

C. determine the treatment options.

D. promote genetic testing to prevent passing on the disease.

3-77 *Which of the following questions does not provide a basis for designating a disease as screenable or not?*

A. Does the significance of the disorder ensure its consideration as a community problem?

B. Can the disease be screened?

C. Should the disease be screened?

D. What is the cost of treatment?

3-78 *To quantify the margin of error in a screening instrument, the measure of validity is divided into two components: sensitivity and specificity. Sensitivity refers to a screening test's ability to*

A. recognize negative reactions or nondiseased individuals.

B. identify persons who actually have the disease.

C. predict populations at risk.

D. give the same result regardless of who performs the test.

3-79 *If a screening test used on 100 individuals known to be free of breast cancer identified 80 individuals who did not have breast cancer while missing 20 of the individuals, the specificity would be*

A. 80%.

B. 60%.

C. 40%.

D. 20%.

3-80 *Mildred, a 92-year-old independent woman, is moving into her daughter's home. Her daughter comes to see you seeking information to help keep her mother from falling. Which of the following interventions would you suggest she do to help prevent Mildred from falling?*

A. Install an intercom system in Mildred's bedroom.

B. Limit the time Mildred is home alone.

C. Hire an aide to assist Mildred 24 hours a day.

D. Remove all loose rugs from floors and install hand grasps in bathtubs and near toilets.

3-81 *The CAGE screening test for alcoholism is suggestive of the disease if two of the responses are positive. What does the E in CAGE stand for?*

A. Every day

B. Eye opener

C. Energy

D. Ego

3-82 *Twenty percent of colorectal cancers can be attributed to which dietary cause?*

A. High-fat diet

B. High-carbohydrate diet

C. Use of alcohol

D. Lack of fiber in the diet

3-83 *For primary prevention of skin cancer, you would recommend a sunscreen with how much ultraviolet (UV) wave protection?*

A. 15

B. 25

C. 30

D. 45

3-84 *Screening test recommendations for HIV infection include*

A. all clients.

B. persons getting married.

C. teenagers who have been sexually active for 1 year.

D. intravenous drug users and clients with high-risk behaviors.

3-85 *When should glaucoma screening be instituted?*

A. When the client is age 65

B. When the client exhibits vision problems

C. At the client's annual exam

D. Starting at age 40

3-86 *When should an African American man start to be screened for prostate enlargement by a digital rectal exam?*

A. Age 60 and then yearly

B. Age 40 and then yearly

C. Age 40 and then every 2 years

D. Age 55 and then yearly

3-87 *Who is the most important source of social support for an adult?*

A. Spouse (if applicable)

B. Parents

C. Close friends

D. Children

3-88 *Which of the following 4-year-olds should not receive an immunization today?*

A. Jerry, who has an upper respiratory tract infection (URI) with a mild fever

B. Timmy, who has otitis media

C. Joan, who needs several other immunizations

D. Joe, who had a previous reaction to egg protein

3-89 *Mark, a 56-year-old man, comes to your practice seeking help to quit smoking. You prescribe Chantix (varenicline), a prescription medication, to aid with his attempt. What instructions do you give Mark regarding how to stop smoking with Chantix?*

A. Start the Chantix today according to the dosing schedule and then quit smoking after the 12-week medication schedule.

B. Start the Chantix today according to the dosing schedule and then pick a date to stop smoking about 7 days after starting Chantix.

C. Pick a date to stop smoking and start Chantix that day according to the dosing schedule.

D. Start Chantix today, take it twice a day for 2 weeks, and then stop smoking.

3-90 *Andrea, a 20-year-old nursing student, never had her second measles, mumps, rubella (MMR) immunization. What test must you do before giving Andrea her second MMR?*

A. Complete blood count

B. Complete metabolic panel

C. Lipid profile

D. Urine pregnancy test

3-91 *The National Cancer Institute recommends that adults eat how many grams of fiber a day?*

A. 10–20 g

B. 20–30 g

C. 30–40 g

D. 40–50 g

3-92 *Postmenopausal women who are not on hormone replacement therapy need how much calcium per day to help prevent osteoporosis?*

A. 1000 mg

B. 1200 mg

C. 1500 mg

D. 1800 mg

3-93 *Margaret, age 29, is of medium build and 5 ft 4 in. tall. You estimate that she should weigh about*

A. 105 lb.

B. 110 lb.

C. 120 lb.

D. 130 lb.

3-94 *Max states that he cannot give up drinking beer, but he will cut down. You suggest that his limit should be*

A. one can of beer a day.

B. two cans of beer a day.

C. three cans of beer a day.

D. four cans of beer a day.

3-95 *Julia, age 18, asks you how many calories of fat she is eating when one serving has 3 g of fat. You tell her*

A. 12 calories.

B. 18 calories.

C. 27 calories.

D. 30 calories.

3-96 *A high sodium intake contributes to the risk of*

A. cancer.

B. heart disease.

C. osteoporosis.

D. hypertension.

3-97 *What is the ultimate goal of crisis intervention?*

A. To help persons function at a higher level than in their precrisis state

B. To help persons eliminate the crisis and get back to where they were

C. To prevent further crises

D. To eliminate stress altogether

3-98 *Martin, an 83-year-old man, is at your office for his yearly physical exam. He has a history of hypertension, hyperlipidemia, cigarette smoking, and chronic obstructive pulmonary disease (COPD). Martin states that he has been feeling increased fatigue with minimal activity but denies any chest pain or shortness of breath. Martin's list of medications includes the following: one* *baby aspirin daily, one ACE inhibitor daily, diuretic daily, and statin medication daily. Martin's physical exam was normal. His blood pressure was 130/68, his heart rate was 88, and his respiratory rate was 22. Observing Martin during your examination, you detect that he utilizes pursed-lip breathing throughout the exam. What medication should he be started on for his COPD?*

A. Inhaled corticosteroid

B. Inhaled anticholinergic and inhaled beta-2 agonists

C. Oral steroids daily

D. Inhaled beta-2 agonists

3-99 *Eileen, a 42-year-old woman, comes to your office with the chief complaint of fatigue, weight loss, and blurred vision. Eileen has a negative past medical history for any chronic medical problems. You obtain a fasting chemistry panel, lipid profile, complete blood count (CBC), and a HgbA_{1c}. The results of the blood work show Eileen's blood sugar to be elevated at 356 mg/dL, total cholesterol elevated at 255, high-density lipoprotein (HDL) cholesterol low at 28, LDL elevated at 167, triglycerides 333, and HgbA_{1c} 12. On questioning Eileen further, you discover that both her grandmothers had adult-onset diabetes mellitus. You diagnose type 2 diabetes mellitus. Your treatment plan should include a cholesterol-lowering agent, an agent that lowers blood sugar, and which other class of medication?*

A. ACE inhibitor

B. Diuretic

C. Weight loss medication

D. Beta blocker

3-100 *You are sharing with your client the idea that he needs to get some counseling to deal with his severe stress because it is affecting his physiological condition. Which of the following hormonal changes occurs during severe stress?*

A. A decrease in catecholamines

B. An increase in cortisol

C. A decrease in antidiuretic hormone

D. A decrease in aldosterone

3-101 *Sal is traveling out of the country and asks for a prescription to prevent traveler's diarrhea. What do you give him?*

A. Trimethoprim with sulfamethoxazole (TMP-SMX) double strength daily

B. Bismuth subsalicylate, 2 tabs qid

C. Nothing, but tell him to "cook it, boil it, peel it, or forget it"

D. Nothing, but tell him to use bottled drinking water

3-102 *Harry is taking his entire family to Central America and is wondering about protection against mosquito bites causing malaria. What advice do you give him?*

A. Use an insect repellent with diethyltoluamide (DEET) for the entire family, applying it sparingly to small children.

B. Make sure the family is in well-screened or indoor areas from dusk to dawn.

C. Use an insect repellent with DEET for adults, and permethrin for children, as well as staying inside from dusk to dawn.

D. Stay inside from dusk to dawn and use an insect repellent with permethrin.

3-103 *Susan is traveling to South America and wonders if she should get a tetanus and diphtheria (Td) vaccination. You tell her that*

A. she needs one if she has not had a Td shot within the past 10 years.

B. she should have tetanus immune globulin administered before departure.

C. she should receive a tetanus shot now.

D. tetanus and diphtheria are no longer a serious problem in South America.

3-104 *When is routine screening for hypothyroidism performed?*

A. When a client reaches age 65

B. Whenever a client exhibits symptoms

C. Never; it is not routinely recommended

D. When a client has a family history of thyroid problems

3-105 *Tuberculin skin testing using the Mantoux test should be considered for*

A. high-risk adolescents, recent immigrants, and homeless individuals.

B. all clients every 2 years.

C. all clients at their annual physical.

D. all children before entrance into first grade.

3-106 *Providers understand the effects of stress on the body. These effects go beyond the skin and can impair hair follicles. Which of the following conditions in a female can be described as hair "coming out in handfuls"?*

A. Telogen effluvium

B. Alopecia areata

C. Female pattern hair loss

D. Androgenic baldness

3-107 *Which program aims to remove racial and ethnic disparities in health by addressing the screening and intervention needs of midlife uninsured women?*

A. Public health screening programs

B. WISEWOMAN projects

C. American Heart Association screening protocols

D. Centers for Disease Control and Prevention

3-108 *Many of the 78 million baby boomers have a hearing loss. In a survey, all of the following statements were reported by baby boomers. Which statement was shared by the greatest percentage?*

A. Hearing loss is affecting the home life of baby boomers.

B. Baby boomers have problems hearing on cell phones.

C. Baby boomers are reluctant to admit the impact of their hearing loss.

D. Hearing loss is affecting the work/jobs of baby boomers.

3-109 *In which of the following situations would you NOT administer the HPV vaccination?*

A. Susie, age 11, who has not had sex yet

B. Janice, age 17, who had a baby 6 months ago and is breastfeeding

C. Alice, age 18, who is in an immunocompromised state

D. Jill, age 19, who is pregnant

3-110 *Which of the following is a major risk factor associated with osteoporosis and fragility fractures?*

A. Body weight <127 lb

B. Alcohol intake >2 drinks/day

C. Estrogen deficiency occurring before 45 years of age

D. Low physical activity

3-111 *The U.S. Department of Health and Human Services recommends which of the following exercise guidelines for Americans to reduce the risk of chronic disease in adulthood?*

A. Participate in 45 minutes of cardiovascular exercise at least three times per week.

B. Walk 1 hour every day.

C. Engage in vigorous intense activity 60 minutes most days of the week.

D. Engage in 30 minutes or more of moderately intense physical activity at least 5 days/week.

Answers

3-1 Answer A

The American Cancer society recommends that mammograms, as a method of screening for breast cancer begin at age 40 for women at average risk of breast cancer and continue yearly. The U.S. Preventive Services Task Force (USPSTF) recommends that screening should be done every two years beginning at age 50 for women at average risk of breast cancer. They also state that there is insufficient evidence that mammogram screening is effective for women age 75 and older.

3-2 Answer D

The tumor marker that is elevated in prostate cancer is prostate-specific antigen (PSA). Determined by a simple blood test, PSA is a tumor marker whose level in the bloodstream becomes elevated with prostate cancer, although it may also become elevated with benign prostatic hypertrophy (BPH). There is no prostate cancer tumor marker (PCTM). Levels of cancer antigen (CA) 125 are increased in the following cancers: epithelial ovarian, fallopian tube, endometrial, endocervical, hepatic, and pancreatic. It is also used to monitor for persistent or recurrent serous carcinoma of the ovary in the postoperative period or during chemotherapy. Measurement of the level of carcinoembryonic antigen (CEA) is used primarily for monitoring persistent, metastatic, or recurrent cancer of the colon after surgery and less frequently for breast or other cancers.

3-3 Answer A

The National Cholesterol Education Program (NCEP), launched by the National Heart, Lung, and Blood Institute, recommends that persons with normal cholesterol levels be tested every 5 years.

3-4 Answer C

The degree of prostate enlargement is based on the amount of projection of the prostate into the rectum. The normal prostate protrudes less than 1 cm into the rectum. Grade 1 enlargement is a protrusion of 1–2 cm, grade 2 is 2–3 cm, grade 3 is 3–4 cm, and grade 4 is greater than 4 cm.

3-5 Answer C

The health belief model follows a paradigm that analyzes factors contributing to a client's perceived state of health or risk of disease and to the client's probability of taking the appropriate health plan of action. Social learning theory assists in explaining, predicting, and influencing behavioral change. The precede-proceed model is a comprehensive planning guide to administering health education programs. The nursing process model is a series of activities that nurses perform as they provide care to clients. The steps include assessment, diagnosis, planning, implementation, and evaluation. Depending on the nursing diagnosis, the plan may be similar to that using the health belief model, but the assessment phase would have to incorporate data related to the client's perceived state of health, at which the health belief model excels.

3-6 Answer B

The two leading causes of death in the United States for all ages are heart disease and cancer. Almost two-thirds of the deaths in the United States every year are from these causes.

3-7 Answer C

The National Cholesterol Education Program recommends that carbohydrates comprise about 55% of total calories, fat no more than 30% of total calories, and proteins about 15%–20% of total calories.

3-8 Answer D

Since 2001, the major public health and safety focus has shifted to safety from the threat of bioterrorism. Nurse practitioners have been answering questions about bacterial and viral infections that they thought were no longer relevant. Other health promotion concerns that are continuing include the threat of cardiovascular disease, cancer, childhood infectious diseases, sexually transmitted diseases, and unintended pregnancies. In addition, clients face problems related to domestic violence, abuse, poverty, and addictions. While nursing education programs have prepared providers to deal with these issues, it wasn't until recently that bioterrorism threats were integrated into curricula.

3-9 Answer C

A conservative, preventive health approach for healthy adults is to recommend limiting salt intake to 6 g or less per day. This includes salt added to food during cooking or at the table, salt added as an ingredient to processed foods, and salt that occurs naturally in foods. Table salt is approximately 40% sodium by weight; therefore, a diet incorporating 6 g of salt contains about 2.4 g of sodium.

3-10 Answer B

Alcohol, especially when used with tobacco, is a dietary factor in cancer of the esophagus. Alcohol is also a factor in liver cancer. Dietary factors related to bladder cancer are unknown. A high-calorie diet (with high fat and low fiber) is a factor in breast cancer.

3-11 Answer C

Rhabdomyolysis is a syndrome that results from destruction of skeletal muscle. It is usually diagnosed from laboratory findings that are characteristic of myonecrosis. Although there are no standard creatine kinase values that establish the diagnosis of rhabdomyolysis, elevations above 10,000 IU/L are usually indicative of clinically significant rhabdomyolysis. The syndrome usually affects muscles used in exercise, but it may present as generalized muscle weakness. It usually resolves on stopping the statin medication, but severe cases may lead to renal failure and death.

3-12 Answer C

Families of persons with Alzheimer's disease (AD) need to know that AD is a progressive disorder of the brain affecting memory, thought, and language. Although the progression of the stages is individual and changes may occur rapidly or slowly over the course of several years, knowing what stage a family member is in helps family members in planning and knowing what to expect. Stage 1 is the onset, which is insidious. Spontaneity, energy, and initiative are decreased; slowness is increased; word finding is difficult; the person angers more easily; and familiarity is sought and preferred. In stage 2, supervision with detailed activities such as banking is needed, speech and understanding are much slower, and the train of thought is lost. In stage 3, personality change is marked and depression may occur. Directions must be specific and repeated for safety, recent memory is poor, disorientation occurs easily, people are incorrectly identified, and the person may be lethargic. In stage 4, apathy is noticeable. Memory is poor or absent, urinary incontinence is present, individuals are not recognized, and the person should not be alone.

3-13 Answer C

Diagnostic criteria for the child with ADHD include frequently blurting out answers before a question is finished, difficulty following directions, engaging in physically dangerous activities (often without thinking of the consequences of actions), tending to talk excessively, and often interrupting others. Behavior in which the child talks very little, but is very restless, is not indicative of ADHD.

3-14 Answer C

An allergy to baker's yeast is a definite contraindication to receiving the hepatitis B vaccine. Yeast is used in making the vaccine and is still present in the vaccine.

3-15 Answer A

White men are at a higher risk for testicular cancer than nonwhite men. Testicular self-examination (TSE), along with early detection and treatment, has decreased the mortality rates appreciably. TSE should be taught to all men beginning in adolescence.

3-16 Answer B

The body mass index (BMI) is an indicator of body fat. It is derived by dividing weight in kilograms by height in meters. It shows a direct and continuous relationship to morbidity and mortality in studies of large populations. The weight/height chart gives a range of what the ideal weight is for each height, but it does not reflect body fat. Anthropometric measurement is the measurement of the size, weight, and proportions of the human body.

3-17 Answer A

The creatinine clearance value is commonly decreased in older adults because of impaired renal function. Serum cholesterol, serum triglyceride, and blood urea nitrogen values are usually increased in older adults.

3-18 Answer C

Anorexia nervosa may occur from prepubescence into the early 30s and occurs most commonly from early to late adolescence. It occurs more frequently in women and may cause bradycardia, arrhythmias, and amenorrhea. Constipation is common in clients with anorexia because of their poor eating habits.

3-19 Answer A

A person with diabetes mellitus type 2 should have a HgbA$_{1c}$ of 6.5 or less and a fasting blood sugar (fbs) less than 120 for optimal control. Because the client's lab results fall in those categories, she is under good control and her medications should stay the same.

3-20 Answer B

Narcolepsy is a disorder characterized by excessive sleep. Narcolepsy with involuntary daytime sleep attacks may begin in adolescence. The person may have symptoms of this problem years before it is diagnosed. Insomnia is the inability to fall asleep or to stay asleep for a sufficient amount of time. Nocturnal myoclonus is a condition characterized by stereotypic kicking movements of the legs during sleep; it is more common in older adults. Cataplexy is often associated with narcolepsy. It is marked by abrupt attacks of muscular weakness and hypotonia triggered by an emotional stimulus such as anger or fear.

3-21 Answer B

The best weapon against infections, such as colds, flu, and respiratory syncytial virus, is prevention, with basic measures of hand washing, good hygiene, and isolation of infected persons. The flu shot augments the basic preventive measures. Although many persons believe taking extra vitamin C and the herb echinacea will shorten the length of a cold, vitamin supplements have not been proved necessary in persons with balanced diets. Rimantadine HCl (Flumadine) is effective against influenza A only if given within 24–48 hours of symptom onset.

3-22 Answer D

Because Susie has not been in for several years, one cannot assume that she will come in next year to get the immunizations that are due between the ages of 4 and 6; therefore, this opportunity to give her immunizations cannot be missed. Between the ages of 4 and 6, a child is due for diphtheria, tetanus, and pertussis (DTP); polio; and measles, mumps, and rubella (MMR) if all other immunizations are up to date.

3-23   Answer C

The only true contraindications to immunizations, according to the American Academy of Pediatrics, are a moderate or severe illness with or without a fever and an anaphylactic reaction to a vaccine or a vaccine constituent. Illnesses themselves are not true contraindications to vaccinations. Early symptoms may be a prodrome of something else; however, risks of the diseases are usually greater than the complications of vaccination. Even a fever of 104.5°F (40°C) with a previous diphtheria, tetanus, and pertussis (DTP) immunization is not a contraindication to a subsequent DTP shot.

3-24   Answer B

Meningitis is one of the most severe manifestations of *Haemophilus influenzae* infection, and the *H. influenzae* type B (HiB) immunization may help prevent its occurrence. The HiB vaccination is especially important for children age 5 years and younger. It should be given at ages 2 months, 4 months, and 6 months, with the fourth dose given between ages 12–18 months. Hepatitis B vaccination is important for all infants to help prevent liver disease as adults. A measles, mumps, and rubella (MMR) vaccination protects against measles, mumps, and rubella (German measles), and varicella vaccination protects against chickenpox.

3-25   Answer B

Prevention of pneumococcal disease in older people is one of the health initiatives of the U.S. government report *Healthy People 2010, National Health Promotion and Disease Prevention Objectives*. The goal for health-care providers is to have 90% of all clients older than 65 years old immunized against pneumococcal disease by the year 2010. The pneumococcal vaccine is a one-time injection that may need to be repeated in 8 years. Gerald does not need a Td booster because his last injection was only 6 years ago, and the CDC recommends a Td booster every 10 years. The influenza injection would not be appropriate at this time. Influenza vaccine is adjusted yearly to address the type of influenza that is thought to be prevalent in that

year. Also, the influenza vaccine is given just before flu season.

3-26   Answer B

Health-care costs for smokers at any given age are as much as 40% higher than for nonsmokers. Although smokers have more diseases than nonsmokers, nonsmokers live longer and can incur more health costs at advanced ages.

3-27   Answer A

The U.S. government report *Healthy People 2010, National Health Promotion and Disease Prevention Objectives* presents measurable objectives organized into 22 priority areas within four broad categories: health promotion, health protection, preventive services, and surveillance and data systems. Obesity, substance abuse, and immunizations are all leading health indicators. Driver education is not considered a leading health-care indicator.

3-28   Answer C

Screening is considered a form of secondary prevention because it seeks to identify the presence of diseases, such as high blood pressure, glaucoma, and diabetes, at early stages when treatment would be most effective.

3-29   Answer B

The broad-based initiative led by the U.S. Public Health Service to improve the health of all Americans through an emphasis on prevention and not just treatment of health problems throughout the next decade was initially called *Healthy People 2000, National Health Promotion and Disease Prevention Objectives*. It took its lead from the 1979 report *Healthy People: The Surgeon General's Report on Health Promotion and Disease Prevention*. Although all the objectives in that report were not achieved, it had such a positive impact that *Healthy People 2000* was conceived. The major difference in the 2000 report was the primary emphasis on health promotion and individual responsibility. The report has since been updated to *Healthy People 2010* to expand the priority areas and objectives.

3-30   Answer D

Performing range-of-motion exercises on a client who has had a cerebrovascular accident (CVA) is an example of rehabilitation prevention. Primary prevention would be eating a healthy diet as a young adult to prevent atherosclerosis, which might precipitate a CVA. Secondary prevention would include taking lipid-lowering drugs to prevent a CVA after having already developed hyperlipidemia. Although it is desirable to prevent any complications from the CVA, there is no level of prevention called complications prevention.

3-31   Answer D

Emily is only 26 years old and has not reached her peak bone mass yet. It has been proved that aerobic exercise increases bone mass. Smoking and soda drinking both have been shown to decrease bone mass. Estrogen replacement therapy is no longer recommended for bone health; it is recommended only for short-term use to alleviate vasomotor symptoms of menopause.

3-32   Answer C

Of all the drug classes, antibiotics cause the most adverse reactions. The other drug classes that cause a high number of adverse drug reactions are, in order, chemotherapeutic agents, cardiovascular agents, antihypertensive agents, anticonvulsants, and antidepressants.

3-33   Answer D

Fatigue for more than 6 months and absence of other clinical conditions that may explain such fatigue are the two major criteria the client must demonstrate to be diagnosed with chronic fatigue syndrome. Other minor criteria include generalized headaches, unexplained generalized muscle weakness, sleep disturbances, sore throat, mild fever or chills, and migratory arthralgias without swelling or redness.

3-34   Answer A

Malignancies (lung, lymphoma, gastrointestinal tract), along with gastrointestinal diseases and psychiatric disorders, are the most common causes of involuntary weight loss. Other less common causes include pulmonary disease, endocrine disturbances, and substance abuse.

3-35   Answer B

The construction industry is responsible for the most injuries (15 injuries per 100 full-time workers per year). Next in line are the agriculture, fishing, and forestry industries, followed by the manufacturing, transportation and utilities, and mining industries.

3-36   Answer D

Skin disorders are the most common type of occupational illness in the United States, accounting for 41,800 illnesses, or 33% of the cases, per year. This is followed by disorders associated with repeated trauma, respiratory conditions, disorders caused by physical agents, poisoning, and dust diseases of the lungs.

3-37   Answer A

Bone loss begins at a rate of 0.5% a year in a woman's mid to late 40s. When menopause occurs, the rate increases to 3% a year. This increase in the rate of bone loss is directly related to the decrease in a woman's estrogen. This high rate of bone loss continues for up to the first 7 years of menopause and then decreases to 0.5%–1% a year until death.

3-38   Answer A

Dehydroepiandrosterone (DHEA) is a hormone that is abundant in the body and is naturally produced from cholesterol by the adrenal glands, with smaller amounts manufactured by ovaries. Taking both DHEA and hormonal replacement therapy (HRT) is not recommended because it is like "double dosing." It is not absolutely contraindicated, but because most clients do not adequately regulate the dosage of over-the-counter medications, the combination therapy may produce excessively high levels of estrogen. Additionally, because almost a third of clients today are taking some sort of herbal therapy, it is essential to ask in the history and physical what other therapies are being used.

3-39   Answer C

Women with HIV infection have a high prevalence of human papillomavirus (HPV) infections. These infections are associated with an increased incidence of squamous intraepithelial lesions in HIV-seropositive women.

3-40   Answer A

Sexually transmitted diseases (STDs) are a cause of anal cancer. For women, other risk factors for anal cancer include an increased number (greater than 10) of sexual partners, having their first sexual experience before age 16, having four or more sexual partners before age 20, and anal intercourse. For men, other risk factors include having more than 10 sexual partners and being homosexual or bisexual.

3-41   Answer A

The risk of sudden death during sports activities from hypertrophic cardiomyopathy may be greatly reduced with a thorough cardiac history and examination. If a child has a relative who died of sudden cardiac disease before age 55, that child could possibly have hypertrophic cardiomyopathy. Family history of asthma is not relevant to this exam question.

3-42   Answer C

Enacting a stress management program is an active strategy of health promotion because it requires individuals to become personally involved. Maintaining clean water, introducing fluoride into the water, and maintaining a sanitary sewage system are all examples of passive strategies—those done for individuals and communities by others.

3-43   Answer A

The best strategy to promote personal health is to instill in people a sense of responsibility for their own health. Until people have made a commitment to assume personal responsibility for their own health, their health-promoting behaviors will not change. One of the nurse practitioner's functions is to effect changes in human behavior. Encouraging the adoption of personal responsibility is one way to do this.

3-44   Answer C

Since the late 1970s, the difference in life expectancy for men and women has narrowed, but women still outlive men by 6–7 years.

3-45   Answer C

The goal of the preparticipation sports exam is to protect the student from injury by identifying health risks and minimizing or curing them so that the student may participate in a sports activity. You might feel pressured by parents or coaches to pass the student regardless of your findings. Your responsibility is to further evaluate any abnormal findings on your exam before clearing the student to participate.

3-46   Answer B

The seventh report of the Joint National Committee on Prevention, Detection, and Treatment of Hypertension (JNC VII) recommends that stage 2 hypertension be treated with a combination of a thiazide diuretic and an ACE inhibitor, ARB, calcium channel blocker, or beta blocker.

3-47   Answer C

The last step in the process of a gay man or lesbian "coming out" is that of identity integration and self-disclosure. The process of discovering and revealing one's sexual orientation can occur at any age and is known as "coming out." Stage theories for coming out have been summarized as a four-step process: (1) awareness of homosexual feelings, (2) testing and exploration, (3) identity acceptance, and (4) identity integration and self-disclosure. If the ultimate costs of self-disclosure are felt to be too high, an individual may become socially isolated or deny gay or lesbian identity.

3-48   Answer C

Ethnocentrism is thinking that ethnic groups other than one's own are inferior. An ethnocentric perspective is a barrier to establishing and maintaining positive relationships with others.

3-49   Answer C

The first step in alleviating the problem of homelessness is to correct the public's perception of homeless persons. Current stereotypical opinions hinder effective delivery of health care, as well as other resources that should be available. Lack of housing for low-income persons, restrictions on public assistance, and inadequate support for deinstitutionalized persons are all factors that have contributed to the problem of homelessness.

3-50   Answer A

Health maintenance organizations (HMOs) deliver comprehensive health maintenance and treatment services to members of an enrolled group who pay a prenegotiated and fixed price. Preferred provider organizations (PPOs) allow persons to go to any doctor in the network, whereas clients of HMOs must choose their doctor ahead of time. Fee-for-service (FFS) independent practices permit an individual to be treated in any facility, with the full fee paid by the client. Exclusive provider organizations (EPOs) limit clients to providers belonging to one organization. Some may be able to use outside providers at an additional out-of-pocket charge.

3-51 Answer A

Acculturation is the process of adapting to a culture belonging to someone else. Biculturalism refers to taking components of both cultures and making them fit one's lifestyle. Cultural relativity refers to the attempt to view the behavior of culturally different individuals within one's own framework. Enculturation is the process of acquiring one's cultural identity as it is transferred down from the older generation.

3-52 Answer D

The American Diabetes Association recommends careful inspection of a diabetic client's feet for corns, calluses, and open lesions to prevent further deterioration into diabetic foot ulcers. The client should wash his or her feet daily with warm soapy water and towel dry them, especially between the toes, to prevent fungal infections. Diabetic clients should see a podiatrist yearly.

3-53 Answer C

The most common adverse reaction to the hepatitis B virus vaccine is pain at the injection site (13%–20% in adults, 3%–9% in children). Other mild, transient systemic adverse effects are fatigue and headache (11%–17% in adults, 8%–18% in children) and temperature elevation (1%–6% of all injections).

3-54 Answer D

A yes answer to any of these questions is of no concern. These are all normal behaviors for preschool children ages 3–6. These are the ways in which children express their concerns and explore their anatomy. Parents should honestly answer questions posed by their children regarding sexuality in terms the children can understand.

3-55 Answer C

More than 90% of all breast abnormalities are first detected by self-examination. All women older than age 20 should examine their breasts monthly, a week after their period. After menopause, women should examine their breasts at the same time each month.

3-56 Answer A

The National Cholesterol Education Program recommends cholesterol screening for persons with no family history of coronary heart disease before age 55. This should start at age 20 and then be done at least every 5 years. Earlier screening—at ages 10–15—should be considered for children with a family history of coronary heart disease that developed before age 55.

3-57 Answer D

A heart-healthy diet should be recommended for all clients regardless of age or risk. It is especially important that children learn healthy eating habits early in life. A heart-healthy diet follows the Dietary Guidelines for Americans as developed by the U.S. Departments of Agriculture and Health and Human Services. It is designed for healthy people older than age 2 to maintain their health. The guidelines include eating a variety of foods; balancing the food you eat with physical activity; maintaining or improving your weight; choosing a diet with plenty of grain products, vegetables, and fruits; choosing a diet low in fat, saturated fat, and cholesterol; choosing a diet moderate in sugars; choosing a diet moderate in salt and sodium; and, if you drink alcoholic beverages, doing so in moderation.

3-58 Answer D

Before drug therapy for hypertension is instituted, nonpharmacological methods such as salt restriction, weight reduction, biofeedback, and exercise should be considered. Aggressive treatment of all clients with a systolic pressure greater than 140 mm Hg and/or a diastolic pressure greater than 90 mm Hg is essential. The client should monitor his or her blood pressure at home and call the health-care provider if it exceeds the parameters discussed. In this case, Harvey should try nonpharmacological methods and monitor his blood pressure at home and then return in 1–2 weeks for follow-up. If his diastolic pressure is still 96 mm Hg after 2 weeks, a diuretic or an ACE inhibitor would be indicated.

3-59 Answer D

Clients with asymptomatic carotid bruits have a 2% incidence of cerebrovascular accidents (CVAs) per year. Although ASA, anticoagulants, and surgery are frequently ordered, there are not sufficient data to prove that these treatments reduce the risk of CVA in clients with asymptomatic carotid bruits. Starting an asymptomatic older woman on ASA therapy may produce more problems, such as skin bruising or gastrointestinal bleeding.

3-60   Answer A

The JNC VII guidelines for treatment of stage 1 hypertension recommend use of a thiazide diuretic as first choice for treatment of hypertension. Lifestyle modification with diet and exercise should already be in place.

3-61   Answer D

A biopsy of the temporal artery is usually required to confirm the diagnosis of temporal arteritis. Color duplex ultrasonography (a combination of ultrasonography and the flow-velocity determinations of a Doppler system) has been shown to examine even small vessels, such as the superficial temporal artery, and show a halo around the inflamed arteries when temporal arteritis is present. Therefore, it is a much less invasive procedure than biopsy. A computed tomography (CT) scan and magnetic resonance imaging (MRI) are done to detect neurological damage from hemorrhage, tumor, cyst, edema, or myocardial infarction. These tests may also identify displacement of the brain structures by expanding lesions. However, not all lesions can be detected by CT scan or MRI. An electroencephalogram is used to evaluate the electrical activity of the brain. It can identify seizure activity, as well as certain infectious and metabolic conditions.

3-62   Answer A

Terazosin (Hytrin) is an alpha-1 adrenergic blocker. It is not a preventive drug, but it does relax smooth muscle in the prostate and bladder neck and allows complete emptying of the bladder, relieving frequent nocturnal urination. Terazosin is begun at 1 mg at bedtime initially and then titrated upward to 10 mg once a day. Doxazosin (Cardura) is also effective as an alpha-1 adrenergic blocker. It is begun initially at 1 mg at bedtime, with the dosage doubled every 1–2 weeks to a maximum of 8 mg per day. Finasteride (Proscar), a 5-alpha reductase inhibitor, decreases the volume of the prostate within about 3 months. At 12 months, it seems to have reached its peak effectiveness. Finasteride is given 5 mg daily for at least 6 months; then the client is reevaluated.

3-63   Answer C

Molly should get an annual flu vaccination because she has a long-term pulmonary problem. Others who should be vaccinated include those older than age 64; nursing home residents; persons with diabetes, blood dyscrasias, suppressed immune systems, and long-term cardiac, urinary, and respiratory problems; and persons who come in close contact with other persons who are vulnerable to influenza.

3-64   Answer A

Clients taking levothyroxine (Levothroid, Synthroid) should avoid foods high in iodine such as brussels sprouts, cabbage, cauliflower, rutabagas, soy, and turnips because these foods, when added to the medication, raise clients' iodine levels.

3-65   Answer D

Head circumference should be measured until a child reaches age 24 months. It should be measured at birth; at 2–4 weeks; and at ages 2, 3, 6, 9, 12, 15, 18, and 24 months. Measuring growth and following its progression over the course of time can help identify significant childhood conditions. In addition to head circumference, height and weight should be measured at ages 3, 4, 5, and 6 months, then every 2 years thereafter.

3-66   Answer D

Children should have their first visual acuity testing at age 3. Visual acuity should be tested using a pictorial wall chart, and strabismus should be tested for using the cover-uncover test. Visual acuity testing should be repeated at age 5 or 6.

3-67   Answer B

The Centers for Disease Control and Prevention recommend that all children be screened for lead poisoning at age 12 months. If resources allow, children should then be screened again at age 24 months. Children ages 3–6 years should be tested for lead levels (using an assessment tool) every 6 months if they have a high risk of lead exposure. Those with normal lead levels should be retested once a year until age 6 years.

3-68   Answer C

A good cardiovascular workout consists of exercising large muscle groups for at least 20 minutes, 3 or more days per week, at an intensity of at least 60%

of the maximum heart rate (220 beats per minute minus age).

3-69   Answer A

There is still debate as to the recommendations for screening for osteoporosis for women. Bone density studies to screen for osteoporosis are recommended for women at age 65. For women younger than 65, the literature supports screening only for perimenopausal women with risk factors that include Caucasian or Asian race, a history of bilateral oopherectomy before menopause, a slender build, smoking or having smoked tobacco, low calcium consumption patterns, a sedentary lifestyle, and a positive family history of the condition. Women who have had a hysterectomy but not an oopherectomy are not considered at particular risk. Alcohol negatively impacts bone health by interfering with the aabsorption and use of calcium and vitamin D and other bone nutrients. Because there are a number of negatives about drinking and bond density, it would be wise for persons with problems with bone loss to decrease or eliminate alcohol.

3-70   Answer B

Pap smears may be discontinued at age 65 if the previous three Pap smears have been normal. For women younger than 65, Pap smears should start at age 18 or at the time of first sexual intercourse and then be repeated every 1–3 years, depending on risk factors, up to age 65. If a woman has had a hysterectomy, there is a need for a Pap smear only if the cervix has been left intact.

3-71   Answer C

Utilization review is a system to monitor diagnosis, treatment, and billing practices. It assists in lowering health-care costs by discouraging unnecessary procedures.

3-72   Answer A

Medicare was established in 1966 by the U.S. government as a federal insurance program to provide funds for medical costs for persons age 65 and older, as well as disabled persons of any age. Medicaid, an amendment to Title XIX of the Social Security Act, went into effect in 1967 to provide basic health services to low-income persons. The Omnibus Budget Reconciliation Act was implemented in 1982, when 20 programs were combined into four block grants.

3-73   Answer A

Medicare Part A is basic hospital insurance. Medicare Part B is supplementary voluntary medical insurance supported by tax revenues and by additional monies paid by the insured to cover physician services, laboratory services, home health care, and outpatient hospital treatments.

3-74   Answer D

A genogram is a diagram that depicts each member of a family and shows connections among the generations, including all members of the extended family for several generations. It includes the health status of each member, including any genetic diseases.

3-75   Answer B

Lewin's change theory involves fundamental shifts in persons' behaviors that evoke and successfully implement change. It is a three-stage process. Stage 1 is unfreezing, in which there is recognition of the need to change and methods are suggested to minimize resistance to the change; stage 2 is the actual changing process, in which the tasks and structure are actually implemented; and stage 3 is refreezing, in which the outcomes are reinforced and results are evaluated.

3-76   Answer B

The primary objective of screening is to detect a disease in its early stages to be able to treat it and change its progression. Treating a disease at the early asymptomatic period can significantly alter the course of the disease.

3-77   Answer D

To designate a disease as screenable or not, several questions are taken into account: Does the significance of the disorder ensure its consideration as a community problem? Can the disease be screened? Should the disease be screened? Questions such as "What is the cost of treatment?" are not taken into account and therefore do not provide a basis for designating a disease as screenable or not.

3-78   Answer B

Sensitivity refers to a screening test's ability to identify persons who actually have a disease (true positives), whereas specificity measures a screening test's ability to recognize negative reactions or nondiseased individuals (true negatives). For example, if a screening tool were used on 100 individuals known to have prostate cancer and it detected 90 persons with prostate cancer, missing 10 of the individuals, the sensitivity would be 90%.

3-79   Answer A

Specificity measures a screening test's ability to recognize individuals who are nondiseased or those with negative reactions (true negatives). It can be represented by a ratio of true negatives to the total number of known true negatives. In this case, the number of true negatives that the test recognized was 80, with the total number of known true negatives being 100. Therefore 80 out of 100 (80/100) equals a specificity of 80%.

3-80   Answer D

The correct answer is to allow Mildred her independence but provide a safe environment by removing loose rugs that she could easily trip over and installing handrails by the toilet and in the bathtub. The rails will provide support for her as she goes from a sitting to a standing position. Hiring an aide 24 hours a day would decrease Mildred's independence. Leaving Mildred home, alone or not, will not change her chance of falling.

3-81   Answer B

The E stands for eye opener, or the need for a drink early in the day. The C stands for cutting down, the A stands for annoyed by criticism of drinking, and the G stands for guilt feelings about drinking.

3-82   Answer D

Twenty percent of colorectal cancers can be attributed to a lack of fiber in the diet. A high-fat diet has also been secondarily implicated.

3-83   Answer A

For primary prevention of skin cancer, a sunscreen with an ultraviolet (UV) wave protection factor of 15 has been shown to be as effective as those with higher numbers. In addition, for primary prevention of skin cancer, all clients should be counseled to avoid UV waves from either the sun or tanning booths and to wear protective clothing.

3-84   Answer D

The Centers for Disease Control and Prevention recommend that all clients with high-risk behaviors be encouraged to be screened for HIV antibodies to identify those who are already infected so that interventions can be started to further halt the spread of the virus.

3-85   Answer D

Glaucoma screening should be instituted starting at age 40 and continue every 5 years until age 60 and then continue every 2–3 years. Glaucoma is an elevated intraocular pressure that is measured with the use of a tonometer.

3-86   Answer B

With respect to African American men, the American Cancer Society recommends that screening for prostate cancer with a digital rectal exam start at age 40 and be done yearly.

3-87   Answer A

The spouse has been shown to be the most important source of social support for an adult. If there is no spouse, family members are the next most important source. Research has shown that support from outside the family cannot compensate for what is missing within the family.

3-88   Answer D

Egg protein is a vaccine component and may cause an anaphylactic reaction; therefore, Joe, who has had a previous reaction to egg protein, should not receive his immunization. To maximize opportunities to vaccinate, every client visit should be assessed for an appropriate vaccination. Clients may receive multiple vaccinations. Mild febrile illnesses, such as upper respiratory tract infection or otitis media, are not contraindications for vaccinations.

3-89   Answer B

Chantix has shown to be more effective in helping smokers quit than Zyban, the only other nonnicotine prescription medicine for smoking cessation. While Chantix contains no nicotine, it works on the same receptors as nicotine. It's the addiction to nicotine inhaled from smoking that makes quitting so hard. The recommended dosing schedule for Chantix is as follows: day one to day three: one tablet per day of 0.5 mg; day four to day seven: one 0.5 mg tablet twice a day (once in the morning and once in the evening); day eight to the end of treatment: one tablet of 1 mg twice per day (once in the morning and once in the evening). Chantix should be taken with a full glass of water after eating. The client should choose a quit date when he/she will stop smoking. Chantix should be taken for 7 days before the quit date. This lets Chantix build up in the body. Smoking should cease on the quit day and Chantix should be continued for up to 12 weeks. If the client has not completely quit smoking by 12 weeks, another 12 weeks may help the client stay cigarette free. The most common side effect is nausea (30%), but not enough to make the client discontinue the medication.

3-90 Answer D

The MMR is a live attenuated vaccine, and therefore a female client must not be pregnant when she receives the vaccination. Female clients must also be informed that they need to refrain from becoming pregnant for the 3 months following MMR vaccination or risk birth defects to the fetus.

3-91 Answer B

The National Cancer Institute recommends that adults eat 20–30 g of fiber a day to prevent colon cancer. The plant kingdom is the only source of fiber-containing foods.

3-92 Answer C

Postmenopausal women who are not taking hormone replacement therapy need 1500 mg of calcium a day to help prevent osteoporosis. Because treatment for osteoporosis is limited, prevention is necessary to reduce the occurrence.

3-93 Answer C

To estimate a client's ideal weight, use the following formula: For women older than age 25, allow 100 lb for the first 5 ft, then add 5 lb for each inch thereafter. For men, allow 106 lb for the first 5 ft, then 6 lb for each inch thereafter. Multiply the number by 110% for a client with a large frame and 90% for a client with a small frame.

3-94 Answer B

The Committee on Diet and Health of the National Research Council recommends that alcohol consumption per day be limited to the equivalent of less than 1 oz of pure alcohol. This equates to two cans of beer, two small glasses of wine, or two average cocktails. This does not apply to pregnant women, who should avoid alcohol altogether.

3-95 Answer C

A gram of fat contains 9 calories, whereas a gram of either carbohydrates or proteins contains 4 calories. In this case, Julie was eating 3 g of fat, or 27 calories of fat (9 calories per gram of fat times 3 g of fat equals 27 calories).

3-96 Answer D

The Food and Drug Administration states that sodium may contribute to the risk of hypertension. Fat and fiber in grains, fruits, and vegetables decrease the risk of cancer, and insufficient calcium contributes to the risk of osteoporosis. Sodium intake should be reduced if there is a family health history of hypertension, diabetes, or any form of cardiovascular disease. Sodium intake should also be reduced if a personal health history indicates hypertension or glucose intolerance. Although hypertension is certainly a factor in heart disease, the best answer is hypertension because not all cardiovascular diseases are affected by the amount of sodium consumption.

3-97 Answer A

The ultimate goal of crisis intervention is to help people function at a higher level than their precrisis state. Eliminating the current crisis and returning people to the functional level where they were before the crisis will put them back in the same situation and make them susceptible to the crisis all over again.

3-98 Answer B

According to the Global Initiative for COPD guidelines, all symptomatic COPD clients should be started on an inhaled anticholinergic drug and a beta-2 agonist. Both are well tolerated by older adults and have few side effects.

3-99 Answer A

Studies have shown the use of ACE inhibitors in clients with diabetes with or without hypertension has slowed the progression of nephropathy. You must monitor the client's creatinine and potassium levels routinely. If the client's renal function does decrease, elevated potassium levels may occur.

3-100 Answer B

During severe stress, the cortisol level increases, allowing mobilization of free fatty acids. This triggers a series of reactions. With the increased cortisol, glucose production from amino acids increases. During severe stress, as glucagon release increases, catecholamine levels increase. The insulin-to-glucagon ratio decreases, glycogen breakdown increases, and glucose production from amino acids increases. The release of antidiuretic hormone also increases during stressful periods, increasing the retention of water, and the level of aldosterone increases, leading to the increased retention of sodium.

3-101   Answer C

Although antibiotics and bismuth subsalicylate are effective in the prevention of traveler's diarrhea, they are not generally recommended because of the potential side effects. Instead, advise clients to "cook it, boil it, peel it, or forget it."

3-102   Answer C

Insect repellents with high concentrations (greater than 35%) of diethyltoluamide (DEET) are effective in preventing mosquito bites; however, DEET is not recommended to be applied to the hands or faces of young children. Permethrin is effective as a scabicide (at 5%) and as a pediculicide (at 1%). It is very effective at a low concentration against malaria-carrying mosquitoes and is safe for all ages. Other preventive measures include remaining in well-screened or indoor areas from dusk to dawn, using mosquito nets, and wearing clothing that covers most of the body.

3-103   Answer A

Because tetanus and diphtheria remain serious problems in South America, it is recommended that all travelers be current (within 10 years) on these vaccinations. Tetanus immune globulin should be administered to persons not previously immunized.

3-104   Answer C

Screening for hypothyroidism is not routinely recommended. Because of the subtle presentation of hypothyroidism, health-care providers should order a thyroid-stimulating hormone level (TSH) test at their discretion. Most clinicians add a T4-level test to routine blood work and, depending on the results, then order a TSH test.

3-105   Answer A

Tuberculin skin testing using the Mantoux test should be considered in high-risk adolescents, as well as recent immigrants and homeless individuals. For high-risk individuals, an induration of 10 mm or greater when read at 48–72 hours is considered positive.

3-106   Answer A

In telogen effluvium, clients usually describe this condition as hair "coming out in handfuls." Stress can cause some hair roots to be pushed prematurely into the resting state. Two months after an extremely stressful event, some clients report losing as much as 70% of scalp hair. The condition may resolve after the stress subsides. This is not the same as gradual genetic hair thinning. Alopecia areata is thought to be an organ-specific autoimmune disease that manifests as round or oval patches of nonscarring hair loss. Female pattern hair loss may be the result of alterations in androgen metabolism at the level of the hair follicle or in systemic hormonal changes. This balding pattern may develop during perimenopause or menopause.

3-107   Answer B

Although the Public Health Department, American Heart Association, and Centers for Disease Control and Prevention all have excellent programs and screening protocols, only the WISEWOMAN program specifically addresses the needs of midlife uninsured women. The Well-Integrated Screening and Evaluation for Women Across the Nation (WISEWOMAN) program aims to remove racial and ethnic disparities in health by addressing the screening and intervention needs of midlife uninsured women. The program consists of 10 projects that have been successful at reaching financially disadvantaged and minority women who are at high risk for chronic diseases.

3-108   Answer C

When the 78 million baby boomers were growing up, television, rock concerts, and other intense audio programs were coming of age. Earplugs were unheard of. This generation does not want to wear hearing aids or anything that marks them as being different or disabled. As a result, baby boomers frequently avoid seeking help from hearing aid professionals. The following statistics are from a national survey of baby boomers: 75% said they find themselves in situations in which people are not speaking loudly or clearly enough or they can't hear the TV, 53% said they have at least a mild hearing loss,

25% said their hearing loss affects their work, and 57% said they have trouble hearing on their cell phone.

3-109   Answer D

HPV vaccination is not recommended for use in women who are pregnant. A contraindication to the HPV vaccines is a history of immediate hypersensitivity to yeast. Women who are lactating or immunocompromised are eligible to receive the vaccine. It is also recommended for females ages 9–25 years, whether or not they have had sex yet and even if the women already have a history of genital warts, a positive HPV test, or an abnormal Pap test.

3-110   Answer A

There are many major risk factors associated with osteoporosis and fragility fractures. The major risk factors are body weight <127 lb, personal history of fracture as an adult, history of fracture in a first-degree relative, oral corticosteroid therapy> 3 months, and current smoking. Minor risk factors include alcohol intake of more than 2 drinks per day, dementia, estrogen deficiency occurring before age 45 years, impaired vision, low lifelong calcium intake, low physical activity, poor health/frailty, and recent falls.

3-111   Answer D

To reduce the risk of chronic disease in adult-hood, engage in 30 or more minutes of moderately intense physical activity at work or at home at least 5 days per week. Greater health benefits may be obtained by participating in activity that is more vigorous in intensity or of longer duration. To help manage body weight and prevent a gradual increase in weight gain, 60 minutes of moderate to vigorous intensity activity may be done on most days of the week without increasing dietary caloric intake.

Bibliography

About Chantix. http://www.chantix.com/content, accessed 5/31/2007.

Dunphy, LM, et al: *Primary Care: The Art and Science of Advanced Practice Nursing*, ed 2. FA Davis, Philadelphia, 2007.

Engel, C: Baby boomers: Poster children for hearing loss? *Healthy Aging*, 89–94, March/April 2007.

Hoffman, R: Vaccine update. http://www.medscape.com/viewprogram/6999_pnt, accessed 5/31/2007.

Licata, A, and Johnston, C. Identifying post-menopausal women at risk for fracture. *The Female Patient* 32:18–25, 2007.

National Heart, Lung, and Blood Institute: *Seventh Report of the Joint National Committee on Prevention, Detection, Evaluation, and Treatment of Hypertension (JNC VII) Express Report*. National Institutes of Health, Bethesda, MD, 2003.

Nettina, SM: Health promotion: More than just cardiovascular risk reduction. *Topics in Advanced Practice Nursing Journal* 2(1), 2002. http://www.medscape.com/viewarticle/ 421467, accessed 5/31/2007.

Rendon, MI: Can stress affect the skin? *Healthy Aging*, 71–76, March/April 2007.

Schmaderer, J, and Unger, J. Dietary guidelines for Americans. *The Female Patient* 31:34–40, September 2006.

Will, JC, et al: Health promotion interventions for disadvantaged women: Overview of the WISEWOMAN projects. *Journal of Women's Health* 13(5):484–502, 2004.

How well did you do?

85% and above, congratulations! This score shows application of test-taking principles and adequate content knowledge.

75%–85%, keep working! Review test-taking principles and try again.

65%–75%, hang in there! Spend some time reviewing concepts and test-taking principles and then try the test again.

Burns, CE, et al: *Pediatric Primary Care*. Saunders-Elsevier, Philadelphia, 2009.

Drachman, DA: Aging of the brain, entropy, and Alzheimer disease. *Neurology* 67:1340–1352, October 2006.

Dunphy, LM, et al: *Primary Care: The Art and Science of Advanced Practice Nursing*, ed 2. FA Davis, Philadelphia, 2007.

Elkind, D: *The Hurried Child, Growing Up Too Fast Too Soon*, ed 3. Da Capo Press, Cambridge, MA, 2001.

Hale, G, et al: Endocrine features of menstrual cycles in middle and late reproductive age and the menopausal transition classified according to the staging of reproductive aging (STRAW) staging system. *The Journal of Clinical Endocrinology and Metabolism* 92(8), 2007.

Havighurst, RJ, Neugarten, BL, and Tobin, SS: Disengagement, personality and life satisfaction in the later years. In Hansen, P (ed), *Age With a Future*. Munksgoard, Copenhagen, Denmark, 1963.

Hockenberry, MJ: *Wong's Clinical Manual of Pediatric Nursing*, ed 6. Mosby, St. Louis, 2004.

Hussain, J, et al: Environmental evaluation of a child with developmental disability. *Pediatric Clinics of North America* 54(1):15–29, 2007.

Jung, C: The stages of life. In *Collected Works: Vol. 8, the Structure and Dynamics of the Psyche*. Pantheon Books, New York, 1960.

Leibson, C, et al: Use and costs of medical care for children and adolescents with and without attention deficit hyperactivity disorder. *Journal of the American Medical Association* 285(1):60–66, 2001.

Marshall, WA, and Tanner, JM: Variations in the pattern of pubertal changes in boys. *Archives of Diseases in Children* 45(239):13–23, 1970.

Marshall, WA, and Tanner, JM: Variations in the pattern of pubertal changes in girls. *Archives of Diseases in Children* 44(235):201–303, 1969.

McDonald, RE, and Avery, DR: *Dentistry for the Child and Adolescent*, ed 6. Mosby, St. Louis, 1994.

Moss, SB, et al: ADHD in adults. *Primary Care Clinics of North America* 34(3), 2007.

Robertson, J, and Shilkofski, N: *The Harriet Lane Handbook*, ed 17. Mosby, St. Louis, 2005.

Tanner, JM: *Growth at Adolescence*. CC Thomas, Springfield, IL, 1955.

How well did you do?

85% and above, congratulations! This score shows application of test-taking principles and adequate content knowledge.

75%–85%, keep working! Review test-taking principles and try again.

65%–75%, hang in there! Spend some time reviewing concepts and test-taking principles and try the test again.

Chapter 6: *Health Counseling*

LYNNE M. DUNPHY
JILL E. WINLAND-BROWN
MARCELLA R. THOMPSON

Questions

6-1 *Jamie, age 7, is most likely to react to her parents' divorce with*

A. sadness, crying, and depression.

B. whining, clinging, and fearful behavior.

C. conflicting loyalties toward her parents.

D. denial and perfect behavior.

6-2 *When you plan health programs, a number of factors are important to take into consideration. Which factor is most critical to successful achievement of a health program?*

A. Convenience

B. Content

C. Using visual images

D. Language

6-3 *You see a 3-year-old child in the office for a mild upper respiratory infection without fever. She is behind on her immunizations. What should you do?*

A. Tell the mother to bring her back when her infection is resolved.

B. Give her the killed-virus vaccines and wait to give the live-virus attenuated vaccines.

C. Give her the appropriate immunizations today.

D. Wait until her next scheduled visit.

6-4 *Marta states that her husband seems depressed lately and she is concerned that he will attempt suicide. In counseling her, you tell her that the risk factors for suicide include all of the following except*

A. a family history of suicide.

B. access to hypnotic medications.

C. a plan for the method of suicide.

D. self-imposed isolation.

6-5 *Gary, a gay male client, age 45, arrives in your office with facial bruises. He states that he injured himself opening a door, but he seems nervous. What do you suspect?*

A. He is manifesting early signs of dementia.

B. His injuries are a result of a hate crime or domestic violence.

C. He engaged in self-mutilation.

D. He injured himself as stated.

6-6 *Mary, age 56, has been on antihypertensive medication. You have switched her regimen more than once. On some occasions when you see her for blood pressure checks, her blood pressure is fine; on other occasions, her blood pressure is out of control. She frequently complains about having to take antihypertensives. She feels she doesn't need them. You suspect she is not taking her medication as ordered. You say,*

A. "Mary, you must take your medication as instructed."

B. "Mary, are you taking your blood pressure medication as prescribed?"

C. "Many people find it difficult to remember to take their medication. During the past week, have you missed any of your pills?"

D. "Mary, let's talk about the side effects of your medication."

6-7 *Nathan, a long-distance runner, says he heard that a high-protein diet would increase his endurance. When you counsel him, which type of diet do you tell him will increase an athlete's endurance?*

A. A fat-and-protein diet

B. A normal mixed diet with fat, protein, and carbohydrates

C. A high-carbohydrate diet

D. A fruit-and-vegetable diet

6-8   *Sam, age 26, likes to enter long-distance bicycle races. He asks you about carbohydrate loading to trick his muscles into storing energy before a competition. You advise him to*

A. eat a high-carbohydrate diet for the first 4 days of the week before the competition, then a moderate-carbohydrate diet for the remaining 3 days.

B. increase his training time for 3 days before the competition to assist in releasing the stored energy.

C. avoid the practice of carbohydrate loading because it is very dangerous to his health.

D. cut back on activity and eat a very high-carbohydrate diet for the 3 days before the competition.

6-9   *In counseling an obese client to lose weight, which of the following is the best recommendation you could make?*

A. "Keep a diet history."

B. "Increase your activity."

C. "Cut down on the foods you eat."

D. "There is nothing to recommend because your obesity is hereditary and you will always be overweight."

6-10   *Mary, who is obese, has started a walking program and wonders how much walking is too much. You tell her she has done too much walking when*

A. her pulse rate increases by 30 beats per minute during the walk.

B. she starts sweating.

C. she still feels fatigued hours after walking.

D. she becomes slightly short of breath.

6-11   *Elyssa, age 69, lives alone. When talking about personal safety activities, you tell her,*

A. "Wear your slippers at all times and don't walk barefoot."

B. "Wear your reading glasses when walking around so you'll have them when you need them."

C. "When smoking in bed, be sure to turn on the light to keep you awake."

D. "Wear wide-base, low-heel shoes with corrugated soles to help prevent slips and falls."

6-12   *Smoking is a risk factor for the top three causes of death. What is your best course of action for dealing with your clients who smoke?*

A. Make your clients aware of the sequelae of smoking.

B. Ask, advise, assess, assist, arrange.

C. Do not bring this topic up unless the client does.

D. Only bring this up if the client has symptoms related to smoking behavior; otherwise, mentioning it is pointless.

6-13   *Sidney has diabetes and asks you why exercise is so essential for him. You tell him that*

A. all persons with diabetes are overweight, and therefore exercise is the one tried-and-true method for weight loss.

B. going for a walk or exercising takes the mind off food, so he will not eat as much.

C. after exercising, people tend to be less hungry and thus do not consume as much.

D. exercising lowers blood sugar and helps the body make better use of its food supply.

6-14   *Gene, who has insulin-dependent diabetes mellitus, is an avid tennis player. When counseling him about insulin and exercise, you tell him,*

A. "When your blood sugar is consistently high, you need to exercise more to try to lower it."

B. "After injection with regular insulin, the peak time to exercise is 2–4 hours later."

C. "Inject the insulin into your arms so that it will be absorbed well while you are playing tennis."

D. "Eat within an hour after exercising."

6-15   *Susan is a new mother and hesitant about vaccinations for her baby. You tell her why they are essential and that by the time her child is 5 years of age, she should receive*

A. 10 vaccines.

B. 15 vaccines.

C. 25 vaccines.

D. more than 30 vaccines.

6-16   *The U.S. Preventive Services Task Force recommends a variety of strategies for motivating clients to* *improve exercise strategies. Which strategy is included in its recommendations?*

A. Stressing the increased mortality associated with not exercising

B. Suggesting a running regimen of 5 days a week for maximum benefit and using a personal trainer

C. Meeting with an exercise physiologist and getting a treadmill for home use and setting specific goals for its use

D. Goal setting by the client; writing an exercise prescription with individually tailored recommendations; follow-up

6-17 *Jill states that she cannot tell when her grandmother is dehydrated and that she never seems to drink much fluid. What do you tell her about fluid and electrolyte changes associated with aging?*

A. Skin turgor is a reliable measure of body fluid levels.

B. Thirst sensation is the best indicator of body fluid balance.

C. Body weight is the best indicator of body fluid balance.

D. Peripheral edema is a reliable indicator of fluid and electrolyte balance in the older adult.

6-18 *Darlene, age 55, is shocked when she is weighed during her visit to your office. "I can't believe that I have gained so much weight! What should I do?" What stage in health behavior change is Darlene in?*

A. Contemplation

B. Preparation

C. Action

D. Maintenance

6-19 *Susan asks you about her husband, who was just told that he has degenerative joint disease (DJD). You know that the most likely joint to be affected by DJD is the*

A. jaw.

B. elbow.

C. hip.

D. ankle.

6-20 *Having routine mammograms after age 50 is an example of*

A. health promotion.

B. disease prevention.

C. screening.

D. tertiary prevention.

6-21 *A smoking cessation program should be initiated when*

A. the client states a readiness to quit.

B. the client is in the hospital.

C. an initial history and physical examination are performed.

D. the client's family convinces the client of the necessity to quit.

6-22 *Which of the following is the primary reason given by health-care professionals as to why inadequate attention is paid to health counseling in the primary care setting?*

A. Lack of motivation because working with clients to achieve behavioral change is difficult and often frustrating for the health professional

B. Skepticism about the effectiveness of health promotion and counseling

C. Uncertainty about which approaches may be most helpful with individual clients and problems

D. The fact that counseling is not "billable" and is therefore not cost effective

6-23 *The most effective interventions available to health-care providers for reducing the incidence and severity of the leading causes of disease and disability in the United States are*

A. screening tests.

B. immunizations.

C. counseling interventions that address the personal health practices of clients.

D. chemoprophylaxes such as the use of drugs and nutritional and mineral supplements.

6-24 *What is the best way to promote a personal behavior change in a client?*

A. Write an order for a treatment plan.

B. Stress compliance with your treatment plan.

C. Prescribe a health promotion regimen.

D. Discuss choices with the client and let him or her decide what will work best.

6-25 *The U.S. Preventive Services Task Force recommends screening which of the following groups for evidence of alcohol dependence, problem drinking, or excessive alcohol consumption?*

A. Individuals whom the provider thinks are abusing alcohol

B. Individuals with altered liver function studies

C. Individuals who have had several recent automobile accidents, regardless of precipitating cause

D. All adult and adolescent clients

6-26 *Which of the following is a four-item screening tool useful in identifying a client who may have a problem with alcohol abuse?*

A. The AUDIT test

B. The CAGE questionnaire

C. The Michigan alcoholism screening test

D. The Problem Drinker/Abuser Test

6-27 *As the nurse practitioner in an outpatient clinic, you will be performing a history and physical on Maria, age 15, whose mother comes to the clinic with her. How would you approach the topic of sexuality with Maria?*

A. Ask Maria's mother if you can discuss this issue with Maria.

B. Ask Maria, with her mother present, if it is OK for you to discuss this issue with them both.

C. Ask Maria's mother to leave the room.

D. When you are alone with Maria, tell her that you want to talk to her about this issue and ask her if she wants her mother to be present.

6-28 *You suspect that Ginger, age 6, has parents who smoke. Ginger is being seen in the office for an acute asthma attack. Her mother is present. How do you approach Ginger's mother about this risk factor?*

A. "You know that smoking is detrimental to Ginger's health."

B. "I hope that you don't smoke in front of Ginger."

C. "Is Ginger ever exposed to cigarette smoke?"

D. "I can smell smoke on your clothes. How many packs do you smoke per day?"

6-29 *Who should have a screening test for skin cancer?*

A. All individuals, starting at adolescence, then every 5 years thereafter

B. All individuals every 2 years

C. Individuals with risk factors for skin cancer

D. All individuals during every health examination

6-30 *Which of the following healthy lifestyle choices has been shown to improve the functioning power of a man's heart?*

A. Improving diet

B. Taking vitamins

C. Doing aerobic exercise

D. Having a restful sleep at night

6-31 *Mike was given three stool cards at the lab and told how to do a fecal occult blood test at home, but he was not counseled as to what foods or drugs to eat or avoid. What do you tell him to do?*

A. Do not take aspirin for 7 days before and during the collection period and avoid red or processed meat for 3 days before and during the collection period.

B. Avoid eating clams and other shellfish.

C. Do not engage in vigorous physical exercise for 5 days prior to the test.

D. Avoid fruit juices.

6-32 *Your client, Casey, a 69-year-old chronic smoker, has called you to find out the result of his recent chest x-ray, which you ordered because of his increasingly troublesome chronic cough. You have seen a large shadow on the chest x-ray that you suspect is a carcinoma. What should you say to Casey?*

A. "I need you to come to the office to discuss your chest x-ray results."

B. "I have seen an area on your chest x-ray that concerns me."

C. "Please let me speak to your wife."

D. "I saw something on your chest x-ray that we need to follow up on, but I am sure it will be all right."

6-33 *Asthma is increasing in all ages of the population. Primary prevention strategies include which of the following?*

A. Screening workers for hypersensitivity to lung irritants and counseling them to avoid jobs where they are exposed to irritants that affect them

B. Providing masks for all industrial workers

C. Providing pulmonary function tests for all industrial workers

D. Providing yearly chest x-rays for all industrial workers

6-34 *Marcie is very depressed because she has fibromyalgia. She states that her husband thinks that she is just lazy. How can you help her deal with this?*

A. Tell her husband that fibromyalgia is a real syndrome, and although it cannot be cured, it can be managed.

B. Have her husband come in with her during her next visit and talk with them together.

C. Have him see a therapist because most husbands do not understand the condition.

D. Tell Marcie that she just has to understand that her husband has made up his mind and will never change.

6-35 *Susan is a 32-year-old woman with chronic headaches. She has come to you specifically for a referral to a neurologist. She has already seen four neurologists but is not satisfied with the answer that any of them has provided. What should you do?*

A. Explain in an empathic way that there is no need to see another neurologist and that you cannot support another referral.

B. Agree to refer her to another neurologist and spend as little time with her as possible so that you can focus on clients who have more immediate concerns.

C. Do a complete history and physical and attempt to find out why the client was dissatisfied with the advice she received from the previous neurological consultations.

D. Rule out any immediate life-threatening problem and tell the client to return in a few weeks. If at that point she still wants the referral, you will provide it.

6-36 *Jane, age 72, is very upset about her stress incontinence. She asks you for advice. What do you tell her?*

A. "Unfortunately, stress incontinence is part of the normal aging process."

B. "There are many new pads on the market that provide an efficacious approach to this common problem, thus preventing social isolation."

C. "A diet that incorporates cranberry juice may be effective in curbing this problem."

D. "Kegel exercises may help."

6-37 *Sandra had a radical mastectomy 20 years ago and asks you why she still cannot have her blood pressure taken on the affected arm. You tell her that*

A. after 20 years with no problem, she can have her blood pressure taken on that arm.

B. she no longer has to worry about injury or infection to that arm.

C. lymphedema can occur for up to 30 years after a mastectomy; therefore, precautions still need to be taken.

D. although she should not have blood drawn from that arm, she may have her blood pressure taken on that arm.

6-38 *Joanne is a second-grade teacher and is frustrated that her students do not seem to be getting any physical exercise at home. She asks you for advice. What do you recommend?*

A. "Advise parents to play outside with their children after dinner."

B. "Tell parents to let their children play outside after school."

C. "Assign homework to students that must be done with their parents and involves physical activity."

D. "Advise parents to turn the TV off for a week to get the children used to doing something else."

6-39 *Janice is recovering from osteomyelitis of her leg. She asks you for advice as to what she can do to promote healing. You tell her to*

A. put weight on the affected leg more frequently to promote increased circulation, oxygenation, and nutrition to the tissues of the wound area.

B. eat foods high in vitamins and calcium and increase her calorie and protein intake.

C. spend time in the fresh air and expose the wound to fresh air and sunlight.

D. be sure to use strict aseptic technique when changing the dressing, which should be kept wet at all times to improve wound healing.

6-40 *Which of the following conditions, which may be detected by a complete blood count, has sufficient prevalence to make early detection beneficial?*

A. Anemia

B. Leukocytosis

C. Thrombocytopenia

D. Leukemia

6-41 *Joe, age 76, has peripheral arterial disease (PAD). You know he does not understand your teaching instructions when he says*

A. "I'll see the podiatrist once a month so he can do my foot care."

B. "I'll soak my feet weekly so my nails will be soft when I trim them."

C. "I'll monitor my BP, and if it really gets out of control, I'll come see you."

D. "I'll cut down on my smoking."

6-42 *It is important to counsel your clients of all ages regarding prevention strategies for cancers of the colon and rectum. These strategies include*

A. fecal occult blood testing on an annual basis after age 50.

B. emphasizing the importance of regular physical exercise and colonoscopy after age 50.

C. stressing the importance of regular physical exercise; a diet rich in vegetables, fruit, and fiber; and regular use of aspirin.

D. weight loss, smoking cessation, and a diet rich in fiber.

6-43 *Henry, age 57, is married and the father of three children. He is overweight and hypertensive and has a sedentary lifestyle. His father died of a myocardial infarction at age 42. Which factor will provide the strongest motivation for Henry to change his lifestyle?*

A. The fear that he will not live to see his daughter get married

B. Feeling "ownership" of the need to change

C. Feeling guilty that his wife might be left alone to raise the children

D. The desire to enjoy his retirement when the time comes

6-44 *Joy wants to stop smoking but is afraid that she will gain weight like all of her friends did when they*

stopped. What might you say to her that will encourage her to stop?

A. "Forget the weight gain; at least you'll live longer."

B. "The average weight gain is 5 pounds; it's worth it."

C. "Let's talk about several strategies you might use to prevent weight gain."

D. "Eat what you want and just exercise more."

6-45 *Alison asks you whether she should do anaerobic or aerobic exercise and what the difference is between them. You tell her that a simple measure of whether or not an exercise activity is aerobic or not is*

A. her heart rate.

B. whether or not she is sweating.

C. her degree of fatigue.

D. whether or not her muscles ache.

6-46 *When counseling a client about low-fat food choices, you recommend which of the following foods as a good choice?*

A. Bluefish

B. Dark-meat chicken

C. Hot dogs

D. Swordfish

6-47 *How do you respond to Trisha, who thinks that skipping breakfast is a way of banking calories for later in the day?*

A. "I do the same thing; that way I feel like I can have a bigger lunch."

B. "That's terrible. Didn't your mother always tell you that breakfast is the most important meal of the day?"

C. "Eating breakfast actually gets your metabolism going."

D. "We all need some essential fatty acids that are obtained only from food."

6-48 *Coconut oil and cocoa butter are examples of which type of fatty acids?*

A. Saturated fats

B. Monounsaturated fats

C. Polyunsaturated fats

D. Both monounsaturated and polyunsaturated fats

6-49 *What is the most common cause of injuries, the leading cause of hospital admissions for trauma, and the* *second leading cause of injury-related deaths for all age groups?*

A. Motor vehicle accidents

B. Falls

C. Bicycle or motorcycle accidents

D. Rollerblading and roller skating accidents

6-50 *Susan asks why her husband developed degenerative joint disease (DJD) when there was no family history. You tell her that a cause of primary DJD is*

A. trauma.

B. obesity.

C. sepsis.

D. a blood dyscrasia.

6-51 *Maury asks for advice on interventions that he can try to alleviate the discomfort of his arthritis. What do you tell him to do?*

A. Apply an ice pack to his stiff joints before exercising to reduce the discomfort.

B. Place a rolled towel under his knees when he lies on his back.

C. Rest frequently throughout the day.

D. Eat more dairy products to increase the amount of calcium in his diet.

6-52 *You are teaching a client about his gout. Which of the following should you include in your teaching?*

A. Once gout is treated, there is no danger of permanent damage.

B. Diet and alcohol may remain the same.

C. He should drink at least 1 quart of fluid per day.

D. Kidney stones and kidney damage may result if gout is not adequately managed.

6-53 *Sylvia has scleroderma and asks for counseling related to measures to help manage its effects. You tell Sylvia to*

A. avoid becoming chilled.

B. cut down on smoking.

C. wear tightly layered clothing to keep the skin warm in winter.

D. begin physical therapy at the first signs of joint stiffness.

6-54 *Martin is marrying Laura, who has a seizure disorder. He asks for advice regarding*

her seizures. Which of the following is most important?

A. Encourage Laura to begin jogging with him.

B. Remind Laura to take her anticonvulsant medication when she is experiencing seizures.

C. Do not let Laura drive for several weeks after she has a seizure.

D. Make sure that Laura wears a medical identification bracelet or necklace stating that she has a seizure disorder.

6-55 *Annie, age 26, has recently been diagnosed with multiple sclerosis. When advising her and her family, you say which of the following?*

A. "You should avoid flying in airplanes because the altitude could trigger an exacerbation of your symptoms."

B. "You should initiate a vigorous exercise schedule to maintain function."

C. "You need to avoid all spicy foods, caffeine, and peppermints."

D. "You need to avoid hot showers."

6-56 *Jill, who is 8 months pregnant, calls you because her father has told her that her mother is gravely ill. Her parents live on the opposite coast of the continental United States from Jill and she would have to take a 4–5 hour flight to see her mother. How would you advise Jill?*

A. Tell her that she should not travel at this point in her pregnancy.

B. Evaluate her risk and make your recommendation on the basis of her risk factors and hemoglobin level.

C. Tell her that it is OK for her to make this flight.

D. Evaluate her risk and make your recommendation on the basis of an electrocardiogram.

6-57 *Helen is 24 weeks pregnant and needs to take a trans-Atlantic flight to attend to a sick parent. What recommendation do you make regarding her plane flight?*

A. Tell her to be sure to eat enough while traveling to avoid any drop in blood sugar.

B. Encourage her to decrease her fluid intake because it may be difficult to use the bathroom facilities and her bladder is overdistended as a result of her pregnancy.

C. Tell her to request an aisle seat so that she can ambulate frequently and advise her to do isometric exercises.

D. She should monitor her blood pressure before and after the flight.

6-58   *Nina has trigeminal neuralgia. She asks you what measures she can take to alleviate some of the nagging problems related to it. You advise her to*

A. chew on the affected side of the mouth to strengthen those muscles.

B. eat and drink hot foods and fluids to help relax the oral mucosa.

C. avoid going to the dentist until the condition is in remission.

D. wear protective sunglasses or goggles when outside.

6-59   *You should advise any client who has received which of the following immunizations to use contraception for the next 3 months to avoid pregnancy?*

A. MMR, yellow fever, or varicella vaccines

B. Rabies postexposure prophylaxis

C. Tetanus-diphtheria

D. Hepatitis B

6-60   *Sam has lumbar spinal stenosis and asks which exercises he should do to help his condition. You advise him to*

A. do any exercise that results in hyperextension of the lumbar spine.

B. do exercises that encourage lumbar flexion and flattening of the lumbar lordotic curve.

C. refrain from exercising.

D. see a surgeon because surgery is the best treatment option.

6-61   *Human papillomavirus (HPV) is detectable in 99% of cervical cancers. Recently, a vaccine has been developed to prevent HPV infection and subsequent cervical intraepithelial neoplasia. What is the ideal time/age to administer this vaccine?*

A. At age 3 months

B. At age 2 years

C. Ideally, before the initiation of sexual activity

D. Shortly after the initiation of sexual activity

6-62   *You must tell Joe that the biopsy results from his lung tumor were positive for lung cancer and that his*

prognosis is poor. Which of the following is the best way to deliver this message?

A. "Whatever I tell you in a moment, I want you to remember that the situation is serious, but there is plenty that we can do. It is important that we work closely together over the next several months. I am sorry, but your tests were positive for lung cancer."

B. "I am sorry, but your test confirmed that you have lung cancer. Although the situation is very serious, there is still plenty that we can do. It is important that we work closely together."

C. "Joe, can I ask that you have a family member or close friend with you when we talk?"

D. "Joe, we need to work together. I am sure that we can provide help for you."

6-63   *Jan states that his ears get plugged up frequently from earwax and asks what he can do. You advise him to*

A. use a cotton-tipped applicator to loosen the wax.

B. flush his ears regularly with water using a bulb syringe.

C. use several drops of mineral oil.

D. irrigate his ears with a commercial preparation and leave it in for 48 hours, using cotton wicks.

6-64   *Bob, age 46, has insulin-dependent diabetes mellitus. He asks your advice about foot care. You tell him to*

A. use alcohol daily to keep his feet dry.

B. soak his feet in warm water daily to keep them from cracking and drying.

C. inspect the bottoms of his feet frequently with a mirror.

D. use emollients to prevent drying and cracking.

6-65   *Mark, age 26, has AIDS. He wants to know why you drew a viral load instead of a CD4 count at his last visit. What do you tell him?*

A. A viral load is a more accurate measure of the progression of the disease.

B. CD4 counts do not contribute any information regarding diagnosis and treatment.

C. A viral load and a CD4 count are similar, but a viral load test is less expensive.

D. Once a person has been given a diagnosis of AIDS, the CD4 count does not change.

6-66   *Cynthia brings her 15-year-old son, David, into the office. She wants some counseling regarding his* *behavior problems. David seems "laid back," quiet, and aloof. All of the information is volunteered by Cynthia. What is the first thing you should do?*

A. Test his urine for drugs.

B. Prescribe an antidepressant medication.

C. Refer David to a psychiatrist.

D. Talk to David about what is concerning him.

6-67   *Melinda brings in her daughter Shirley, age 2, with an ear infection. She asks why Shirley gets such frequent infections. You respond that*

A. Shirley must be putting something in her ear.

B. a high-fat diet results in higher cerumen production; the cerumen traps bacteria, causing the infection.

C. her eustachian tubes are horizontal, which does not allow drainage.

D. Melinda must dry Shirley's ears more thoroughly after bathing.

6-68   *Ilene brings in her 14-year-old daughter, Tracie, because she fears that Tracie may be sexually active. What do you do?*

A. Start her on medroxyprogesterone acetate (Depo-Provera) immediately.

B. Perform a vaginal exam.

C. Ascertain in private from Tracie if she is contemplating becoming or is sexually active.

D. Call child protective services.

6-69   *Phil, 14 years old, reluctantly tells you that he thinks he has something seriously wrong with him because he has awakened in the morning with a wet sheet around his penis. What do you do?*

A. Perform a test to rule out a sexually transmitted disease.

B. Tell him that this is a normal part of his sexual development.

C. Ask him if he is emptying his bladder before he goes to bed.

D. Tell him that this is abnormal and you want to refer him to a urologist.

6-70   *Which of the following most commonly cause(s) intentional, nonoccupational poisoning deaths in adults?*

A. Heroin and cocaine

B. Antidepressants and tranquilizers

C. Motor vehicle exhaust

D. Barbiturates

6-71   *You are counseling the parents of a 2-year-old about accidental poisoning. What do you instruct them to administer if their child should accidentally ingest something poisonous?*

A. Burnt toast

B. Tea

C. Ipecac syrup

D. Milk of magnesia

6-72   *Your neighbors are building a swimming pool and have two children, ages 2 and 8. What is the best recommendation you could make to them to prevent an accidental drowning of the 2-year-old?*

A. Install a fence around the pool.

B. Have the 8-year-old learn cardiopulmonary resuscitation.

C. Never let the children out of your sight.

D. Keep the entrances to the backyard locked at all times.

6-73   *You suspect that a client is being physically abused by her husband because she has had unexplainable ecchymotic areas on her face and upper arms in her past two visits to the office. You would like to raise the issue of abuse. Which of the following statements might prompt the best response from the client?*

A. "These bruises are very unusual. Is your husband hurting you?"

B. "How did you get these bruises?"

C. "Would you like to talk about what's going on?"

D. "Do you frequently get a lot of bruises?"

6-74   *Melanie wants to start working on a tan before her Caribbean cruise. You warn her about the hazards of sun exposure, but she is still insistent about getting a tan. What do you recommend?*

A. Brief tanning periods using a sunscreen

B. Use of a tanning salon for several weeks before the cruise

C. Use of a self-tanning lotion or cream

D. Intervals of a half hour in the sun and a half hour out of the sun

6-75 *When you are performing a history and physical examination on Jason, age 16, he tells you that although he does not smoke, he uses snuff (smokeless tobacco). He says that he wants the nicotine "high" but does not want it to become a habit like cigarette smoking. What should you tell him about smokeless tobacco?*

A. It may lead to mouth or throat cancer.

B. Smokeless tobacco has no effect on teeth and gums.

C. Smokeless tobacco will increase his appetite.

D. It is less dangerous than cigarette smoking.

6-76 *While examining Marcia, age 12 months, you notice that her teeth are in very poor condition. What is the most appropriate question to ask the parents?*

A. "Does Marcia go to bed with a bottle at night?"

B. "Have you been cleaning Marcia's teeth with a piece of gauze around your finger every day?"

C. "What kinds of foods does Marcia eat?"

D. "Does Marcia chew on her toys?"

6-77 *Tim, age 66, has chronic obstructive pulmonary disease (COPD). He comes in for counseling regarding a flu shot. He states that he thinks he needs one but has heard some horror stories about the shot related to Guillain-Barré syndrome. What do you tell him?*

A. "You have to weigh the advantages against the disadvantages."

B. "Your chances of getting the flu are 10 to 1 and your chances of getting Guillain-Barré are 1,000,000 to 1."

C. "If you are worried, you shouldn't receive the flu shot."

D. "There is no relationship between the flu shot and neurological complications."

6-78 *Jake, age 10, comes to your primary care office with his mother. You are in a rural area. What is a priority area for health counseling?*

A. Assessing the physical education program provided in Jake's school

B. Finding out whether the family has any pets

C. Determining whether Jake is able to swim

D. Asking about the occupation of the family, and if it is farming, providing adequate health counseling

6-79 *Olive has gastroesophageal reflux disease (GERD). She asks for advice as to what she can do to help her condition. You tell her to*

A. take NSAIDs for the discomfort.

B. cut down on smoking.

C. monitor stools for steatorrhea.

D. avoid caffeine and chocolate.

6-80 *Mandy is pregnant with her first baby. She asks you what the safest drug to use in pregnancy is. What do you suggest?*

A. Acetylsalicylic acid (aspirin)

B. Acetaminophen (Tylenol)

C. Erythromycin (E-Mycin, Eryc)

D. Tetracycline (Achromycin, Sumycin)

6-81 *Martha is concerned because her 6-year-old daughter wets the bed almost every night. Appropriate counseling statements include which of the following?*

A. "Enuresis is a common problem, and it may have a physiological basis. It also may be inherited."

B. "This problem has serious repercussions for the child and must be dealt with on a variety of levels."

C. "Nighttime enuresis is not an inherited problem."

D. "A self-help group for clients may prove helpful in dealing with this recalcitrant behavior."

6-82 *You suspect that Tania, age 16, is depressed. Her mother states that she exhibits many behaviors that suggest this. Which of the following would not be of concern?*

A. A change in weight or eating habits

B. Refusal to talk about death

C. Insomnia or hypersomnia

D. A drop in school performance

6-83 *Smoking cessation strategies are more effective when the health-care educator*

A. stresses the importance of not smoking and the disease sequelae if smoking continues.

B. encourages persons to stop immediately.

C. conducts follow-up reinforcement sessions.

D. involves the entire family in the process.

6-84 *Primary prevention measures for sexually transmitted diseases and unwanted pregnancies should be* based on an understanding of which of the following psychosocial determinants?

A. Informing adolescents of disease risk is an essential component of primary prevention.

B. There must be multiple approaches and these should begin in middle childhood.

C. Working for personality change encourages adolescents to give up destructive behaviors.

D. Handing out latex condoms and showing people how to use them is the best defense against sexually transmitted diseases and unwanted pregnancies.

6-85 *Your client, whom you recently treated for a sexually transmitted disease, has returned with a reinfection. At this point, you*

A. reeducate.

B. stress the importance of "safe sex" in more emphatic terms.

C. instruct the client to avoid all sexual contacts.

D. expect that the client will need to come back for more than one visit.

6-86 *When is it appropriate to discuss smoking cessation techniques with a client who smokes?*

A. When the client presents with a smoking-related disease

B. At every visit

C. When the client indicates a readiness to stop smoking

D. Only when the client asks about them

6-87 *James, a 32-year-old medical student, received two of three hepatitis B vaccinations last year. He is wondering if he needs to start the schedule all over again. What do you tell him?*

A. "We'll give the third dose now because it's been at least 4 months since the first dose."

B. "Yes, all three vaccinations need to be repeated if it's been longer than 1 year."

C. "No, but we'll need to repeat the second injection."

D. "If the third injection wasn't given within 6 months after the first one, all three will have to be repeated."

6-88 *Sydney, age 15, has anorexia nervosa. Her mother is seeking nutrition counseling. You refer*

her to a specialist, but in the meantime you recommend

A. that rewards be linked to every pound Sydney gains.

B. that Sydney drink caffeinated sodas after meals to avoid filling up before meals.

C. that Sydney take liquid supplements in addition to solid foods.

D. that Sydney eat three meals a day, plus a bedtime snack.

6-89 *Nelda wants some counseling regarding her stepdaughter, age 18, whom she suspects has bulimia nervosa. You ask her if her stepdaughter exhibits*

A. frequent urinary tract infections (UTIs), dental caries, and bruised or cut hands.

B. dental caries; dizziness; and dry, sparse hair.

C. amenorrhea, weakness, and sleep disturbances.

D. hyperactivity and bizarre behaviors around food.

6-90 *Which of the following foods would be the best choice for a client recovering from bulimia nervosa?*

A. Rice

B. Baked potato

C. Pasta

D. French fries

6-91 *John is 52 years old and has decided to take up tennis. What are some areas of health counseling that may help prevent injury?*

A. Advising him to eat before playing tennis so he does not become dehydrated

B. Suggesting a narrow grip size for the tennis racket and making sure the strings are tight

C. Suggesting a wide grip and working with a professional to assess how tight the strings should be

D. Discouraging him from beginning a competitive sport like tennis because of the high risk of injury

6-92 *Chloe is chronically tired. During a telephone conversation, she asks you for advice. What do you recommend?*

A. To not nap during the day and establish a routine for sleep at night

B. To add iron to her diet

C. To take a vitamin supplement with iron

D. To make an appointment

6-93 *Raymond presents with bleeding gums and broken capillaries under his skin. What vitamin deficiency do you suspect he has?*

A. Vitamin A

B. Vitamin B_{12}

C. Vitamin C

D. Vitamin D

6-94 *Marvin has just been given a diagnosis of diabetes. To increase his adherence to a healthful lifestyle, you*

A. initially have him come in every week for a urinalysis and fingerstick blood glucose test to see how he's doing.

B. tell him you will do a glycohemoglobin test every 3 months to assess his control of his blood sugar.

C. instruct him on self-monitoring of blood sugar.

D. tell him to call a nutritionist.

6-95 *George, age 52, is taking a diuretic to control his blood pressure. What foods should he be eating in addition that might help?*

A. Bananas and milk

B. Ribs and coleslaw

C. Avocados and soda

D. Popcorn and peaches

6-96 *Sam asks about saturated fats or "bad" fats, as he calls them. Which of the following is not a saturated fat?*

A. Soybean oil

B. Coconut oil

C. Palm oil

D. Cocoa butter

6-97 *Alicia, age 22, is in your office for her first prenatal visit. Recommended preventive services for all pregnant women include*

A. blood typing and HIV and hypertensive screening.

B. assessment of height and weight and screening for HIV and asymptomatic bacteriuria.

C. *chlamydia* screening, hypertension screening, and Rh(D) incompatibility screening with blood typing.

D. screening for syphilis, *chlamydia*, hepatitis B, alcohol and tobacco abuse, asymptomatic bacteriuria, and Rh(D) incompatibility; blood typing; and discussing the importance of breastfeeding.

6-98 *Ralph, age 66, comes to your office with concerns regarding declining sexual function. He states that it takes him much longer to get an erection and sometimes he cannot get or maintain an erection. He has also noticed a diminished desire for sexual activity. He denies any change in his relationship with his wife of 35 years, with whom he has always enjoyed a satisfying sexual relationship. What do you do?*

A. Explain that you must investigate possible underlying causes of his problem, some of which are reversible and some of which are not.

B. Explain that diminished sexual desire and function are natural sequelae of aging.

C. Advise sexual counseling and prescribe Viagra.

D. Suggest that Ralph may be suffering from a low-grade depression and prescribe an antidepressant.

6-99 *Thomas, age 10, is sent home from school with pediculosis. You tell his mother that the cheapest and easiest remedy is to*

A. use regular shampoo on his hair three times a day.

B. apply petroleum jelly (Vaseline) to the scalp and hair.

C. apply mayonnaise to the scalp and hair.

D. cut the hair very short or shave the head.

6-100 *Wes, age 60, wants advice regarding what to look for as signs of skin cancer. You tell him to observe any lesions he has and do which of the following?*

A. He should alert you if he observes a lesion with asymmetrical borders, a multicolored lesion, a lesion greater than 6 mm in diameter, or a change in the appearance of a nevus or mole.

B. He should alert you if he observes a new papule that is 2 mm in size.

C. He should have any crusty-appearing lesion evaluated immediately.

D. He should not be concerned if there is no change in any lesion; he does not need formal screening.

6-101 *Betty brings her 2-year-old in for a routine visit and mentions that her husband has a gun at home for protection. In counseling her, which is most appropriate?*

A. Tell her that you are obliged to report this to the police.

B. Recommend that the bullets and gun be kept separately, discuss other home protection devices, and suggest a combination lock on the trigger.

C. Ask her, "Why on earth would you keep a gun in the house with a 2-year-old?"

D. Tell Betty that you must speak to her and her husband together about this situation.

6-102   *Mary is caring for her 83-year-old father at home. He has dementia and is unsteady on his feet. You recommend that Mary*

A. put her father in a nursing home so that she can have a life of her own.

B. take in another elderly person so that her father can have company.

C. get information on home safety and community resources.

D. lock her father's bedroom door at night so that he will not wander into the street.

6-103   *Shelley, 55 years old, sees you for the first time. She has demonstrated osteopenia on a bone density test, and you have prescribed the appropriate medication for her. What additional lifestyle changes should you counsel for this client?*

A. She should begin a rigorous swimming program to actively build bone.

B. She should cut down on coffee, but tea is OK.

C. She needs to take a multivitamin every day.

D. She should begin weight training.

6-104   *Mr. Green is a vigorous 70-year-old who comes for early assessment of dementia. He wants to "work" to keep up his mental capacities. You counsel that he should*

A. make sure he gets enough rest because cells need time to regenerate as a result of the stress of the aging process.

B. begin taking a calcium supplement.

C. consider a hobby that challenges his mental capacity, like building model ships or airplanes.

D. play bridge (or any group card game) several times a week.

6-105   *You see a 19-year-old college student, Melissa, who is listless and speaks in monosyllabic language. Her affect is flat. Her mother has brought her to your primary care office because she is concerned about her. You know that risk factors for depression include which of the following?*

A. Being a college student

B. Believing oneself to be incapable, helpless, a victim, or hopeless

C. Having the summer free from school

D. Not having a car or transportation available

6-106   *As you speak with Melissa and her mother, you ascertain more signs and symptoms that contribute to a clinical picture of depression. These include*

A. sad, discouraged, irritable mood and feelings of loneliness.

B. going on a spending spree.

C. obsessively exercising.

D. constant hand washing.

6-107   *In counseling Melissa on dealing with her depression, you are aware of the successful strategies in managing a depressive illness. Apart from pharmacological interventions, some suggested strategies include*

A. more exposure to daylight; rethinking one's situation.

B. stressing the importance of rest.

C. doing complete blood work on Melissa and recommending a multivitamin and vitamin E.

D. recommending St. John's wort, an herbal remedy, because Melissa does not want to take antidepressants.

6-108   *Mr. Kent is a 60-year-old man who has a variety of cardiac risk factors. When you evaluate his risk profile, which of the following should be taken into consideration?*

A. Past surgeries

B. Number of children

C. Temperament

D. Economic advantage

6-109   *What is one specific intervention that might help Mr. Kent deal with his underlying coronary artery disease (CAD)?*

A. Frequent rest periods

B. Drinking at least one glass of red wine a day

C. Having a pet

D. Practicing relaxation exercises daily

6-110   *A new mother is refusing to vaccinate her infant because she is concerned about mercury in vaccines. What do you advise her?*

A. The risk of dying from childhood disease is greater than the health risks of thimerosal.

B. If thimerosal were dangerous, there would be an FDA warning on the label.

C. Thimerosal is not used as a preservative in routinely recommended childhood vaccines except the influenza vaccine.

D. She should not be concerned about this.

6-111   *A client who is an engineer flies frequently to Asia from the United States. Why should you educate him/her about deep vein thrombosis (DVT)?*

A. Because Asian food is linked to DVT

B. Because the Asian time zone is 11 hours ahead

C. Because Asia is known to have endemic disease

D. Because an Asia/U.S. flight takes more than 8–10 hours

6-112   *Your client has a hearing loss, probably a result of exposure to noise when working as a machine operator. What do you advise him/her?*

A. There is no need to wear hearing protection because there is already a hearing loss.

B. Stay out of work; noise-induced hearing loss is reversible with time.

C. Continue to wear hearing protection at work.

D. Wear hearing protection whenever exposed to loud noise.

6-113   *Which of the following seafoods do you not recommend for women who might become pregnant, are pregnant, or are nursing?*

A. Swordfish, albacore tuna

B. Light white tuna, salmon

C. Haddock, halibut

D. Shrimp, pollock

6-114   *Your new client is a woman in her 80s who has a chronic cough that is progressively worsening. As part of your initial assessment, you ask about her occupational history. She states that she was a stay-at-home wife/mother. Why do you ask her about her husband's employment history and his workplace exposures?*

A. Her husband could have been exposed to tobacco smoke at work.

B. Her husband may have had an infectious disease like tuberculosis.

C. Her husband may have retiree benefits that will pay for her health care.

D. Her husband could have brought home contaminated work clothes to which she would have been exposed.

6-115   *A client has questions about the chemicals at his/her workplace. Which initial action would you recommend?*

A. Obtain a sample of the chemical(s) for laboratory analysis.

B. Request a material safety data sheet (MSDS) from the employer.

C. Terminate employment as soon as possible.

D. Call the local fire department.

6-116   *You are working in the emergency room when a firefighter arrives directly from the fire scene with increasing chest pain and shortness of breath. For which chemical exposure would you recommend biological monitoring?*

A. Carbon monoxide (CO)

B. Carbon dioxide (CO_2)

C. Hydrogen cyanide (HCN)

D. Methane (CH_4)

6-117   *You are conducting a preplacement examination of a female disabled client who has been offered a job as a secretary. You recommend that she request accommodation for her disability under the Americans with Disabilities Act (ADA). Which federal agency has jurisdiction?*

A. Occupational Safety and Health Administration

B. Department of Justice

C. Equal Employment Opportunity Commission

D. Department of Labor

6-118   *You counsel the mother of 2-year-old twins who live near a hazardous waste site that exposure to pesticides, polychlorinated biphenyls (PCBs), and dioxins has been linked to*

A. endocrine disruption.

B. autism.

C. asthma.

D. leukemia.

6-119   *A client has incurred a work-related back injury. What can you tell the client about his/her rights under workers' compensation?*

A. An employer pays work-related medical expenses only if there is lost time from work.

B. An employer pays for all work-related medical expenses.

C. An employee can sue his/her employer.

D. An employee must prove the employer was negligent before he or she can qualify for workers' compensation benefits.

Answers

6-1 Answer A

Young school-age children (age 6–8) usually react to their parents' divorce with sadness, crying, and depression. They also have guilt and often blame themselves for the divorce. They long for the absent parent and have increased behavior problems. The preschool-age child (age 3–5) has a fear of abandonment and reacts with whining, clinging, and fearful behavior, or is in denial with perfect behavior. The older school-age child (age 9–11) sees the divorce as the parents' problem but needs to find blame or a reason and reacts with conflicting loyalties toward the parents.

6-2 Answer A

Health programs must be convenient if they are to be effective. This includes convenience in location—someplace easily accessible, for example—convenience in times, and convenience and comfort in participating in the program. A friendly, culturally appropriate, "user-friendly" style is critical. Although the content, language, and visual images of the health information presented are important, nothing is more important than getting the participants to the program. No matter how excellent the content, if no one is there to participate, it is meaningless.

6-3 Answer C

Even though a child has a mild upper respiratory infection, if the child does not have a fever, immunizations should be administered. Missed opportunities for immunizations are lost forever. The contraindications for administering immunizations include anaphylactic reactions to egg ingestion (for live vaccines) and a moderate to severe infection with a fever.

6-4 Answer D

Self-imposed isolation is not a risk factor for suicide. In fact, most depressed persons isolate themselves.

Risk factors for suicide include a family history of suicide; access to hypnotic medications or other means of self-destruction, such as a handgun; and a plan for the method of committing suicide.

6-5 Answer B

There is no reason to suspect dementia related to the data presented in the question. Self-mutilation is not likely; this behavior usually manifests itself at a younger age and there would be a pattern of this behavior and usually concurrent behavioral problems. It is possible that the injuries are a result of the stated injury, but Gary's "nervousness" should cause you to consider domestic violence, alcohol or drug abuse, and Gary being the victim of a "hate crime." Contrary to some popular beliefs, battery of lesbians and gay men by their partners exists, although the prevalence is not known. Gay men may find it more difficult to find services related to battery. All gay and lesbian clients should be screened for domestic violence, and just as with heterosexuals, this should be openly discussed. When clients present with nervousness and anxiety or symptoms of depression, you should consider violence, including hate crimes, as possible correlates. Perpetrators of hate crimes may include family members and community authorities. The incidence of alcohol and drug abuse among homosexuals is reported to be slightly higher than among their heterosexual counterparts. Substance abuse should therefore also be explored in a client presenting with Gary's symptoms.

6-6 Answer C

When asked, approximately 50% of noncompliant clients will admit to not taking their medication as ordered. Clients who admit to missing medication generally overestimate the amount of medication they do take. Although the direct approach may be effective, it is often more productive to inquire in such a way as to allow the client to save face. Any questioning should be done in a nonthreatening and nonjudgmental manner.

6-7 Answer C

A high-carbohydrate diet will increase an athlete's endurance. A fat-and-protein diet provides 95% of total calories from fat and 5% from protein; a normal mixed diet with fat, protein, and carbohydrates provides 55% of total calories from carbohydrates; and a high-carbohydrate diet provides 83% of total calories from carbohydrates. Although fruits and vegetables should be a component of all diets, they should not make up the entire diet. A fruit-and-vegetable diet would not maximize an athlete's endurance time. In a study related to these diets and an athlete's maximum endurance time, a fat-and-protein diet gave 57 minutes of maximum endurance, a normal mixed diet gave 114 minutes, and a high-carbohydrate diet gave 167 minutes.

6-8   Answer D

Carbohydrate loading tricks muscles into storing extra glycogen before a competition. In training, a high-carbohydrate diet should be eaten regularly. During the first 4 days of the week before the competition, the individual should train moderately hard (1–2 hours per day) and eat a diet moderate in carbohydrates. During the 3 days before the competition, the individual should cut back on activity and eat a diet very high in carbohydrates. This practice can benefit an athlete who must keep going for 90 minutes or longer.

6-9   Answer B

The best recommendation when counseling an obese client to lose weight is to advise the client to increase activity. Because obese persons usually eat more and exercise less than nonobese persons, simply increasing energy expenditure may result in weight loss. Diet histories from obese persons have shown that their intakes are similar to, or even less than, those of nonobese persons. Although a diet history may not be totally accurate, it will show the types of food the person is eating. Heredity does play a major factor; if both parents are obese, there is an 80% chance that the children will be obese. However, most experts conclude that overweight persons simply eat more and exercise less than nonobese persons.

6-10   Answer C

Fatigue for hours after exercising or feeling sore and stiff means the exercise has either been done for too long or incorrectly. A person should never feel exhausted after the cool-down period of exercising. If that happens, the person should slow down and take it easier next time.

6-11   Answer D

For the promotion of personal safety, advise clients to wear wide-base, low-heel shoes with corrugated soles to help prevent slips and falls. Slippers or flimsy or slippery-soled shoes should not be worn. No one should walk around with glasses that are meant only for reading; they should be taken off before moving. Smoking should never take place in bed.

6-12   Answer B

Although the development of physiological symptoms related to smoking behavior may provide a "teachable moment," and although the client indeed will *not* stop smoking until ready, it is your job to assist that process. Simply informing your client of the dangers of smoking and the health-related consequences is not enough. The Agency for Healthcare Research and Quality (AHRQ) recommends the following "A's." (1) **Ask:** At every visit, ask about tobacco use. (2) **Advise** to quit *now* through clear, personalized messages. (3) **Assess:** Assess willingness to quit. (4) **Assist:** If a client is ready to quit, ask him or her to set a "quit date" and provide self-help materials and possibly pharmacological intervention. If a client is not ready to quit, provide motivational readings, discuss the dangers of exposing others to secondhand smoke, and indicate willingness to help when he or she is ready to quit. (5) **Arrange** follow-up visits. Make a follow-up appointment for 1 week after the quit date and assess smoking status; explore reasons for not stopping if the client has not been successful. Congratulate those that are successful, identify high-risk situations that they may encounter in the future, and provide coping strategies for those situations.

6-13   Answer D

Exercise provides several benefits for persons with diabetes. The most significant benefit is that exercise usually lowers blood sugar and helps the body to use its food supply better. Exercise also helps insulin work better; lowers cholesterol and triglyceride levels; improves blood flow through small vessels; increases the heart's ability to pump; helps burn excess calories; and relieves tension, anxiety, and depression.

6-14   Answer D

When counseling clients about diet and exercise, advise them, regardless of their blood sugar level, that they should eat within an hour after exercising. If they are not able to eat a full meal, they should have a high-carbohydrate snack, such as 6 oz of fruit juice or half a bagel. If more intensive exercise is planned, they should consume a little more, such as half a meat sandwich and a cup of low-fat milk. Advise clients to avoid exercise when their blood sugar is consistently high and ketones are present in the urine. Exercise should be avoided at the peak action time of insulin—for example, 2–4 hours for short-acting insulin, 12 hours for intermediate-acting insulin, and 16 hours for long-acting insulin. In addition, insulin should never be injected into parts of the body that are being used during exercise, such as the arms for tennis players or the legs for joggers, because it will be absorbed into the bloodstream too quickly.

6-15   Answer C

All children will receive approximately 25 vaccines by the time they reach 5 years of age. During early childhood, infants and children are immunized with a wide variety of vaccines, including hepatitis B (hep B); diphtheria, acellular pertussis, and tetanus (DTaP); inactivated polio vaccine (IPV); *Haemophilus influenzae* type b (HIB); measles, mumps, and rubella (MMR); varicella vaccine (VZV); pneumococcal conjugate vaccine (PCV); and influenza, pneumococcal, and meningococcal vaccine. After the age of 5, they will continue to receive a tetanus diphtheria (Td) every 10 years. They may also continue to receive an influenza vaccine yearly depending on their medical history. The immunization schedules change rapidly, so to obtain the most current information, go to http://www.cdc.gov/vaccines/recs/acip/default.htm, which offers current immunization guidelines for children and adults.

6-16   Answer D

The U.S. Preventive Services Task Force recommends goal setting by clients, individually tailored physical activity regimens, and telephone follow-up by specially trained staff for motivating clients to improve their exercise habits.

6-17   Answer C

In older adults, there is a decline in all parameters of renal function, including decreased renal concentrating capacity, impaired sodium conservation, decreased glomerular filtration rate, altered acid-base regulation (decreased ammonia production), and reduced response to antidiuretic hormone. Skin turgor is poor in older adults, so it is not a reliable measure of body fluids. Older adults are usually not thirsty, and edema in an older adult does not necessarily indicate

pathology or fluid and electrolyte imbalance. The best indicator of body fluid balance is body weight. In older adults, there is a decrease in the amount of total body water. This is attributable to an increase in body fat relative to a decline in lean body mass as intracellular water decreases.

6-18   Answer B

A frequently cited model describes five stages in health behavior change: precontemplation, contemplation, preparation, action, and maintenance. Precontemplation is described as the stage in which the individual is not even considering the idea of change; contemplation is the stage when people begin to actively think about the health risk but no action is planned; preparation occurs when the individual begins to actively plan and move into early action—for example, by developing a plan or joining a self-help group; action is marked by observable changes in health-related behavior (there may be relapses, but this is part of the process); and maintenance is when the new health action is firmly consolidated as a permanent lifestyle. Prevention of relapse is critical.

6-19   Answer C

Degenerative joint disease (DJD), also called osteoarthritis, is characterized by the degeneration and loss of articular cartilage in synovial joints. The joint most likely to be affected is the hip. DJD is the leading cause of disability in the older adult, affecting 20 million to 40 million adults in the United States. By age 40, almost 90% of adults show changes characteristic of DJD in the weight-bearing joints, particularly the hips. Other joints affected include the knees, lumbar and cervical vertebrae, proximal and distal interphalangeal joints of the fingers, first carpometacarpal joint of the wrist, and first metatarsophalangeal (big toe) joint of the foot.

6-20   Answer C

Epidemiologists have identified three stages of the disease process at which preventive actions can be effective: primary prevention, secondary prevention, and tertiary prevention. Health promotion programs usually begin at the primary prevention level, which aims at keeping a disease from beginning or a trauma from occurring. Primary prevention programs aim to reach the widest possible population group that is or might be at risk for a given health problem. Immunization is an example of primary prevention. Health promotion programs aimed at increasing exercise are another example of primary prevention of problems; their goal is to avert problems such as coronary artery disease and diabetes mellitus.

Secondary prevention involves early detection and early intervention against disease before it fully develops. Screening for potential disorders is considered secondary prevention. Mammography is an example of a strategy to detect breast cancer in its early stages. Pap smears are another example of secondary prevention, aimed at detecting cervical cancer in its early stages.

Tertiary prevention takes place after a disease or injury has occurred. Cardiac rehabilitation programs are an example of tertiary prevention. These programs are aimed at improving heart function and reducing the risk of subsequent damage to the heart.

6-21   Answer A

A smoking cessation program should be initiated when the client states a readiness to quit. Any smoking cessation program will have limited success when used to treat a highly dependent smoker who is not interested in smoking cessation. Therefore, the first crucial step is to assess a client's readiness to quit before initiating a smoking cessation program.

6-22   Answer A

There are many reasons why health-care professionals give inadequate counseling for behavioral change in the primary care setting. The primary reason is a lack of motivation because facilitating behavioral change in clients may be difficult and frustrating. Another reason is that health-care providers are skeptical about the benefits of counseling: Do clients really listen, or are they present only to receive treatment of their chief complaint? The fact that providers are not used to discussing risk factors and health promotion behaviors and counseling regarding self-care activities is another reason why information is withheld. The U.S. Preventive Services Task Force examined more than 200 clinical preventive services and suggested health counseling and self-care activities that providers can recommend to their clients.

6-23   Answer C

The most effective interventions available to health-care providers for reducing the incidence and severity of the leading causes of disease and disability in the United States are those counseling interventions that address the personal health practices of clients. This is the first type of clinical preventive service that providers should use, according to the U.S. Preventive Services Task Force. These counseling interventions address use of tobacco, diet, physical activity, sexual practices, and injury prevention. Other interventions that should be used include screening tests, immunizations, and chemoprophylaxis.

6-24   Answer D

The best way to promote a personal behavior change in a client is to discuss choices with the client and let him or her decide what will work best. Because medicine is moving away from the paternalistic model, health-care providers are changing their way of thinking and are involving clients in a shared decision-making model that results in a discourse between providers and clients. Under this shared decision-making model, clients—because of a vested interest in their health and the way information is expressed—tend to listen to the information, make informed choices, and actually practice improved health promotion activities. Providers should use the words *choices* rather than *orders*, *client initiative* rather than *compliance*, and *partnership* rather than *prescription*.

6-25   Answer D

The U.S. Preventive Services Task Force recommends screening all adult and adolescent clients for evidence of alcohol dependence, problem drinking, or excessive alcohol consumption. A client's self-report of the quantity and frequency of alcohol use does not usually provide accurate information. Responses such as "I only drink socially" need to be explored. By screening all adult and adolescent clients, you will screen the other individuals mentioned in answers A–C as well.

6-26   Answer B

The CAGE questionnaire is a four-item screening tool that is useful in identifying a client who may have a problem with alcohol abuse. C stands for "Have you ever felt you ought to cut down on your drinking?"; A for "Have people annoyed you by criticizing your drinking?"; G for "Have you ever felt guilty or bad about your drinking?"; and E for "Have you ever had a drink first thing in the morning (<u>e</u>ye opener) to steady your nerves or get rid of a hangover?" The AUDIT test and the Michigan alcoholism screening test are also useful in identifying a client who may have a problem with alcohol abuse, but they are not quite as short and easy to remember or administer. There is no Problem Drinker/Abuser Test.

6-27   Answer D

The U.S. Preventive Services Task Force and other groups advise health-care providers to take a complete sexual history on all adolescent and adult clients. Because of the sensitive nature of the topic, the provider needs to emphasize its importance to the client and state the relevance to a total history and physical. The client who is present with another in the room needs to be asked in private if he or she would be more comfortable addressing this topic alone or with the other person present.

6-28   Answer C

Asking "Is Ginger ever exposed to cigarette smoke?" is less threatening to a parent who may interpret the other questions as indictments of his or her parenting skills. Most parents know they should not smoke around a person with a respiratory problem, and making them feel guilty does not address the problem of how they can stop smoking or how the risk factor can be eliminated from their child's environment.

6-29   Answer C

Individuals with risk factors for skin cancer should have a screening test for skin cancer. Although the U.S. Preventive Services Task Force has not found sufficient evidence to recommend for or against routine screening by primary care providers, other groups, such as the Canadian Task Force on the Periodic Health Examination and the American Academy of Family Physicians, recommend complete skin examinations of adolescents and adults who have risk factors for skin cancer. These risk factors include a personal or family history of skin cancer; clinical evidence of precursor lesions, such as dysplastic nevi, actinic keratoses, or certain congenital nevi; and increased occupational or recreational exposure to sunlight.

6-30   Answer C

Researchers in a study on the strength of hearts in men and women found that men's hearts lose

20%–25% of their power from ages 20–70 while the power of women's hearts essentially remains unchanged. These researchers found that 70-year-old men who did regular aerobic exercise had the same functioning power of the heart as 20-year-old men. The study helps to illustrate the fact that although men's hearts can, with aging, lose some of their power or strength, aerobic exercise can help to prevent this loss. This is another example of how encouragement of healthy lifestyle choices (ie, regular aeroblc exercise) can enhance or preserve health. Certainly diet and good sleep habits are important but not as much as exercise for improving overall heart functioning.

6-31   Answer A

To get an accurate result when collecting fecal occult blood samples, the following should be avoided: aspirin or aspirin-containing drugs for 7 days before and during the collection period; red or processed meat and raw fruits and vegetables for 3 days before and during the collection period; and vitamin C or multivitamins containing more than 250 mg of vitamin C per day during the collection period. Clients may have fruit juices and other beverages they normally drink, cooked vegetables or fruits, breads, cereal, fish, chicken, pork, and popcorn. They do not need to avoid shellfish, nor do they need to avoid vigorous exercise.

6-32   Answer B

Although it is always best to give bad news in person, if the client asks for the news over the telephone, it is best not to lie. Instead, begin a dialogue that provides basic information. News should always be conveyed directly to the client and not through a family member. False reassurance, even if bad news is still premature, never builds trust in the long run.

6-33   Answer A

Screening for hypersensitivity to lung irritants is primary prevention of asthma because you are screening individuals before the development of disease and the commencement of counseling for it. Primary prevention for asthma includes cessation of tobacco smoking and the removal of environmental tobacco smoke left by smokers. The use of newer technologies to precipitate industrial air pollutants before they reach human air space is another emerging strategy. The use of masks has not been shown to be effective as a primary preventive strategy. Screening yearly with pulmonary function tests is secondary prevention, as are chest x-rays.

6-34   Answer B

Understanding that the pain and fatigue of fibromyalgia are real will enable the client, family, and friends to work with the health-care provider to offer support and education that might assist the couple in dealing with this chronic condition. The couple should be seen together so that they may be counseled about the chronicity of the syndrome and how it may be managed. Support groups and educational classes are a source of help for clients with fibromyalgia.

6-35   Answer C

The correct course of action is to do a complete history and physical examination and try to determine the cause of the client's discontent with the neurology consults. It may be that what this client needs is someone to listen to her and help her deal with her chronic headaches in a different manner. Conversely, there may still be some other underlying, undiscovered cause of her chronic headaches. Requests for repeated referrals are not uncommon.

6-36   Answer D

Stress urinary incontinence is not a normal part of the aging process. It may be controlled or alleviated in many women. The diagnosis must be confirmed first to rule out other causes of incontinence. Nonsurgical treatment options include drug therapy with estrogen vaginal cream, pelvic floor electrical stimulation, imipramine, Kegel exercises with biofeedback, pessaries, and occlusive devices. Very often, a combination of several of these will benefit the client. Surgery may be indicated, depending on which structure needs repairing. For example, if a cystocele is producing the symptoms, repair of the anterior vaginal wall prolapse is indicated. Pads may prove helpful, but the underlying causes must first be investigated. There is no evidence that cranberry juice helps curb stress incontinence.

6-37   Answer C

Lymphedema, a lifelong potential complication of breast and axillary node surgery and radiation, has been documented up to 30 years after surgery.

Practicing good limb care is essential for managing and preventing lymphedema. You should advise the client of the following measures to prevent lymphedema: Protect the affected arm from extreme heat and burns (including sunburn), avoid constriction of the affected arm (including by blood pressure cuffs), avoid carrying heavy purses on the affected side, avoid injury and infection of the affected arm (venipunctures are contraindicated), wear gloves when gardening and cleaning, care for minor injuries on the affected arm promptly, and keep regular appointments for follow-up care.

6-38   Answer C

To encourage physical activity along with parental involvement, advise teachers to assign homework to the students that must be done with their parents and involves physical activity, such as having the parents count how many times in 2 minutes the child can hop on one foot. Recommending play outside may not be safe, depending on the neighborhood. Turning off the TV is a good idea, but children may then substitute some other sedentary method of play, such as computer games.

6-39   Answer B

To help Janice recover from osteomyelitis and promote healing, advise her to do the following: Do range-of-motion and strengthening exercises; eat foods high in vitamins and calcium; and increase caloric and protein intake, as well as fluid intake, which helps minimize the risks of kidney damage, yeast infections, and adverse gastrointestinal effects. You do not have enough history in the stem of the question to determine if the client should bear weight. Likewise, it is unclear if exposing the wound to open air would be helpful or if wet dressings should be applied.

6-40   Answer A

Anemia, which may be detected by a complete blood count (CBC), is sufficiently prevalent to justify screening, and it is a condition for which early detection may be beneficial. A CBC is often ordered as a routine screening test. It can detect anemia, leukocytosis, thrombocytopenia, and leukemia, as well as other hematological disorders. Anemia is the only condition with sufficient prevalence for which early detection may be beneficial.

Anemia is present in nearly 4 million Americans. Iron-deficiency anemia is easily treated and may be harmful in certain populations, such as young children and pregnant women.

6-41   Answer D

Clients who have been diagnosed with PAD or chronic venous insufficiency should be counseled about the modification of risk factors. Clients need to stop smoking completely, not merely cut down. Stating that "I'll cut down on my smoking" means that Joe has not understood your teaching instructions. It is essential to control hypertension and diabetes, if present. Dietary control must include limitation of fat and salt intake. Clients must be taught to do meticulous daily foot care that includes inspecting feet daily for sores, ulcers, and abrasions, including the use of a mirror to check the soles of the feet. Clients should not walk barefoot and should wear well-fitting supportive shoes. They should not soak their feet and should be careful trimming their nails. All clients should be taught to watch for the signs and symptoms that might indicate progressive ischemia, such as increased pain, increased pallor or cyanosis, and rest pain.

6-42   Answer C

Colonoscopy is not a preventive strategy but rather a form of secondary (screening) prevention, as is routine annual testing for fecal occult blood after age 50. Obesity is a weak risk factor for colon and rectal cancer, so weight loss is not the most valuable preventive strategy. No correlation between cigarette smoking and colon and rectal cancer has been discovered. However, the preventive power of regular physical exercise has been established as a protective factor against colon cancer and also against rectal cancer, but to a lesser degree. Likewise, a healthy diet rich in vegetables, fruits, and fiber has been shown to have protective effects against colon and rectal cancer. The effect of regular aspirin use as a protector against colon cancers has been replicated in several studies. Aspirin inhibits the growth of colonic and rectal polyps, perhaps by means of inhibiting prostaglandin synthesis.

6-43   Answer B

To change behaviors successfully, clients need to feel "ownership in" the need for change. Internal motivation has been shown to be predictive of successful treatment programs. To recognize that a change needs to take place and actually make the move to initiate a change, most clients need to feel that there is more to gain than to lose. The pleasure, comfort, or other gains the client receives from overeating, smoking, and other undesirable behaviors need to be outweighed by the gains the client values and believes are attainable. Although Henry wants to attend his daughter's wedding in the future and be able to enjoy his retirement when the time comes, they are temporary motivators that may not give him the needed impetus because they are far in the future. He needs to take ownership of the problem and start today to make changes that will enable him to enjoy his future.

6-44   Answer C

The appropriate response to a client who is concerned about gaining weight after smoking cessation is to suggest several strategies that the client might use to prevent a weight gain. Many clients who have stopped smoking and gain weight resume smoking. Therefore, this is an important area to address when the client is considering smoking cessation so that it can be dealt with before the weight is gained. The average amount of weight gained after smoking cessation is about 5 lb. Two strategies to be used are avoiding high-calorie foods (while keeping low-calorie foods available to satisfy the urge to eat) and increasing exercise.

6-45   Answer A

A simple measure of whether an exercise activity is aerobic is the client's heart rate. If the pulse reaches or exceeds a level of 60% of the maximum normal pulse, the exercise is considered aerobic. This only roughly measures the true degree of increased oxygen uptake by the muscles and is more accurate for measuring the intensity of exercise in beginners than in conditioned athletes. The formula to use is 220 minus the person's age times 0.6 (or 60% of the theoretical maximum normal pulse). This means that for a person 63 years old to have aerobic exercise, the heart rate must reach at least 94 bpm ($220 - 63 = 157; 157 \times 0.6 = 94$). One can usually assume that exercise is aerobic if breathing is deep and sweating occurs in mild to cold temperatures, but this is not as reliable measure as heart rate. For exercise to be beneficial in reducing the long-term risk for coronary artery disease, it must be aerobic, although any exercise is beneficial for weight loss.

6-46   Answer A

Low-fat varieties of fish include bluefish, Dover sole, bass, albacore tuna, cod, haddock, northern pike, flounder, grouper, halibut, and red snapper. It should be noted that tuna, red snapper, and swordfish also have high levels of mercury. High-fat meats include sausages, hot dogs, luncheon meats (unless made from low-fat poultry), hamburger, and steak. Better choices of meat include flank steak, pork tenderloin, and loin lamb chops. All visible fat should be trimmed off meat before cooking. Poultry choices should include white meat rather than dark meat, and the skin and all visible fats should be trimmed, preferably before cooking.

6-47   Answer C

Eating breakfast and eating at regular intervals are elements of a successful weight-loss program that can be as important as the content of the meals. Eating breakfast actually gets the metabolism going so that one will be able to digest all the essential nutrients. Saying "We all need some essential fatty acids that are obtained only from food" is unrelated to the fact that Trisha skips breakfast. The other responses are inappropriate and critical.

6-48   Answer A

Coconut oil, cocoa butter, and palm and palm kernel oils are all examples of saturated fat, a type of fatty acid. Olive oil is an example of a monounsaturated fatty acid. Corn, cottonseed, soybean, and safflower oils are all types of polyunsaturated fatty acids. There are no combinations of monounsaturated and polyunsaturated fats.

6-49   Answer B

Falls are the most common cause of injuries, the leading cause of hospital admissions for trauma, and the second most common cause of injury-related deaths for all age groups (about 12,000 annually). About 1 out of 20 persons receives emergency room care for injuries sustained in falls. Children typically fall from buildings or other elevated structures, whereas older adults are more likely to fall during normal household activities. Adult falls are usually a result of gait instability, decreased proprioception and muscle strength, or vision problems. Falls cause nearly 90% of all fractures among older adults. Motor vehicle and bicycle accidents are a cause of death in 1 out of 6 school-age children.

6-50   Answer B

A primary cause of degenerative joint disease (DJD) is obesity. Repetitive mechanical joint overuse is also a risk factor for DJD and can be seen in athletes such as tennis players and baseball pitchers. Arthritis also occurs in joints that have previously been operated on or injured. The etiology of the primary form of the disease is unknown, although genetic and immunological factors appear to play a role in its development.

6-51   Answer C

Encourage the client with arthritis to rest frequently throughout the day to help alleviate discomfort and pain. Other interventions include applying heat to painful joints, usually in the form of warm packs or warm baths; applying splints to the affected joint to help maintain the joint in correct alignment; using good body mechanics and proper posture to reduce the stress on the affected joints; and losing weight (if overweight) to take stress off the affected joint.

6-52   Answer D

When teaching clients about gout, include the following information: Although the initial attack of gout causes no permanent damage, recurrent attacks may lead to permanent damage and joint destruction. Kidney stones and kidney damage may result if the gout is not managed adequately. Clients should drink at least 3 quarts of fluid per day to help prevent kidney stones and damage to the kidneys from hyperuricemia, and they should avoid alcohol. Other potential effects of continued hyperuricemia include tophaceous deposits in subcutaneous and other connective tissues.

6-53   Answer A

To help manage the effects of scleroderma, advise clients to avoid becoming chilled, which could trigger episodes of Raynaud's phenomenon; maintain good skin care; perform physical therapy, particularly of the hands and face, to help maintain mobility; wear loose, warm clothing, gloves, and warm stockings in the winter; and stop smoking altogether (because of the vasoconstrictive effect of nicotine, as well as the respiratory effects of the disease).

6-54   Answer D

Martin should make sure that Laura is wearing a medical identification bracelet or necklace, such as those made by MedicAlert, stating that she has a seizure disorder. This will alert others in case she is not responsive. If a person has a seizure disorder, alcoholic beverages should be avoided completely and caffeine intake should be limited. The importance of continuing to take anticonvulsant medications should be stressed even when no seizures are experienced. State and local laws differ regarding persons with seizure disorders. Usually, driving a motor vehicle is prohibited for 6 months to 2 years after a seizure episode.

6-55   Answer D

Hot showers may transiently exacerbate symptoms. There is no evidence that flying exacerbates multiple sclerosis. Exercise is important to maintain function and flexibility, but it needs to be balanced with rest to avoid excessive fatigue. There is no need to avoid spicy foods, caffeine, and peppermint because of multiple sclerosis.

6-56   Answer B

Most airlines do not allow pregnant women to travel if they are at more than 35 to 36 weeks' gestation without a letter from their physician or health-care provider. Commercial aircraft cruising at high altitude are able to pressurize only up to 5000 to 8000 ft above sea level. Women with moderate anemia (hemoglobin <8.5 g/dL) or with compromised oxygen saturation may need oxygen supplementation. Women with sickle cell disease may experience a crisis during the desaturation. Other medical risk factors include congenital or acquired heart disease, history of thromboembolic disease, hemoglobin <8.5 g/dL, chronic lung disease such as asthma, and medical disease requiring ongoing assessment and medication.

Obstetric risk factors include history of miscarriage, threatened abortion or vaginal bleeding during the present pregnancy, history of ectopic pregnancy (rule out with ultrasound before flying), primigravida older than 35 or younger than 15 years of age, history of diabetes with pregnancy, hypertension, toxemia, multiple gestation in present pregnancy, incompetent cervix, history of infertility, or difficulty becoming pregnant. An electrocardiogram would be indicated only related to a specific risk factor, whereas it would be essential to check the hemoglobin level in making your decision. Even those with sickle cell trait may experience hematuria or renal microthrombosis during desaturation. The fetal circulation and

fetal hemoglobin protect the fetus against desaturation during flight.

6-57   Answer C

An alteration in clotting factors and venous dilation during pregnancy may predispose pregnant women to superficial and deep venous thrombosis, or "economy class syndrome." Pregnant women have a rate of acute iliofemoral venous thrombosis that is six times greater than that of nonpregnant women. The pregnant traveler should request an aisle seat and should walk in the aisles at least once an hour during long airplane flights whenever it is safe to do so. General stretching and isometric leg exercises should be encouraged on long flights. Pregnant women should also be encouraged to drink nonalcoholic beverages to maintain hydration and to wear seat belts low around the pelvis throughout the entire flight. They should avoid heavy eating because intestinal gas expansion can be particularly uncomfortable for the pregnant traveler. Monitoring of blood pressure is not essential unless there is an identified underlying risk factor.

6-58   Answer D

Clients with trigeminal neuralgia should always wear protective sunglasses or goggles when outside, working in dusty areas, mowing the lawn, or using any type of spray material. They should also use artificial tears and an eye patch at night. Clients should be counseled to chew on the unaffected side of the mouth and avoid eating or drinking hot foods or fluids. They should also have regular dental examinations because they will not be able to feel pain associated with gum infection or tooth decay.

6-59   Answer A

Delay pregnancy for 3 months following vaccines for measles, mumps, and rubella (MMR); yellow fever; or varicella. These are all live attenuated vaccines. The others are not.

6-60   Answer B

For the client with lumbar spinal stenosis, exercises that encourage lumbar flexion and flattening of the lumbar lordotic curve are particularly helpful. Also, exercises that strengthen the abdominal muscles and promote mobility of the lumbar paraspinal muscles can help minimize lordosis of the lumbar spine. Lumbar extension worsens the radiculopathy by increasing the laxity of the ligamentum. Any exercise that results in hyperextension of the lumbar spine should be avoided. Swimming and walking against the resistance of the water in a swimming pool promote healthful cardiovascular function while maintaining lumbar flexion. Surgery may be necessary for clients who have severe neurological dysfunction and pain.

6-61 Answer C

To achieve optimum protection, vaccination should ideally occur before the initiation of sexual activity. An estimated 33% of high school freshmen and 62% of seniors engage in sexual intercourse. An estimated 7.4% of students engage in sexual intercourse for the first time before age 13 years. Currently there is controversy over the age at which this vaccine should be administered.

6-62 Answer A

When delivering bad news, the following framework may prove helpful: (1) preparation (forecast possibility of bad news); (2) setting (give news in person if possible with privacy and adequate time); (3) delivery (give the news clearly but present the hopeful message first and then identify important feelings and concerns); (4) emotional support (remain with client and use empathic statements); (5) information (use clear words and summarize; use handouts as needed); and (6) closure (make a plan for the immediate future and schedule a follow-up appointment). Do not provide false reassurance. Allow time for silence throughout. The specific rationale for providing the hopeful message first is that typically clients remember very little after hearing the distressing news.

6-63 Answer C

Several drops of mineral oil can be used to soften earwax. The adage of "never insert anything smaller than your elbow in your ear" still applies, even with cotton-tipped applicators. Flushing the ears using a bulb syringe should be avoided because the vacuum pressure may be excessive and rupture the tympanic membrane. Commercial preparations can be used to irrigate, but they should never be left in longer than directed because they can cause local irritation.

6-64 Answer C

Clients with diabetes mellitus should be taught proper foot care, especially the use of a mirror to help them inspect the bottoms (soles) of their feet because peripheral neuropathy may prevent them from feeling any foreign bodies or cuts. Preparations such as alcohol should be avoided because they tend to dry and crack the feet, allowing microorganisms to enter. Soaking the feet in water and use of emollients should also be avoided because they help to keep the feet moist and thus become a good medium for the growth of bacteria.

6-65 Answer A

For clients with AIDS, a viral load test is a more accurate measure of the progression of the disease than a CD4 count. The CD4 count is a surrogate marker that provides important, but indirect, measures of the state of a client's HIV disease and immunosuppression. The prognostic information it provides is useful, but incomplete, because the CD4 count can fluctuate depending on the status of the immune system, such as when the client has a cold, or as a result of dietary intake. A CD4 count is still recommended every 6 months, but a viral load test is more accurate.

6-66 Answer D

When an adolescent appears "laid back," quiet, and aloof, measures must be taken to ascertain from the teen what is concerning him or her. It may be appropriate to do a drug test, but first you should share that information with the client and ask if a urine test is necessary—is he or she, in fact, taking recreational drugs, or is there something else going on? You may still want to do a urine test if you do not think the client is credible, but certainly give the client the opportunity to talk. Eventually, the client may need to be referred to a counselor or psychiatrist or started on antidepressant medication, but this should not be the initial action.

6-67 Answer C

Children younger than the age of 7 years often experience frequent ear infections. The eustachian tubes of children this age are horizontal and do not allow the drainage of infecting organisms—viral or bacterial. An infection in the nasopharynx may ascend to a child's horizontal eustachian tube and then into the middle ear by impairing local host defenses or by eustachian tube dysfunction. By age 7, 35% of children experience six or more episodes of acute otitis media. As the child grows, the eustachian tube angles more and is no longer horizontal. If Shirley inserted a foreign body into her ear and it remained in place occluding the canal, she could develop an infection, but the mother is asking about frequent infections, which are more common than infections induced by foreign bodies. A high-fat diet will not affect cerumen production. The mother cannot be expected to dry her daughter's ears completely after bathing. She should be drying the external canal with a cloth or tissue, nothing smaller.

6-68   Answer C

If a mother brings in her daughter because she thinks her daughter is sexually active, you should not take as fact the mother's belief. You should find out directly from the daughter. If the daughter admits to being sexually active, you may want to do a vaginal examination and discuss contraception methods or counseling. Notification of a child protective services agency may be warranted if the daughter admits to, or if you suspect, sexual abuse or an incestuous relationship with her father, stepfather, or other male relative given the age of the child and state law on statuatory rape, even if sexual activity is consensual and nonfamilial.

6-69   Answer B

If an adolescent boy tells you he thinks he has something seriously wrong with him because he has awakened in the morning with a wet sheet around his penis, tell him that this a normal progression in his sexual development. In this case, Phil may be embarrassed to ask his friends about this and not realize that "wet dreams" are a normal progression in sexual development. Ejaculation occurs in the early morning hours during an erection while sleeping and is referred to as a nocturnal emission. Phil should be assured that this is perfectly normal.

6-70   Answer C

The most common agent of intentional, nonoccupational poisoning deaths in adults is motor vehicle exhaust (25%), followed by cocaine and heroin (11%), antidepressants and tranquilizers (10%), and barbiturates (2%).

6-71   Answer C

When counseling parents about accidental poisonings in children, instruct the parents to administer ipecac syrup to induce vomiting if their child accidentally ingests something poisonous. In some instances, however, inducing vomiting is harmful because the chemical ingested may be irritating to the gastrointestinal mucosa as it ascends. When in doubt about inducing vomiting, advise the parents to contact their local emergency room, which will put them in contact with the poison control hotline. If the parent is unable to get to a telephone, less damage will be done by administering ipecac syrup and inducing vomiting than by waiting. Of all poisoning cases, 85% involve children, and 70% of those children are younger than 5 years of age. Families should have a bottle of ipecac syrup to administer on the way to the hospital because many toxins are absorbed rapidly. Burnt toast, tea, and milk of magnesia are old-fashioned home remedies that should be replaced with ipecac syrup.

6-72   Answer B

Studies have shown that siblings are usually present when a brother or sister becomes a drowning victim. To help prevent an accidental drowning, young children (even as young as 8 years old) can learn cardiopulmonary resuscitation (CPR). A large number of swimming pool drowning deaths could have been prevented by immediate CPR. Children are very creative and can unlock doors and climb or go around fences. It is impractical to keep the backyard entrances locked at all times because the 8-year-old could certainly unlock them. It is almost impossible for a parent to keep a child in view 24 hours a day. Parents should learn CPR.

6-73   Answer A

Although stating, "These bruises are very unusual. Is your husband hurting you?" sounds very forthright, studies have shown that such a statement is what the client needs and is willing to respond to. Most clients who have been abused have been waiting to be confronted in a matter-of-fact manner rather than an accusatory tone or one that makes the client seem like the victim. If asked, "How did you get these bruises?" or "Would you like to talk about what's going on?" a client will usually continue the silence, denial, and victimization. Another common approach is to link the question to information that the client has already provided in the encounter, such as, "You said that one bad thing about working opposite shifts is that you frequently argue about child rearing. Does your husband ever hurt you during these arguments?" Another approach is to normalize the problem, such as, "Many of my clients have told me that their husbands hit them; they complain of being abused. Is this how it is for you?"

6-74   Answer C

Self-tanning lotions or creams are a safe alternative to tanning from natural sunlight, tanning beds, or lamps. These substances contain dihydroxyacetone, a substance approved by the Food and Drug Administration, which binds to the epidermis and chemically produces a skin color resembling a sunlight-induced tan. Self-tanning does not affect melanocytes or melanogenesis, does not increase melanin levels, and does not depend on ultraviolet light. However, it is unrealistic to think that young women will take your advice and avoid the sun completely. While recommending a self-tanning lotion to Melanie, you should also stress that if she insists on getting a tan naturally, she should have brief tanning periods using a sunscreen with a skin protection factor (SPF) of 15 or higher.

6-75   Answer A

Almost 20% of teenage boys in the United States use smokeless tobacco. It is more common in rural areas than in urban settings. Long-term use is addictive; may lead to mouth or throat cancer; and can cause gum recession, which can lead to the loss of teeth. Smokeless tobacco does not affect appetite. All clients who use tobacco in any form should be counseled to stop because of the risks to oral and general health.

6-76   Answer A

Baby bottle tooth decay (BBTD) can occur when a child goes to bed with a bottle containing anything but water. Some parents use milk sweetened with sugar, sugared water, fruit juices, or carbonated or noncarbonated beverages. Even milk-based baby formula, because of its lactose content, is a potential promoter of BBTD. Some parents may use a sweetened pacifier at night, and this is also a contributing factor in BBTD. The child should be switched to a plain water bottle or weaned from the practice altogether.

6-77   Answer D

Although Guillain-Barré syndrome was associated with the use of the "swine flu" vaccine in 1976, studies done every year since have not shown a clear association between influenza vaccination and neurological complications. Tim is a definite candidate for a flu shot because he is older than age 65 and has pulmonary disease. A flu shot is recommended for residents and employees of nursing homes and other chronic care facilities; for clients with diabetes mellitus, renal dysfunction, hemoglobinopathy, and immunosuppression; and for health-care personnel.

6-78   Answer D

Agriculture continues to rank as the most dangerous industry in the United States. It is important for the health-care provider to provide anticipatory guidance related to farm safety. Various groups such as the National Committee for Childhood Agricultural Injury Prevention (NCAIP) and Farm Safety 4 Just Kids provide resources for farm safety information, including age-appropriate publications such as storybooks and coloring books, as well as a rural health and safety kit that includes games, puzzles, and brochures. Still, farm-related injuries and fatalities continue to occur. Contributing factors include lack of parental supervision, operator fatigue, and children performing tasks inappropriate for age. Education and health counseling is a high priority for all members of the farming family.

6-79   Answer D

Clients with gastroesophageal reflux disease should avoid caffeine and chocolate, as well as mints, citrus products, alcohol, aspirin, and other NSAIDs. They should discontinue smoking altogether because it interferes with the action and effectiveness of H_2-receptor antagonists and be advised to report worsening of symptoms, such as tarry stools, fever, sore throat, or hallucinations.

6-80   Answer C

Erythromycin (E-Mycin, Eryc) has been found to be the safest drug to use in pregnancy because it has no teratogenic effects on the fetus. Acetylsalicylic acid (aspirin) alters platelet function and can cause maternal and newborn bleeding; acetaminophen (Tylenol) can be toxic to the liver; and tetracycline (Achromycin, Sumycin), if given to a pregnant mother between the fourth month of pregnancy and delivery, will cause abnormalities in tooth development, including brown spotting and unusual shape.

6-81   Answer A

Usually no serious physical problem is present with nighttime enuresis, although the child may have a small or immature bladder. When counseling the parents of a child with nighttime enuresis, tell them that it is a common problem that is often inherited. Stress the idea that the parents are not at fault. A family plan for dealing with the wet bed may include deciding who strips the bed and where the sheets should go. The child needs to play a major role in this plan, and positive reinforcement should be given when the child remains dry through the night.

6-82   Answer B

Adolescents who are depressed may have a preoccupation with death. They exhibit the following behaviors: a change in weight or eating habits; insomnia or hypersomnia; a drop in school performance; fatigue; a change in motor activity, presenting as either inactivity or hyperactivity; loss of interest in usual activities; and strong feelings of self-reproach or guilt.

6-83   Answer C

The health counselor must work with the client because smoking cessation will not be effective unless the smoker is ready to quit. Follow-up reinforcement sessions are essential. The client should be followed first weekly, then monthly, and then quarterly for a year. Treatment for smoking cessation is most effective when the health-care counselor is perceived as being understanding and when the expression of feelings and concerns is encouraged. If a client is smoking more than 20–30 cigarettes per day, he or she should be encouraged to start a tapering-off program; persons who smoke fewer than 20 cigarettes per day should be encouraged to set a "quit date." The client should announce the quit date to family and friends and all should provide additional support during this time. It is not necessary for the health counselor to meet with family, although strategies may be shared if the family requests.

6-84   Answer B

Although many sources do cite the condom as the most essential form of primary prevention against sexually transmitted diseases and unwanted pregnancies, in reality the best prevention tool is the brain. For this reason, an adequate understanding of psychosocial and cultural determinants underlying sexual behaviors is essential to individualize counseling approaches depending on the client. Teaching

should begin before puberty. Middle childhood is a "rationale period" for children. Sex education has vocal opposition in many subcultures. However, preventive teaching and participatory discussion need not focus on sex specifically. Teaching can be centered on making positive future choices and impulse control. This teaching should address girls in particular because of the lifelong consequences of unintended pregnancy and sexually transmitted diseases in women. Although sharing disease-specific information may help, it is only one prong of what should be a multipronged approach to prevention. Likewise, your job as a health counselor is not to change your client's personality or world view, nor to solve their deep conflicts; rather, you should offer better and healthier ways for clients to get what they want.

6-85   Answer D

When counseling clients, practice the "art of the possible." Your goal is not to increase the client's knowledge, but rather to effect behavioral change. Be realistic. For example, a client should not be asked to stop all intercourse. Clients who are not adequately helped the first time will be back again and again. It is practically impossible to counsel clients in this area adequately in one session. Personal connection, repeated messages, praise of progress, and negotiation are the name of the game. Even commercial sex workers, for example, might learn to be more restrictive by insisting on practicing only safe sex, or by avoiding high-risk situations such as working with belligerent or drugged clients.

6-86   Answer B

With a client who smokes, it is appropriate to discuss smoking cessation techniques at every visit. Because family practitioners see about 70% of the smokers in the United States during the course of each year, these encounters present excellent opportunities for providers to deliver smoking cessation advice to clients who smoke. This should be done at each visit, regardless of the reason why the client is being seen. *Healthy People 2010* includes an objective to increase to at least 75% the proportion of health-care providers who routinely advise their clients who smoke to quit.

6-87   Answer A

If the hepatitis B vaccine schedule is interrupted, it should be continued. If interrupted after the first dose, the second dose should be given as soon as possible; the third dose can be given 2 months after the second dose and at least 4 months after the first dose. This client's normal schedule would have been a series of three immunizations, with the second and third doses administered 1 month and 6 months, respectively, after the first dose. If a period longer than 6 months has elapsed, a titer must be drawn to evaluate need for further vaccine.

6-88   Answer C

Principles of nutrition intervention in anorexia nervosa include using liquid supplements in addition to solid food when the client cannot achieve the desired intake with solid food. Linking rewards to food energy intake and not to weight gain; reducing excessive caffeine intake; increasing food energy intake slowly by adding 200 kcal/week; giving multiple vitamin and mineral supplements at recommended daily allowance levels; enhancing elimination with dietary fiber from grain sources; and reducing sensations of bloating with small, frequent feedings are also recommended.

6-89   Answer A

Signs and symptoms of bulimia nervosa include frequent urinary tract infections, which usually result from fluid and electrolyte imbalance; more than the average number of dental caries for the person's age and erosion of the teeth, usually as a result of vomiting, which can also cause irritation and infection of the pharynx, esophagus, and salivary glands; bruised or cut hands, which usually result from contact with the teeth when inducing vomiting; and injury to the lower intestinal tract from frequent use of strong laxatives. Bizarre behavior around food; hyperactivity; amenorrhea; and dry, sparse hair are all more typical of anorexia nervosa than bulimia.

6-90   Answer B

For the person with bulimia nervosa, foods that can be naturally divided into portions, such as a baked potato, should be given rather than rice, pasta, or French fries.

6-91   Answer C

Technological changes have made tennis rackets lighter, creating racket head speed and velocity. To compensate for this, suggest a wide grip, which may distribute forces more evenly to the forearm and elbow. Extremely tight strings accelerate

velocity. For a new player, this may be dangerous and can increase the amount of force and impact transmitted to the forearm, elbow, and shoulder. An experienced racket professional may be best suited to assist a new player in making the best selection and equipment adjustments. You should not discourage John from taking up this sport because physical activity is good.

6-92   Answer D

A person who is chronically tired should see a health-care provider rather than self-prescribe. Many self-diagnose iron-deficiency anemia and self-prescribe an iron supplement, which will relieve tiredness only if the cause of the tiredness is iron-deficiency anemia. If the cause is a folate deficiency, taking iron will prolong the tiredness. Taking a vitamin supplement with iron may cure a vitamin deficiency. However, the symptoms of fatigue may have a nonnutritional cause. If the cause of the tiredness is actually a hidden blood loss because of cancer, the diagnosis may not be picked up as early as it could be. When tiredness is caused by a lack of sleep, no nutrient or combination of nutrients can replace a good night's sleep. If nutritional causes and blood loss or other disease process is ruled out as the cause of the fatigue, then a nursing measure that may be beneficial is a discussion of sleep-promoting behaviors.

6-93   Answer C

Two of the most notable signs of a vitamin C deficiency are bleeding gums and broken capillaries under the skin that occur spontaneously and produce pinpoint hemorrhages. Other signs of vitamin C deficiency include failure to promote normal collagen synthesis, which causes further hemorrhaging; degeneration of muscles, including the heart muscle; rough, brown, scaly, and dry skin; and wounds that fail to heal because scar tissue will not form. Signs of vitamin A deficiency do not appear until after stores are depleted, which takes 1 to 2 years or less in a growing child. A deficiency of vitamin A affects the bones and teeth, with cessation of bone growth and painful joints; affects the blood with anemia; affects the eyes with night blindness; and affects the skin by plugging hair follicles with keratin, which forms white lumps (hyperkeratosis). Most vitamin B_{12} deficiencies reflect inadequate absorption, not poor intake. Inadequate absorption typically occurs for one of two reasons: a lack of hydrochloric acid or a lack of intrinsic factor. Many people older than age 60 develop atrophic gastritis, a condition characterized by inadequate hydrochloric acid. In vitamin D deficiency, production of the calcium-binding protein in the intestinal cells slows so that even when calcium is adequate in the diet, it passes through the gastrointestinal tract unabsorbed, leaving the bones undersupplied. The symptoms of a vitamin D deficiency are those of calcium deficiency: rickets and osteomalacia.

6-94   Answer C

Instructing Marvin on self-monitoring of his blood sugar makes him an active participant in his own health care, which, in turn, will improve his adherence to the plan of care. Although you may want him to call a nutritionist, he may never get around to this or may be in denial. Initially you will have Marvin come in frequently for a urinalysis and will monitor glycohemoglobin levels every 3 months, but making him a participant in his care is one way to encourage ownership of the problem, which leads to an active approach.

6-95   Answer A

Foods high in potassium and calcium, such as bananas and milk, help to lower blood pressure. Also, a low-sodium diet is recommended to help reduce the amount of retained water, which, in turn, helps to lower blood pressure. In addition, some diuretics deplete serum potassium, which bananas will help to replace.

6-96   Answer A

Polyunsaturated fats ("good fats"), such as soybean oil, are liquid at room temperature and come from vegetables. Saturated fats ("bad fats"), such as coconut and palm oils and cocoa butter, harden at room temperature and are found in meat and dairy products made from whole milk or cream, as well as in solid and hydrogenated shortening.

6-97   Answer D

The U.S. Preventive Services Task Force recommends the following for all pregnant women: screening for *chlamydia*, syphilis, hepatitis B, and asymptomatic bacteriuria; interventions to reduce alcohol abuse with screening and behavioral counseling; counseling to prevent tobacco use and tobacco-caused disease; blood typing and assessment for Rh(D) incompatibility; and behavioral interventions to promote breastfeeding.

6-98   Answer A

You must investigate the underlying causes of this new change in sexual function and desire. Although testosterone deficiency is a common cause of low desire and is more common in older adults, this change in sexual function is not a natural consequence of aging and should not be treated as such. It is too soon to send this client for sexual counseling as you must first attempt to ascertain the underlying reason behind the problem. You do not have enough data to presume depression, although depression is a common component of low sexual desire. Also, prescribing serotonin reuptake inhibitors (SSRIs), a type of antidepressant, may create other forms of sexual dysfunction, typically delayed or absent orgasm. You may end up sending this client for counseling and/or prescribing Viagra, but more investigation should be completed first.

6-99   Answer C

The cheapest and easiest remedy for pediculosis (head lice) is to apply mayonnaise or White Rain conditioner to the scalp and hair. The solution smothers the live lice and loosens nits to facilitate their removal from the hair shaft. Although petroleum jelly (Vaseline) also works, it is extremely difficult to remove from the hair. Cutting the hair very short or shaving it should not be necessary.

6-100   Answer A

When advising clients what to look for in skin cancer and melanoma, tell them to look for the ABCDs: A for asymmetrical border, B for border irregularity, C for color variations, and D for diameter greater than 6 mm. A papule that is 2 mm in size sounds harmless, depending on the border and color. A crusty-appearing lesion may be an actinic keratosis and is not a medical emergency that needs to be seen immediately. It is overbroad to say that the absence of change in any lesion will negate the need for follow-up.

6-101   Answer B

Although you might like to report a gun in the house to the police, especially a gun in a house with a young child, this is not required; the gun may, in fact, be registered. What you do want to do is to stress the need to keep the gun in a locked place, where the child has no access to it, with a combination lock on the trigger, and to keep the ammunition and gun in separate places. You might also want to talk about other home safety devices, such as alarms, if the client feels that his or her home is not safe. Unfortunately, your personal bias and views on this situation, as expressed in options C and D, are not pertinent. You should not pass judgment; it is an ineffective strategy for behavioral change. Additionally, you cannot require a meeting with both parents regarding this issue.

6-102   Answer C

If a client is caring for an elderly parent with dementia, recommend that the client get information on home safety and community resources. In this case, Mary should be put in touch with support services for herself and given information about respite care. She should also receive information about resources regarding home safety that can be implemented so that she will not have to worry constantly about her father injuring himself. Mary should be encouraged to keep her father at home as long as possible because changing his environment may tend to worsen his dementia. However, she should not be made to feel guilty if she reaches the decision that she can no longer care for him at home. An elderly person's door should never be locked at night to keep him or her from wandering because there would be no way of escaping in case of a fire.

6-103   Answer D

Swimming greatly benefits the heart and lungs but does not help osteoporosis. All caffeine is a risk factor for osteoporosis. Cutting down on coffee is a good first step, but black (regular) tea also contains caffeine. Herbal tea or decaffeinated coffee are better recommendations. Shelley needs an adequate calcium intake, not just a multivitamin. Regular exercise, especially weight-bearing exercise that includes walking and running, is recommended. This is because these types of exercises put the body's weight on the bones, pressing calcium into the bone matrix. Additionally, strengthening the leg muscles helps prevent falls; therefore, simply standing is more beneficial than sitting.

6-104   Answer D

Regular interaction with others exercises social and language skills, and playing a card game like bridge reinforces memory, providing a form of cognitive

"exercise." Along those same lines, doing crossword puzzles and jigsaw puzzles helps exercise the mind. The benefits of video games and simulations are being researched at present. Although working on model ships or airplanes may provide some stimulation, the solitary nature of these hobbies over time makes them not as beneficial as an activity like card playing that demands social interaction in addition to mental effort. Engaging in rigorous physical activity, not resting, is considered protective of mental abilities. An older adult would do better to take a daily multivitamin, not just calcium, as a mental protective strategy. Research has also shown that a longer education as a youth is a protective factor. Maintaining a sense of self-efficacy—the belief, faith, and action that "I can do it"—and a "use it or lose it" approach are keys to effective mental functioning in older age.

6-105   Answer B

Although being a college student and lacking structure and transportation over a summer break might contribute to an ongoing depression, they are not risk factors in and of themselves. Believing oneself to be incapable, however, is a risk factor for depression. Other risk factors include being female, living in poverty or a powerless social position, having a severe physical illness, experiencing a severe stressor such as death or loss of a close person, and having a first-degree biological relative with a depressive mood disorder.

6-106   Answer A

Signs and symptoms of depression include sad mood, crying spells, loss of interest in activities and people, slowed movements, disturbed sleep cycle, trouble concentrating, and thinking about death. There may be an increase in alcohol or drug use. Comorbidity is common, with anxiety symptoms accompanying depression in perhaps 70% of episodes (this figure differs in different cultural groups). This may bring on restlessness, fidgeting, worrying, and the inability to relax. Going on a spending spree is more indicative of a manic-depressive mood disorder; obsessively exercising is more consistent with anorexia nervosa; and obsessive hand washing is more typical of an obsessive-compulsive disorder.

6-107   Answer A

Physical exercise, more daylight, and rethinking one's situation ("cognitive restructuring") are all important interventions for depression. Rest will not help, and although having a nutritionally sound diet is recommended, it is not as important as the other suggested strategies. St. John's wort, initially heralded as an important adjuvant treatment of depression, has in later studies proved to be virtually ineffective for depression.

6-108   Answer C

Past surgeries and number of children are not documented risk factors for coronary artery disease (CAD). Economic disadvantage, rather than economic advantage, is a risk factor. Temperament, however, is a risk factor. Studies from several industrialized nations suggest that people experiencing stressful situations who show their emotions are less likely to develop sustained high blood pressure, although their blood pressure may temporarily rise during the stressor. Social disadvantage, such as race, is another often-overlooked documented risk factor. Those who are discriminated against or who are poor face uncertain life situations and must constantly be vigilant. Both of these are risk factors for CAD. There are five documented psychosocial risk factors for CAD: uncertain life situation, lack of experience to learn which behavioral response will solve a given problem, the possibility of serious harm, the fact that flight or fight reactions are unlikely to help, and the need for sustained mental vigilance. Air traffic controllers, for example, experience all of the above except for lack of experience. These risk factors, as well as temperament, are often overlooked.

6-109   Answer D

Various relaxation exercises and yoga practices have been shown to lower blood pressure both acutely and chronically. If exercise and/or yoga reduces blood pressure, the client taking antihypertensive drugs may be able to lower the dosage and experience fewer side effects. Although rest may be important, physical activity is even more important, and rest, if not of a relaxed nature, may create a more sedentary lifestyle, which is counterproductive. Although some studies have shown a glass of red wine every day to be cardioprotective, the evidence is not unequivocal, and in the case of a client who has a tendency to drink more alcohol than recommended, this practice is not advisable. Likewise, some studies have shown that a pet can reduce blood pressure, but the evidence is less conclusive than the evidence supporting relaxation practices.

6-110   Answer C

Thimerosal is a preservative that contains ethyl mercury 50% by weight. Though the risk of dying from childhood disease is greater than any potential health risks associated with thimerosal, this first answer does not address the parent's concern about thimerosal specifically. The U.S. Food and Drug Administration (FDA) can and does issue directives to drug manufacturers concerning label warnings; however, to date, the FDA has not issued such a directive about thimerosal because it has not been adequately demonstrated that thimerosal contributes to or causes autism or any other neurodevelopmental disorder. Concerned parents should ensure that all currently used vaccine is thimerosal free as there may be 'old' stock still in circulation. In the United States, thimerosal is no longer added as a preservative to routinely recommended childhood vaccines, except inactivated influenza vaccine. Concerned parents can request thimerosal-free vaccines. Always address parents' concerns.

6-111   Answer D

Asian food is not associated with an increased risk of DVT. The time difference is immaterial to risk of DVT; jet lag is not associated with DVT. DVT is neither an infectious disease nor an endemic disease. Asia/U.S. flights take more than 8–10 hours; long periods of immobility and dehydration are risk factors for deep vein thrombosis.

6-112   Answer D

Wearing hearing protection whenever exposed to loud noise, whether work related or not, can prevent further hearing loss. Noise-induced hearing loss is irreversible because it destroys the nerve receptors in the inner ear.

6-113   Answer A

The Environmental Protection Agency/Food and Drug Administration (EPA/FDA) recommends that pregnant women not eat swordfish, tilefish, shark, or king mackerel and no more than 6 oz per week of albacore tuna because of moderate to high levels of methyl mercury found in these fish. All seafood contains some amount of this environmental contaminant. Light white tuna, salmon, haddock, halibut, shrimp, and pollock have much lower amounts of methyl mercury. These fish are excellent sources of protein and contribute to healthy fetal neurodevelopment. Women should be encouraged to eat these types of fish.

6-114 Answer D

Her husband could have brought home work clothes that were contaminated with harmful chemicals, including lead, asbestos, and pesticides. As a result, she would have been exposed to these contaminants. After a long latency period, these hazardous substances are known to be a significant contributing factor to lung diseases/cancers. Secondhand smoke can also contribute to lung disease. However, there is no direct mechanism for her being exposed to secondhand smoke unless either her husband and/or someone who resided with her smoked. Tuberculosis is a potential contributing factor to lung disease, and coughing is a symptom of TB. However, an occupational history addresses exposures to a broader range of hazards associated with pneumoconiosis than just tuberculosis. Retiree health-care benefits are inconsequential to this question about the origin of the client's cough.

6-115 Answer B

To adequately address the client's questions, specific and accurate information is required. The client should request a material safety data sheet (MSDS) from his employer. Today, many manufacturers have MSDSs for their products online and publicly available. Regardless, employees and health-care professionals have the legal right to request an MSDS from (their clients') employers per OSHA Hazard Communication Standard 29CFR1910.1200 (published by Occupational Safety and Health Administration in 1999). Additionally, health-care professionals have the legal right to access trade secret information if necessary. If the employer refuses, contact the local Occupational Safety and Health Administration (OSHA) office. It is premature and may be unnecessary to request/obtain a chemical sample for laboratory analysis. To recommend terminating employment is unwarranted at this time. The local fire department has chemical-related information for emergency planning and response purposes.

6-116 Answer A

You should recommend biological monitoring of the firefighter's exposure to carbon monoxide. This particular situation states the firefighter came directly from fighting the fire (fire suppression). Byproducts of combustion include carbon dioxide (CO_2) and carbon monoxide (CO). Carbon dioxide is a simple asphyxiate (displaces oxygen in a room); carbon monoxide is a chemical asphyxiate (structurally binds with hemoglobin). CO poisoning it not readily reversible and can result in myocardial infarction and death. Diagnosis of CO poisoning is determined by analyzing a blood sample. Often during fire overhaul—that is, after the fire is "out" when firefighters continue to look for "hidden fire" inside attics, walls, and so on—they typically do not wear respiratory protection. As a result, they may be exposed to other dangerous gases, including hydrogen cyanide (HCN). If the firefighter came from the scene after the fire was out, HCN poisoning should be considered. Methane is an explosive gas and could have been the cause of the fire.

6-117 Answer C

The Equal Employment Opportunity Commission (EEOC) has jurisdiction over the enforcement of the Americans with Disabilities Act (ADA). The Occupational Safety and Health Administration (OSHA) has jurisdiction over workplace safety and health. OSHA is under the umbrella of the Department of Labor. State workers' compensation laws are under the jurisdiction of the states' Department of Justice.

6-118 Answer A

Hazardous chemicals present at hazardous waste sites can leach into groundwater and/or soil and subsequently into drinking water and the food chain. Exposure to pesticides, polychlorinated biphenyls (PCBs), and dioxins has been linked to disruption of the endocrine system. Exposure to these chemicals has not been linked to autism specifically, though it has been linked to neurodevelopment generally. These chemicals are not leukemogenic substances; such substances include solvents such as benzene. For infants, toddlers, and young children, secondary ingestion (hand to mouth) of environmental chemicals is the primary route of entry. As a result, toddlers should not be allowed to play in any area where hazardous environmental chemicals may be present. These chemicals would have to become airborne to be inhaled and play a role in the development of asthma. Insects are potential asthmagens, an exposure that can occur in the home and near a hazardous waste site.

6-119 Answer B

Under the states' workers' compensation laws, an employer must pay all medical expenses for a work-related injury/illness. In addition to medical expenses, if an employee is out of work as a result of his/her work-related injury or illness, employers must pay for lost wages if the work absence exceeds a specified waiting period (usually a few days). Under these statutes, an employee forfeits his/her right to sue the employer. Workers' compensation is a "no-fault" insurance; the negligence of employer and/or employee is not at issue with respect to a worker's right to receive benefits under these statutes.

Bibliography

Albohm, MJ: Getting the right fit. *Healthy Aging,* 31–34, January/February 2007.

Armour, S: Exposing family members to toxins. *USA Today,* October 5, 2000. http://www.usatoday.com/money/bighits/toxin3.htm, accessed 12/15/07.

Armour, S: Workplace toxins can kill at home. *USA Today,* October 11, 2000. http://www.usatoday.com/money/bighits/toxin1.htm, accessed 12/15/07.

Centers for Disease Control and Prevention: http://www.cdc.gov/od/science/iso/concerns/thimerisol.htm, Mercury in vaccines, October 23, 2007, accessed 12/15/07.

Conway, AE: Down on the farm: Preventing farm accidents in children. *Pediatric Nursing* 1(33): 45–48, 2007.

Dunphy, LM, et al: *Primary Care: The Art and Science of Advanced Practice Nursing,* ed 2. FA Davis, Philadelphia, 2007.

Feldman, MD, and Christensen, J: *Behavioral Medicine in Primary Care,* ed 2. Appleton & Lange, Stamford, CT, 2002.

Goolsey, MJ: *Nurse Practitioner Secrets.* Hanley & Belfus, Philadelphia, 2002.

Guirguis-Blake, J, and Yawn, BP: The United States Preventive Services Task Force: Putting recommendations into practice. *The Female Patient,* 34–44, May 2006.

Horan, D, and McMullen, M: Assessment and management of the woman with lymphedema after breast cancer. *Journal of the American Academy of Nurse Practitioners* 10:4, 1998.

Jankovic, J, et al: Environmental study of firefighters. *Annals of Occupational Hygiene (Brit.)* 35(6):581–602, 1991.

Jenkins, CD: *Building Better Health: A Handbook of Behavioral Change.* Pan American Health Organization Scientific and Technical Publication No. 590, Washington, DC, 2003.

Job Accommodation Network: http://www.jan.wvu.edu/links/adalinks.htm, ADA Hot Links and Document Center, May 21, 2007, accessed 12/15/07.

Jong, EC, and McMullen, R: The *Travel and Tropical Medicine Manual,* ed 3. WB Saunders, Philadelphia, 2003.

Miles-Richardson, S: Endocrine disruption: Is there cause for concern? *Hazardous Substances & Public Health* 12(2), Summer 2002. http://www.atsdr.cdc.gov/HEC/HSPH/v12n2-2.html#endocrine, accessed 12/15/07.

Nagler, W, and Hausen, HS: Conservative management of lumbar spinal stenosis. *Postgraduate Medicine* 103:4, 1998.

National Institute of Environmental Health Sciences: http://www.niehs.nih.gov/health/topics/agents/endocrine/index.cfm, Endocrine disruptors, July 27, 2007, accessed 12/15/07.

National Institute for Occupational Safety and Health: http://www.cdc.gov/niosh/docs/2007-133/pdfs/2007-133.pdf, *Preventing Fire Fighter Fatalities Due to Heart Attacks and Other Sudden Cardiovascular Events,* June 2007, accessed 12/15/07.

National Travel Health Network and Centre: http://www.nathnac.org/pro/factsheets/documents/TravellersthrombosisrevisedApril2007.pdf, *Travel Related Deep Vein Thrombosis,* April 2007, accessed 12/15/07.

Occupational Safety and Health Administration: http://www.osha.gov/pls/oshaweb/owadisp.show_document?p_table=INTERPRETATIONS&p_id=22830, Employee access to MSDSs required by 1910.1200 vs. 1910.1020, December 7, 1999, accessed 12/15/07.

Occupational Safety and Health Administration: http://www.osha.gov/pls/oshaweb/owadisp.show_document?p_table=INTERPRETATIONS&p_id=22377, Employee safety and the laundering of contaminated clothing, April 1, 1997, accessed 12/15/07.

Occupational Safety and Health Administration: http://www.osha.gov/Publications/osha3074.pdf, *Hearing Conservation*, 2002, accessed 12/15/07.

Rabinowitz, PM: Determining when hearing loss is work related. *Update* 17(3), Fall 2005. http://www.caohc.org/updatearticles/fall05.pdf, accessed 12/15/07.

Stellar, MA: Universal human papillomavirus vaccination. In the hot seat. *The Female Patient* 32:47–48, May 2007.

Thunder, T: Hearing conservation in the U.S.—A road less traveled. *Update* 17(2), Summer 2005. http://www.caohc.org/updatearticles/summer05.pdf, accessed 12/15/07.

U.S. Department of Labor, Office of Workers' Compensation Programs, Division of Federal Employees' Compensation Web site: http://www.dol.gov/esa/regs/compliance/owcp/fecacont.htm, accessed 12/15/07.

U.S. Environmental Protection Agency: http://www.epa.gov/waterscience/fish/, Fish advisories, October 14, 2007, accessed 12/15/07.

U.S. Environmental Protection Agency: http://www.epa.gov/waterscience/fish/files/MethylmercuryBrochure.pdf, *What You Need to Know About Mercury in Fish and Shellfish*, 2004, accessed 12/15/07.

U.S. Equal Employment Opportunity Commission: http://www.eeoc.gov/policy/ada.html, *The Americans with Disabilities Act of 1990 (Pub. L. 101-336), Titles I and V*, accessed 12/15/07.

U.S. Federal Aviation Administration: http://www.faa.gov/pilots/safety/pilotsafetybrochures/media/DVT_07182005.0pdf, *Deep Vein Thrombosis and Travel*, July 18, 2005, accessed 12/15/07.

U.S. Food and Drug Administration: http://www.fda.gov/cber/vaccine/thimerosal.htm, Thimerosal in vaccines, September 6, 2007, accessed 12/15/07.

U.S. Preventive Services Task Force: *The Guide to Clinical Preventive Services 2006: Recommendations of the U.S. Preventive Services Task Force* (AHRQ Publication No. 06-0588). Agency for Healthcare Research and Quality, Silver Spring, MD.

Woolf, SH, et al: *Health Promotion and Disease Prevention in Clinical Practice*, ed 2. Lippincott Williams & Wilkins, Baltimore, 2002.

How well did you do?

85% and above, congratulations! This score shows application of test-taking principles and adequate content knowledge.

75%–85%, keep working! Review test-taking principles and try again.

65%–75%, hang in there! Spend some time reviewing concepts and test-taking principles and then try the test again.

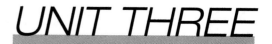

ASSESSMENT AND MANAGEMENT OF CLIENT ILLNESSES

Chapter 7: *Neurological Problems*

JILL E. WINLAND-BROWN
LYNNE M. DUNPHY

Questions

7-1 *Which cranial nerve do you test when you apply a small amount of sugar or salt to the anterior two-thirds of the tongue?*

A. Facial

B. Trigeminal

C. Abducens

D. Glossopharyngeal

7-2 *How is cranial nerve XI tested?*

A. Ask the client to say "ah."

B. Have the client shrug his or her shoulders while you resist the movement.

C. Have the client stick out his or her tongue and move it from side to side.

D. Touch the pharynx with a cotton-tipped applicator.

7-3 *Alternately touching the nose with the index finger of each hand and repeating the motion faster and faster with the eyes closed tests*

A. cranial nerve X.

B. cranial nerve XI.

C. cranial nerve XII.

D. cerebellar function.

7-4 *During a mental status exam, which question might you ask to assess remote memory?*

A. "How long have you been here?"

B. "What time did you get here today?"

C. "What did you eat for breakfast?"

D. "What was your mother's maiden name?"

7-5 *During a mental status exam, which question might you ask to assess abstraction ability?*

A. "What does 'a rolling stone gathers no moss' mean?"

B. "Start with 100 and keep subtracting 7."

C. "What do you think is the best treatment for your problem?"

D. "What would you do if you were in a restaurant and a fire broke out?"

7-6 *Which assessment tool rates the level of consciousness by assigning a numerical score to the behavioral components of eye opening, verbal response, and motor response?*

A. Mini-Mental State Examination

B. Brudzinski sign

C. Glasgow Coma Scale

D. CAGE questionnaire

7-7 *Sam, age 29, has lost his sense of smell. You would document this as*

A. hyposmia.

B. anosmia.

C. ageusia.

D. agnosia.

7-8 *Jim, age 45, has two small children. He states that his wife made him come to this appointment because she thinks he has been impossible to live with lately. He admits to being stressed and depressed because he is working two jobs, and he says he sometimes takes his stress out on his family. About twice a week he complains of palpitations along with nervous energy. What is the most important question to ask him at this time?*

A. "How is your wife handling stress?"

B. "Have you thought about committing suicide?"

C. "Do you and your wife spend time alone together?"

D. "Tell me more about what you think is causing this."

7-9 *Obsessive-compulsive disorder symptoms usually occur*

A. before age 15.

B. during midlife crises.

C. during late adolescence and early adulthood.

D. in later life.

7-10 *What is the medication of choice for obsessive-compulsive disorders?*

A. Alprazolam (Xanax)

B. Carbamazepine (Tegretol)

C. Clomipramine (Anafranil)

D. Buspirone (Buspar)

7-11 *Which of the following tests is highly specific and fairly sensitive for myasthenia gravis?*

A. Electromyography nerve conduction tests

B. Magnetic resonance imaging scan of the brain and brainstem

C. Serum acetylcholine receptor antibody level

D. Lumbar puncture

7-12 *Current pharmacological therapy for chronic relapsing-remitting multiple sclerosis involves*

A. high-dose steroids.

B. baclofen (Lioresal) or diazepam (Valium).

C. interferon B (Betaseron).

D. benzodiazepines.

7-13 *Which of the following interventions can significantly slow the decline in performing activities of daily living (ADLs) in clients with Alzheimer's disease living in a nursing home?*

A. A simple exercise program

B. *Ginkgo biloba*

C. Doing crossword puzzles

D. Improving nutritional state

7-14 *Deficiency of which nutritional source usually presents with an insidious onset of paresthesias of the hands and feet that are usually painful?*

A. Thiamine

B. Vitamin B_{12}

C. Folic acid

D. Vitamin K

7-15 *Jim, a 45-year-old postal worker, presents for the first time with a sudden onset of intense apprehension, fear, dyspnea, palpitations, and a choking sensation. What is your initial diagnosis?*

A. Anxiety

B. Panic attack

C. Depression

D. Agoraphobia

7-16 *The persistent and irrational fear of a specific object, activity, or situation that results in a compelling desire to avoid the dreaded object, activity, or situation is defined as*

A. depression.

B. obsession-compulsion.

C. agoraphobia.

D. phobia.

7-17 *Marie, age 17, was raped when she was 13. She is now experiencing sleeping problems, flashbacks, and depression. What is your initial diagnosis?*

A. Depression

B. Panic disorder

C. Anxiety

D. Post-traumatic stress disorder

7-18 *Mark, age 29, tells you that he has thought about suicide. Which should you say next?*

A. "How long have you felt this way?"

B. "Tell me more about it."

C. "Do you have a plan?"

D. "Have you told anyone else?"

7-19 *In the depressed client, antidepressants are most effective in alleviating*

A. suicidal feelings.

B. interpersonal problems.

C. sleep disturbances.

D. anxiety disorders.

7-20 *What are the two most common causes of dementia in older adults?*

A. Polypharmacy and nutritional disorders

B. Alzheimer's disease and vascular disorders

C. Metabolic disorders and space-occupying lesions

D. Infections affecting the brain and polypharmacy

7-21 *What does a carotid bruit heard on auscultation indicate?*

A. A normal finding in adults recovering from a carotid endarterectomy

B. An evolving embolus

C. A narrowing of the carotid artery because of atherosclerosis of the vessel

D. A complete occlusion of the carotid artery

7-22 *The typical perpetrator in a domestic violence situation is one who*

A. has a history of being a victim of abuse.

B. has a criminal record.

C. is involved in a new relationship.

D. is on a lower socioeconomic scale.

7-23 *Karen Ann, age 52, has four children and a very stressful job. After you perform her physical, which was normal, she tells you she has insomnia. You make several suggestions for lifestyle changes that might assist in promoting helpful sleep. You know she misunderstands when she states which of the following?*

A. "I'll wind down before bedtime by taking a warm bath or by reading for 10 minutes."

B. "I'll try some valerian extract from the health food store."

C. "I'll exercise in the evening to tire myself out before bed."

D. "I won't read or watch television while in bed."

7-24 *June, age 79, comes to your office with a recent onset of depression. She is taking several medications. Which medication is safe for her to take because depression is not one of the side effects?*

A. Antiparkinsonian agents

B. Hormones

C. Cholesterol-lowering agents

D. Antihypertensive agents

7-25 *Which of the following symptoms related to memory indicates depression rather than delirium or dementia in the older adult?*

A. Inability to concentrate, with psychomotor agitation or retardation

B. Impaired memory, especially of recent events

C. Inability to learn new material

D. Difficulty with long-term memory

7-26 *The older adult with delirium would present with which of the following behaviors?*

A. Fatigue, apathy, and occasional agitation

B. Agitation, apathy, and wandering behavior

C. Agitation and restlessness

D. Slowness and absence of purpose

7-27 *Dave, age 76, is brought in by his wife, who states that within the past 2 days Dave has become agitated and restless, has had few lucid moments, slept very poorly last night, and can remember only recent events. Of the following differential diagnoses, which seems the most logical from this brief history?*

A. Depression

B. Dementia

C. Delirium

D. Schizophrenia

7-28 *Which of the following is characteristic of a manic episode?*

A. Weight loss or gain

B. Insomnia or hypersomnia

C. Diminished ability to think or concentrate

D. Grandiose delusions

7-29 *Bob, age 49, is complaining of recurrent, intrusive dreams since returning from his Marine combat training. You suspect*

A. depersonalization.

B. schizophrenia.

C. post-traumatic stress disorder.

D. anxiety.

7-30 *Ed, age 50, has a chronic, episodic headache. He states that it can wake him up at night, lasts 15 minutes to 3 hours, and has occurred daily over a period of 4–8 weeks. You suspect a*

A. tension headache.

B. migraine headache.

C. cluster headache.

D. potential brain tumor.

7-31 *A thymectomy is usually recommended in the early treatment of which disease?*

A. Parkinson's disease

B. Multiple sclerosis

C. Myasthenia gravis

D. Huntington's chorea

7-32 Which peripheral nervous system disorder usually follows a viral respiratory or gastrointestinal infection?

A. Cytomegalovirus

B. Herpes zoster

C. Guillain-Barré syndrome

D. Trigeminal neuralgia

7-33 Lynne, age 72, presents for the first time with her daughter. Her daughter describes some recent disturbing facts about her mother. How can you differentiate between depression and dementia?

A. You might be able to pinpoint the onset of dementia, but the onset of depression is difficult to identify.

B. A depressed person has wide mood swings, whereas a person with dementia demonstrates apathetic behavior.

C. The person with dementia tries to hide problems concerning his or her memory, whereas the person with depression complains about memory.

D. The person with dementia has a poor self-image, whereas the person with depression does not have a change in self-image.

7-34 Clients with senile dementia of the Alzheimer's type often die of

A. pneumonia.

B. suicide.

C. pressure sores.

D. malnutrition.

7-35 Clients with spinal cord injuries often have bowel incontinence and need to have a bowel program instituted. What is the most effective way to stimulate the rectum to evacuate in the quadriplegic client?

A. Administer stool softeners every night.

B. Insert a rectal suppository and then eventually perform digital stimulation.

C. Administer laxatives every other night.

D. Administer enemas on a regular basis.

7-36 Which of the following lab results would indicate a specific infection in the central nervous system?

A. Cerebrospinal fluid (CSF) glucose of 35 mg/dL

B. A CSF pressure of 250 mm of water

C. A CSF red blood cell count of 25/mm^3

D. A serum white blood cell count of 12,000/mm^3

7-37 A rhizotomy may be performed for the client with

A. Bell's palsy.

B. tic douloureux.

C. Parkinson's disease.

D. myasthenia gravis.

7-38 What is the first line of protection against an increase in anxiety?

A. Mental defense mechanisms

B. An increase in the level of serotonin

C. A panic attack

D. Denial

7-39 Barbara, age 36, presents with episodic attacks of severe vertigo, usually with associated ear fullness. Her attacks usually last several hours and she feels well before and after the attacks. To what might you attribute these symptoms?

A. Ménière's disease

B. Vestibular neuronitis

C. Benign paroxysmal positional vertigo

D. Otosclerosis

7-40 Janice, age 14, is markedly obese and has a poor self-image. How do you differentiate between compulsive eating and bulimia?

A. Bulimia results in irregular menstruation.

B. A compulsive eater does not induce vomiting.

C. A compulsive eater has tooth and gum erosion.

D. A compulsive eater does compulsive exercising.

7-41 Sigrid, age 83, has postherpetic neuralgia from a bout of herpes zoster last year. She has been having daily painful episodes and would like to start some kind of therapy. What do you recommend?

A. A tricyclic antidepressant

B. A beta blocker

C. A systemic steroid

D. An NSAID

7-42 Persistent, excessive, or unreasonable fear of a specific object or situation, such as dogs or *injections, is a description of which major anxiety disorder?*

A. Panic disorder

B. Agoraphobia

C. Phobia

D. Obsessive-compulsive disorder

7-43 *Which of the following risk factors for a stroke can be eliminated?*

A. Hypertension

B. Carotid artery stenosis

C. Smoking

D. Hyperlipidemia

7-44 *What is the first symptom seen in the majority of clients with Parkinson's disease?*

A. Rigidity

B. Bradykinesia

C. Rest tremor

D. Flexed posture

7-45 *What is the main overall goal of therapy for the client with Parkinson's disease?*

A. To halt the progression of the disease

B. To keep the client functioning independently as long as possible

C. To control the symptoms of the disease

D. To ease the depression associated with the disease so that the client will be compliant with other therapies

7-46 *Decreased facial strength indicates a lesion of which cranial nerve?*

A. Cranial nerve III

B. Cranial nerve V

C. Cranial nerve VII

D. Cranial nerve VIII

7-47 *With which of the following movements might a client with a cerebellar problem have difficulty?*

A. Inserting a key into the narrow slot of a lock

B. Driving a car with a standard shift

C. Walking up stairs

D. Eating

7-48 *Sophie is 82 and scores 25 on the Mini-Mental State Examination (MMSE). What is your initial thought?*

A. Normal for age

B. Depression

C. Early Alzheimer's disease

D. Late Alzheimer's disease

7-49 *In which syndrome does the client often undergo multiple invasive procedures with negative findings?*

A. Masochist syndrome

B. Malingering syndrome

C. Munchausen syndrome by proxy

D. Munchausen syndrome

7-50 *Naloxone (Narcan) is the antidote for an overdose of*

A. acetaminophen.

B. benzodiazepines.

C. narcotics.

D. phenothiazines.

7-51 *What is the most sensitive diagnostic test for identifying an alcoholic client?*

A. Aspartate transaminase (SGOT)

B. Mean corpuscular volume

C. Alkaline phosphatase

D. γ-glutamyltransferase (GGT)

7-52 *If you suspect that your client abuses alcohol, the most appropriate action would be to*

A. confront the client.

B. obtain further confirmatory information.

C. consult with family members.

D. suggest Alcoholics Anonymous (AA).

7-53 *When a client is in the precontemplation stage of smoking cessation, which question should the health-care provider ask?*

A. "What would it take for you to consider quitting?"

B. "What would it take for you to quit now?"

C. "What technique do you think will work best for you?"

D. "What do you think will be your biggest challenge to quitting?"

7-54 *How often does the Agency for Health Care Policy and Research recommend that providers ask clients about their tobacco-use status?*

A. At every visit

B. At least every 6 months

C. Once a year

D. At the initial history and physical examination

7-55 *Which drug has been shown to be an effective aid to smoking cessation?*

A. Oxazepam (Serax)

B. Clorazepate dipotassium (Tranxene)

C. Varenicline (Chantix)

D. Alprazolam (Xanax)

7-56 *Urine drug screening tests, often performed in the workplace, are frequently effective in finding a person who smokes marijuana because a urine test will be positive for marijuana for up to how long after a person stops smoking the drug?*

A. 24 hours

B. 1 week

C. 2 weeks

D. 30 days

7-57 *Susan has a slipped lumbar disk. When assessing her Achilles tendon, what would you expect her reflex score to be?*

A. 1+

B. 2+

C. 3+

D. 4+

7-58 *You are performing some neurological assessment tests on Daniel. When you ask Daniel to lie supine and flex his head to his chest, what are you assessing?*

A. Brudzinski sign

B. Kernig's sign

C. Decorticate posturing

D. Decerebrate posturing

7-59 *When you move a client's head to the left and the eyes move to the right in relation to the head, this is referred to as*

A. extraocular eye movements.

B. oculomotor degeneration.

C. doll's eyes.

D. decerebrate posturing.

7-60 *Which type of intracranial hematoma is the most common and has the clinical manifestations of headache, drowsiness, agitation, slowed thinking, and confusion?*

A. Epidural

B. Subdural

C. Intracerebral

D. Meningeal

7-61 *Which statement is inaccurate regarding a client who is at highest risk for an eating disorder?*

A. The client is female.

B. The client is usually 12–24 years of age.

C. The client has high self-esteem.

D. The client has a perfectionist personality.

7-62 *Julie, age 15, is 5 ft tall and weighs 85 lb. You suspect anorexia and know that the best initial approach is to*

A. discuss proper nutrition.

B. tell Julie what she should weigh for her height and suggest a balanced diet.

C. speak to her parents before going any further.

D. confront Julie with the fact that you suspect an eating disorder.

7-63 *Don, age 62, calls to complain of a severe headache. With which of his following statements are you most concerned?*

A. "It hurts whenever I turn my head a specific way."

B. "It's the worst headache I've ever had."

C. "Nothing I do seems to help this constant ache."

D. "I'm so worried. Can you do a CT scan?"

7-64 *The Hallpike maneuver is performed to elicit*

A. a seizure.

B. vertigo.

C. syncope.

D. a headache.

7-65 *In the stages of Elisabeth Kübler-Ross' anticipatory grieving, which stage follows that of anger?*

A. Denial

B. Bargaining

C. Depression

D. Acceptance

7-66 *Which of the following screening instruments is quick and easy to use and has a high level of diagnostic accuracy to detect alcohol abuse?*

A. The CAGE questionnaire

B. The HEAT instrument

C. The DRINK tool

D. MMSE

7-67 *How do you respond when Mavis, age 32, who is taking ergotamine tartrate (Ergostat), asks you about rebound headaches?*

A. "It's a headache that comes back if you don't take a sufficient dose of the medication."

B. "A daily or 'rebound' headache may occur if you take medication for a headache more than three times per week."

C. "A 'rebound' headache is another symptom indicating central nervous system involvement."

D. "Rebound headaches don't occur with ergotamine."

7-68 *Which of the following cardiac drugs is used to treat migraine headaches?*

A. Beta blockers

B. Nitrates

C. Angiotensin-converting enzyme inhibitors

D. Alpha-adrenergic blockers

7-69 *In teaching a client with multiple sclerosis, the provider should emphasize all of the following points except*

A. taking a daily hot shower to relax.

B. exercising to maintain mobility.

C. getting plenty of rest.

D. seeking psychological and emotional support.

7-70 *Which appropriate test for the initial assessment of Alzheimer's disease provides performance ratings on 10 complex, higher-order activities?*

A. MMSE

B. CAGE questionnaire

C. FAQ

D. Holmes and Rahe Social Readjustment Scale

7-71 *Bell's palsy affects which cranial nerve?*

A. Cranial nerve V

B. Cranial nerve VI

C. Cranial nerve VII

D. Cranial nerve VIII

7-72 *Sally, age 52, presents with a rapidly progressive weakness of her legs that is moving up the trunk. She also has absent reflexes and no sensory change. What do you suspect?*

A. Peripheral neuropathy

B. Guillain-Barré syndrome

C. Myasthenia gravis

D. Radiculopathy

7-73 *What is the most common cause of cerebellar disease?*

A. Hypothyroidism

B. Use of drugs such as 5-fluorouracil or phenytoin

C. Cerebellar neoplasm

D. Alcoholism

7-74 *Of the four types of strokes, which one is the most common and has a gradual onset?*

A. Thrombotic

B. Embolic

C. Lacunar

D. Hemorrhagic

7-75 *Which of the following complications is the leading cause of death shortly after a stroke?*

A. Septicemia

B. Pneumonia

C. Pulmonary embolus

D. Ischemic heart disease

7-76 *Generalized absence seizures usually occur in which age group?*

A. Children

B. Adolescents

C. Middle-aged adults

D. Older adults

7-77   When you ask a client to walk a straight line placing heel to toe, you are assessing

A. sensory function.

B. cerebellar function.

C. cranial nerve function.

D. the proprioceptive system.

7-78   When you place a key in the hand of a client whose eyes are closed and ask him to identify the object, what are you assessing?

A. Stereognosis

B. Graphesthesia

C. Two-point discrimination

D. Position sense

7-79   When assessing a client's deep tendon reflexes, you note they are more brisk than normal. You document them as

A. 3+.

B. 2+.

C. 1+.

D. 0.

7-80   Jonas, age 62, experienced a temporary loss of consciousness that was associated with an increased rate of respiration, tachycardia, pallor, perspiration, and coolness of the skin. How would you describe this?

A. Lethargy

B. Delirium

C. Syncope

D. A fugue state

7-81   Jeff, age 12, injured his spinal cord by diving into a shallow lake. He is in a wheelchair but can self-transfer. He can use his shoulder and extend his wrist but has no finger control. At what level of the spinal cord was the damage?

A. C4

B. C5

C. C6

D. C7

7-82   Diane, age 35, presents with weakness and numbness of the left arm, diplopia, and some bowel and bladder changes for the past week. She states that the same thing happened last year and lasted for several weeks. What diagnosis is a strong possibility?

A. Multiple sclerosis

B. Subdural hematoma

C. Pituitary tumor

D. Myasthenia gravis

7-83   You assess for cogwheel rigidity in Sophia, age 76. What is cogwheel rigidity a manifestation of?

A. Alzheimer's disease

B. Parkinson's disease

C. Brain attack

D. Degenerative joint disease

7-84   Which of the following conditions is most responsible for developmental delays in children?

A. Cerebral palsy

B. Fetal alcohol syndrome

C. Down syndrome

D. Meningomyelocele

7-85   Which of the following drugs used for parkinsonism mimics dopamine?

A. Anticholinergics

B. Levodopa (l-dopa)

C. Bromocriptine

D. Tolcapone

7-86   Mattie, age 52, has a ruptured vertebral disk with the following symptoms: pain in the midgluteal region, as well as the posterior thigh and calf-to-heel area; paresthesias in the posterior calf and lateral heel, foot, and toes; and difficulty walking on her toes. Which intervertebral disks are involved?

A. L4–L5

B. L5–S1

C. C5–C6

D. C7–T1

7-87   Sandra has a ruptured intervertebral disk and is not responding to conservative management. She is requesting surgery for relief of her pain. She is going to have an enlargement of the opening between the disk and the facet joint to remove the bony overgrowth *compressing the nerve. This describes which surgical procedure?*

A. Laminectomy

B. Diskectomy

C. Foraminotomy

D. Chemonucleolysis

7-88   *Grace, age 82, has Alzheimer's disease. Her daughter states that she is agitated, has time disorientation, and wanders during the afternoon and evening hours. How do you describe this behavior?*

A. Alzheimer's dementia

B. Sundowning

C. Deficits of the Alzheimer's type

D. Senile dementia

7-89   *Marian, age 39, has multiple sclerosis (MS). She tells you that she heard that the majority of people with MS have the chronic-relapsing type of disease and that she has nothing to live for. How do you respond?*

A. "The majority of people have this response to MS."

B. "There are many different clinical courses of MS and the chronic-relapsing type is only one of them."

C. "The chronic-relapsing type of MS is in the minority."

D. "There is an even chance that you have this type."

7-90   *Some providers have successfully induced remission in clients with multiple sclerosis by using adrenocorticotropic hormone therapy or other pharmacological therapy along with*

A. chelation therapy.

B. plasmapheresis.

C. bone marrow transplantation.

D. intravenous lipids.

7-91   *Morrison exhibits extrapyramidal side effects of antipsychotic medications. Which of the following symptoms would lead you to look for another diagnosis?*

A. Akathisia

B. Dystonia

C. Parkinsonism

D. Hallucinations

7-92   *Doris has extrapyramidal side effects from taking medications for her Parkinson's disease. Which of the following drugs that Doris is taking will not help her extrapyramidal symptoms?*

A. Benztropine (Cogentin)

B. Trihexyphenidyl (Artane)

C. Methylphenidate (Ritalin)

D. Amantadine (Symmetrel)

7-93   *What is the most sensitive indicator of increased intracranial pressure and the first symptom to change as the pressure rises?*

A. Dilation of the pupil

B. Hyperventilation

C. Altered mental status

D. Development of focal neurological signs such as hemiparesis

7-94   *Mary, age 82, appears without an appointment. She is complaining of a new, moderately diffuse headache; fever; and muscle aches. She denies any precipitating event. On further examination, you note that her erythrocyte sedimentation rate is over 100 mm/min. What do you suspect?*

A. Temporal arteritis

B. Meningitis

C. Subarachnoid hemorrhage

D. Intracerebral hemorrhage

7-95   *George, age 52, has a recurring headache every Monday morning. What do you plan to order?*

A. An EEG

B. A CT scan

C. An MRI

D. An NSAID

7-96   *Which of the following may immediately follow a stroke in the older adult and be the body's attempt to maintain perfusion?*

A. Bradycardia

B. Tachycardia

C. Hypotension

D. Hypertension

7-97   *Gary, age 5, has a diagnosis of encopresis. After the diagnosis, what would be your next action?*

A. Order extensive lab work.

B. Send Gary to a psychologist.

C. Rule out a neurological disorder.

D. Bring Gary's parents in for counseling.

7-98   *James, age 58, has had several transient ischemic attacks. After a diagnostic evaluation, what medication would you start him on?*

A. Ticlopidine (Ticlid)

B. Aspirin

C. Warfarin (Coumadin)

D. Nitroglycerin (Nitro-Dur)

7-99   *Jessie, age 29, sees flashing lights 20 minutes before experiencing severe headaches. How would you describe her headache?*

A. Migraine without aura

B. Classic migraine

C. Tension headache

D. Cluster headache

7-100   *Which headache preparation has gastrointestinal distress as a side effect?*

A. Sumatriptan (Imitrex)

B. Nadolol (Corgard)

C. Naproxen sodium (Anaprox DS)

D. Ergot preparations (Cafergot)

7-101   *Major depression occurs most often in which of the following conditions?*

A. Parkinson's disease

B. Alzheimer's disease

C. Myocardial infarction

D. Stroke

7-102   *Dan, age 82, recently lost his wife to breast cancer. He presents with weight loss, fatigue, and difficulty sleeping. What should your first response be?*

A. "Do you have a history of thyroid problems in your family?"

B. "Do you think a sleeping pill might help you sleep at night?"

C. "Things might look up if you added nutritional supplements to your diet."

D. "Have you thought of suicide?"

7-103   *Which of the following gaits in older adults includes brusqueness of the movements of the leg and stamping of the feet?*

A. Gait of sensory ataxia

B. Parkinsonian gait

C. Antalgic gait

D. Cerebellar gait

7-104   *Ivy, age 73, presents with limb paralysis, nystagmus, vertigo, nausea, slurred speech, and cerebellar ataxia. You suspect an occlusion of which part of the brain?*

A. Occipital and temporal lobes, dorsal surface of thalamus, upper part of cerebellum, midbrain

B. Anterior cerebral surfaces

C. Posterior cerebral surfaces

D. Parts of medulla

7-105   *Which type of encephalitis is the most common?*

A. Microbial

B. Herpes simplex virus

C. Viral

D. Pneumococcal

7-106   *Herbert, age 58, has just been diagnosed with Bell's palsy. He is understandably upset and has questions about the prognosis. Your response should be*

A. "Although most of the symptoms will disappear, some will remain but can usually be camouflaged by altering your hairstyle or growing a beard or mustache."

B. "Unfortunately, there is no cure, but you have a mild case."

C. "The condition is self-limiting, and most likely complete recovery will occur."

D. "With suppressive drug therapy, you can minimize the symptoms."

7-107   *In the Physicians' Health Study, middle-aged men who suffer from migraine headaches are 42% more likely to have which condition when compared with nonsufferers?*

A. Congestive heart failure

B. Peripheral vascular disease

C. Abdominal aortic aneurysm

D. Myocardial infarction

7-108 *Which of the following objective data are associated with significantly better long-term outcomes in children born with open spina bifida?*

A. A higher APGAR score

B. Presence of Babinski's reflex

C. Perineal sensation

D. A higher score on the Glascow Coma Scale

7-109 *Jessica, a retired nurse, is contemplating surgery for severe sciatica and asks you for your opinion. How do you respond?*

A. "If you continue with conservative treatment for a while, your pain will be relieved faster."

B. "If you have surgery early, rather than continue with conservative therapy, your rate of pain relief and recovery will be faster."

C. "The 1-year outcomes related to pain relief and recovery are the same for both early surgery and conservative therapy."

D. "What has your doctor told you?"

7-110 *Which medication should be avoided in clients with Alzheimer's disease who have concurrent vascular dementia or vascular risk factors?*

A. Acetycholinesterase inhibitors like donepezil (Aricept)

B. N-methyl-D-aspartate (NMDA) receptor antagonists

C. Anxiolytics like bupirone (Buspar)

D. Atypical antipsychotics like risperidone (Risperdal)

7-111 *David is exhibiting the following signs and symptoms of cerebral occlusion: limb paralysis, nystagmus, vertigo, nausea, slurred speech, and cerebellar ataxia. Which specific vessels are involved and what area of the brain do those vessels supply?*

A. Internal carotid artery: anterior cerebral surfaces

B. Vertebrobasilar system: posterior cerebral surfaces

C. Vertebral arteries: parts of the medulla

D. Basilar artery branches: occipital and temporal lobes, dorsal surface of thalamus, upper part of cerebellum, and midbrain

7-112 *Which type of meningitis is a more benign, self-limited syndrome caused primarily by viruses?*

A. Aseptic

B. Bacterial

C. Chronic

D. Inflammatory

Answers

7-1 Answer A

The facial nerve (cranial nerve [CN] VII) is tested by applying a small amount of sugar or salt to the anterior two-thirds of the tongue. Sensory function of the trigeminal nerve (CN V) is tested by tactile and pain sensation in all three divisions on the face. The motor function is tested by feeling the two masseter muscles as the client bites down. The abducens nerve (CN VI) is tested by extraocular eye movements. The motor portion of the glossopharyngeal nerve (CN IX) is tested by touching the pharynx with a cotton-tipped applicator, and the sensory portion is tested by taste on the posterior third of the tongue.

7-2 Answer B

Cranial nerve XI is the accessory nerve. It is tested by having the client shrug his or her shoulders while you resist the movement. Having the client say "ah" tests CN X, the vagus nerve. Having the client stick out his or her tongue and move it from side to side tests CN XII, the hypoglossal nerve. Touching the pharynx with a cotton-tipped applicator tests CN IX, the glossopharyngeal nerve.

7-3 Answer D

Alternately touching the nose with the index finger of each hand and repeating the motion faster and faster with the eyes closed tests cerebellar function, which integrates muscle contractions to maintain posture. Cranial nerve (CN) X is assessed by eliciting the gag reflex and observing for uvula movement, CN XI by checking for the strength of the trapezius muscles, and CN XII by assessing tongue movement.

7-4 Answer D

Remote memory is verbalized after hours, days, or years and may be assessed by asking a client his or her mother's maiden name. Asking questions about things that happened today, such as how long the client has been at your office, what time the client arrived, and what he or she ate for breakfast, tests recent memory.

7-5 Answer A

Asking the client the meaning of a familiar proverb assesses abstraction ability. It must be kept in mind that many proverbs are culturally derived, and the client may not have heard them before. Asking the client to subtract numbers tests computational ability. Asking clients what they think is the best treatment for their problem elicits information about their mental representation or beliefs about the illness. Asking clients what they would do if a fire broke out in a restaurant assesses their judgment.

7-6 Answer C

The Glasgow Coma Scale is an assessment tool that rates the level of consciousness by assigning a numerical score to the behavioral components of eye opening, verbal response, and motor response. The Mini-Mental State Examination (MMSE) tests orientation, registration, attention and calculation, recall, and language. The Brudzinski sign tests nuchal rigidity, which indicates meningeal irritation. The CAGE questionnaire is a screening tool for alcoholism.

7-7 Answer B

Anosmia is the inability to smell. Hyposmia is a diminished sense of smell. Ageusia is the loss of the sensation of taste or the ability to discriminate sweet, sour, salty, and bitter tastes. Agnosia is the inability to discriminate sensory stimuli.

7-8 Answer B

Although all the questions are important, suicidal ideation is an emergency situation, and if it is present, the client needs immediate admission, preferably to a psychiatric hospital. The next most appropriate question would be to ask him what he thinks is causing the problem, but certainly assessing suicide risk takes priority.

7-9 Answer A

Obsessive-compulsive disorder symptoms usually occur before age 15. Young people in their early teens with obsessive-compulsive disorder are inflexible, lack spontaneity, are ambivalent, and are in a constant

state of conflict while harboring hostile feelings. The condition is manifested in this age group when parents of these individuals expect their children to live up to their expectations and condemn them if they fail to achieve the imposed standards of conduct.

7-10 Answer C

The medication of choice for obsessive-compulsive disorders is clomipramine (Anafranil), a tricyclic antidepressant. It seems to have a much better effect than alprazolam (Xanax), an antianxiety agent; carbamazepine (Tegretol), an anticonvulsant; or buspirone (Buspar), a nonbenzodiazepine anxiolytic.

7-11 Answer C

Of clients with generalized myasthenia gravis, 80%–90% have antibodies to acetylcholine receptors. Electromyography nerve conduction tests are a way to categorize peripheral neuropathies as being demyelinating or axonal. A magnetic resonance imaging scan of the brain and brainstem is useful in helping to diagnose amyotrophic lateral sclerosis. A lumbar puncture is crucial in diagnosing suspected bacterial meningitis.

7-12 Answer C

Interferon B (Betasseron) was approved in 1993 for the treatment of multiple sclerosis because it decreases the frequency of exacerbations in clients with the relapsing-remitting type of multiple sclerosis. Before 1993, high-dose steroids were used for acute exacerbations, and baclofen (Lioresal) or diazepam (Valium) was used for excessive spasticity and spasms. Benzodiazepines are ordered in a small dosage for anxiety.

7-13 Answer A

A simple exercise program, 1 hour twice a week, has been shown to significantly slow the decline in performing ADLs in persons living in a nursing home. While *Ginkgo biloba* and doing crossword puzzles may possibly affect the decline of brain function, they don't affect ADLs. Improving nutritional status has not been shown to slow the decline in the ability to perform ADLs.

7-14 Answer B

Deficiency of vitamin B$_{12}$ usually presents with an insidious onset of paresthesias of the hands and feet that are usually painful. A thiamine deficiency, commonly seen with chronic severe alcoholism or malabsorption, results in Wernicke-Korsakoff syndrome, which manifests as confusion, involuntary eye movements, and gait instability or ataxia. A folic acid deficiency results in neural tube defects in the fetus. A vitamin K deficiency results in coagulation disorders.

7-15   Answer B

A panic attack is characterized by its episodic nature. It is manifested by the sudden onset of intense apprehension, fear, or terror and the abrupt development of some of the following symptoms: dyspnea, palpitations, chest pain or discomfort, choking or smothering sensations, dizziness, a feeling of being detached, diaphoresis, trembling, and nausea. All of these peak within 10 minutes. Anxiety is manifested for longer periods of time. Although depression may involve some psychomotor agitation—either irritability or anxiety—usually there is decreased energy, lack of motivation, fatigue in the morning, and depressed affect. Agoraphobia is fear of leaving the house because of the association of panic attacks with associated environmental cues.

7-16   Answer D

A phobia is the persistent and irrational fear of a specific object, activity, or situation that results in the compelling desire to avoid the dreaded object, activity, or situation. A depressed person has feelings of hopelessness and helplessness and has no energy to "fight off" the cause of the fear. An obsession is a recurrent and persistent thought or desire, whereas a compulsion is an uncontrollable urge to perform some repetitive and stereotyped action. Agoraphobia is fear of leaving the house or of open spaces.

7-17   Answer D

Clients with post-traumatic stress disorder (PTSD) have experienced some severe catastrophic event (in this case, rape) and reexperience the event by having recurrent, often intrusive images of the trauma and recurrent dreams or nightmares of the event. Clients frequently have combinations of symptoms of PTSD, panic disorder, and major depression, all relating to the initial traumatic stress event.

7-18   Answer C

A client's intent or commitment to the act of suicide by means of a plan suggests a high risk of

actually committing the act. A client is at high risk if he or she has a definite plan, considers using more than one method at a time, and has made preparations for death. Also at high risk is the client who is impulsive, psychotic, or frequently intoxicated.

7-19   Answer C

In the depressed client, antidepressants are most effective in alleviating sleep and appetite disturbances. Psychotherapy is most effective in dealing with suicidal feelings and interpersonal problems.

7-20   Answer B

The two most common causes of dementia in older adults are dementia of the Alzheimer type (Alzheimer's disease) and vascular disorders such as hypertension, atherosclerosis, vasculitis, embolic disease, and cardiac disease. Polypharmacy, nutritional disorders, metabolic disorders, space-occupying lesions, and infections affecting the brain are all additional causes of dementia that can be removed or reversed.

7-21   Answer C

A carotid bruit heard on auscultation indicates a narrowing of the carotid artery as a result of atherosclerosis of the vessel. Bruits and heart murmurs have similar characteristics and are both caused by turbulent blood flow; however, they arise from different causes. In this case, the turbulent flow is heard as a bruit because the vessel is narrowed as a result of atherosclerotic changes. Auscultation alone cannot diagnose an evolving embolus. If a complete occlusion of the carotid artery were present, no sound would be heard.

7-22   Answer A

The typical perpetrator in a domestic violence situation is one who has a history of being a victim of abuse. Domestic violence abusers may or may not have a criminal record, are typically in a long-term relationship, and are from all socioeconomic backgrounds.

7-23   Answer C

Suggestions for making lifestyle changes that might assist a client in promoting helpful sleep include advising the client to wind down before bedtime by taking a warm bath or by reading for 10 minutes, to try some valerian extract (obtainable from a health food store), and not to read or watch television while in bed. Exercising before going to bed is stimulating, but evidence suggests that an afternoon workout improves sleep quantity and quality. In a large study, people fell asleep twice as fast and slept an extra hour once they began going for brisk walks in the afternoon. Bed should be a place for sleep and sex only. In a recent study of valerian extract, it was found to help troubled sleepers drop off faster and stay asleep longer.

7-24   Answer C

The diagnosis of depression in an older adult is especially difficult when a medical illness is present. Antiparkinsonian agents, hormones, and antihypertensive drugs all have depression as a possible side effect. Cholesterol-lowering agents do not cause depression. Other drugs that also have depression as a possible side effect include analgesics, anti-inflammatory drugs, antianxiety agents, anticonvulsants, antihistamines, antimicrobials, antipsychotics, cytotoxic agents, and immunosuppressants.

7-25   Answer A

The prevalence of depression (5%–10%) does not change with age, but depression is often overlooked in the older adult. The diagnosis requires a depressed mood for 2 straight weeks and at least four of the following eight signs (which can be remembered using the mnemonic SIG E CAPS [like prescribing energy caps]): S for sleep disturbance, I for lack of interest, G for feelings of guilt, E for decreased energy, C for decreased concentration, A for decreased appetite, P for psychomotor agitation or retardation, and S for suicidal ideation.

Dementia and delirium often coexist with depression. Delirium is a confusional state characterized by inattention, rapid onset, and a fluctuating course that may persist for months if untreated. The person with delirium has memory impairment, such as the inability to learn new material or to remember past events. With dementia, there is a cognitive deterioration with little or no disturbance of consciousness or perception; attention span and short-term memory are impaired, along with judgment, insight, spatial perception, abstract reasoning, and thought process and content.

7-26   Answer C

The older adult with delirium would present with agitated and restless behavior. The older adult with depression would be fatigued, apathetic, and occasionally agitated, whereas the person with dementia would be agitated and apathetic and exhibit wandering behavior. Slow and purposeless behavior may indicate either depression or dementia.

7-27   Answer C

The key phrase is the time of onset of the symptoms. Dave's wife stated that her husband's complaints occurred within the past few days, which is characteristic of delirium. In a depressive state, the onset may be weeks to months, whereas with dementia, the onset is usually insidious and gradual.

7-28   Answer D

Grandiose delusions refer to exaggerated beliefs of one's importance or identity, one of the criteria for a manic episode. Criteria for a major depressive episode include weight loss or gain, insomnia or hypersomnia, and diminished ability to think or concentrate. Others may include feelings of worthlessness, excessive or inappropriate feelings of guilt, indecisiveness, recurrent thoughts of death, and suicidal ideation.

7-29   Answer C

Although Bob is experiencing anxiety with his unpleasant dreams, they are a component of post-traumatic stress disorder (PTSD). One of the specific diagnostic criteria of PTSD is reexperiencing the traumatic event in recurrent, intrusive, and distressing images, thoughts, or perceptions. Depersonalization can be seen in depression and schizophrenia but not PTSD. With schizophrenia, there may or may not be a history of a major disruption in the person's life, but eventually gross psychotic deterioration is evident.

7-30   Answer C

Middle-aged men get cluster headaches more frequently than women. Ed's presentation (a chronic, episodic headache that can wake up the client at night; lasts 15 minutes to 3 hours; and occurs daily over a period of 4–8 weeks) is a classic instance of a cluster headache. A tension headache may also be chronic and episodic, but it usually lasts from 30 minutes to 7 days. A migraine headache may last from 4–72 hours. Organic disease, such as a brain tumor, would be ruled out once the practitioner looked for signs or symptoms of organic disease, such as abnormal vital signs, altered consciousness, unequal pupils, weakness, and reflex asymmetry.

The headache pain in a person with a brain tumor is constant because of increased intracranial pressure.

7-31 Answer C

A thymectomy is performed in approximately 75% of clients with myasthenia gravis because of dysplasia of the thymus gland. It is usually recommended within 2 years after diagnosis. The thymus gland is usually inactive after puberty, but in about 75% of clients with myasthenia gravis, the gland continues to produce antibodies because of hyperplasia of the gland or tumors. The thymus is a source of autoantigen that triggers an autoimmune response in clients with myasthenia gravis.

7-32 Answer C

Guillain-Barré syndrome (GBS) is an acute demyelinating disorder. It is a peripheral nervous system disorder that usually follows a viral respiratory or gastrointestinal infection. Cytomegalovirus, herpes zoster, and sometimes general anesthesia have been associated with the development of GBS. Trigeminal neuralgia is a chronic disease of the trigeminal cranial nerve.

7-33 Answer C

To help differentiate between depression and dementia, keep in mind that the person with dementia tries to hide problems concerning memory, whereas the person with depression complains about memory and discusses the fact that there is a problem with memory. Also, with depression there is usually a time-specific onset, and affected clients tend to be apathetic and withdrawn and have a poor self-image.

7-34 Answer A

Clients with senile dementia of the Alzheimer's type (SDAT) commonly die of pneumonia (the most common cause of death of clients with Alzheimer's disease). Clients with late-stage Alzheimer's disease have problems related to immobility and usually develop pressure sores. They also have a poor nutritional status and may develop malnutrition. Depressed clients are at more risk for suicide than demented clients.

7-35 Answer B

With the quadriplegic client, the most effective program to stimulate the rectum to evacuate is to insert a rectal suppository and then eventually perform digital stimulation. The rectum will expel a rectal suppository along with the contents of the sigmoid colon. The bowel can be trained by using this stimulus and eventually all that will be needed will be a digital stimulus. Occasionally, digital evacuation may be necessary. Increasing fluids and roughage in the diet are also part of a bowel program, along with occasional stool softeners or laxatives and, rarely, an enema.

7-36 Answer A

A low cerebrospinal fluid (CSF) glucose level may indicate a specific central nervous system infection such as meningitis. The normal CSF glucose level is 45–80 mg/dL, which is about 20 mg/dL less than the serum glucose level. An elevated CSF pressure may be the result of several problems, not specifically a central nervous system (CNS) infection. A few red blood cells in the CSF may be a result of the procedure of the lumbar puncture. Elevated white blood cell levels may be the result of any number of infections, not specifically one in the CNS.

7-37 Answer B

A rhizotomy, the surgical severing of a nerve root, performed on the trigeminal nerve, may be performed for the client with tic douloureux (trigeminal neuralgia) if pharmacological treatment is not successful. There is no evidence that surgical decompression of the facial nerve is helpful in Bell's palsy. Surgical implantation of adrenal medullary or specific fetal tissue into the caudate nucleus has been tried in Parkinson's disease with mixed results. A thymectomy is performed in 75% of the clients with myasthenia gravis.

7-38 Answer A

Mental defense mechanisms are the first line of protection or defense against an increase in anxiety. Serotonin is the central mood regulator neurotransmitter. A panic attack is the highest anxiety level. Immature, ineffective defenses such as denial reduce anxiety but undermine effective coping.

7-39 Answer A

A client with Ménière's disease presents with episodic attacks of severe vertigo, usually with associated ear fullness or hearing loss. The duration of the attacks is usually several hours, and the client is well before and after the attack unless hearing loss progresses and persists. The diagnosis is based on a typical history with recurrences. Treatment involves a low-sodium diet, diuretics, and possibly surgery. Vestibular neuronitis has an acute onset with severe vertigo and sometimes follows a viral respiratory infection. Benign paroxysmal positional vertigo is paroxysmal, brief, and purely positional vertigo. Otosclerosis involves progressive hearing loss, sometimes with intermittent vertigo.

7-40   Answer B

A compulsive eater engages in uncontrolled eating, like the client with bulimia, but does not purge (induce vomiting). Clients with anorexia have an absence of or irregular menstruation. Clients with bulimia have tooth and gum erosion from frequent exposure to gastric enzymes through vomiting. Clients with anorexia and bulimia have compulsive exercising habits; compulsive eaters do not. It is important to distinguish among the types of eating disorders because their treatment differs.

7-41   Answer A

Although systemic steroids have been shown to possibly prevent the development of postherpetic neuralgia if given early in the course of herpes zoster, once postherpetic neuralgia is present, tricyclic antidepressants such as amitriptyline (Elavil) have been shown to be effective in relieving the pain. Beta blockers and NSAIDs offer minimal relief.

7-42   Answer C

A phobia is a persistent, excessive, or unreasonable fear of a specific object or situation such as elevators, airplanes, dogs, injections, and so on. A panic disorder presents as a discrete episode of intense anxiety that begins abruptly and reaches a peak in about 10 minutes. Agoraphobia occurs in crowds, or being in a place from which the individual cannot escape. Obsessive-compulsive disorder is an occurrence of recurrent thoughts, images, or impulses that are intrusive and inappropriate and that cause anxiety—the "obsessions"—along with repetitive behaviors aimed at allaying the anxiety—the "compulsions."

7-43   Answer C

The best way to prevent a stroke is to identify at-risk clients and control as many risk factors as

possible. Some risk factors, such as smoking, may be eliminated and others, such as hypertension, carotid artery stenosis, and hyperlipidemia, can be controlled or treated to reduce the risk of stroke.

7-44   Answer C

Although rigidity, bradykinesia, and flexed posture are associated with Parkinson's disease, rest tremor is usually the first symptom seen. Rest tremor disappears with action but recurs when the limbs maintain a posture.

7-45   Answer B

The main overall goal of therapy for the client with Parkinson's disease is to keep the client functioning independently as long as possible. There is no drug or surgical approach that will prevent the progression of the disease. Treatment is aimed at controlling symptoms. Depression occurs in more than 50% of clients with Parkinson's disease, and it is undetermined whether it is a reaction to the illness or a part of the illness itself.

7-46   Answer C

Decreased facial strength indicates a lesion of cranial nerve (CN) VII. A CN III lesion would cause diplopia, a CN V lesion would cause decreased facial sensation, and a CN VIII lesion would cause dizziness and deafness.

7-47   Answer A

Although the client with a cerebellar problem may have difficulty driving a car with a standard shift, walking up stairs, and eating, inserting a key into the narrow slot of a lock requires the most finely coordinated movement and therefore would be the most difficult.

7-48   Answer A

The total possible score on the MMSE is 30. The median score for persons ages 18–59 is 29. For persons ages 80 and older, the median score is 25. A score of 20–25 indicates early Alzheimer's disease; a score of 10–19 indicates middle-stage Alzheimer's disease. Someone with late-stage Alzheimer's disease may score below 10.

7-49   Answer D

Munchausen syndrome, named after a fictional German baron and storyteller, is a psychiatric condition, occurring more frequently in women, in which the history often includes multiple invasive procedures with negative findings. When the client is someone other than the person requesting the procedure or causing the problem, it is called Munchausen syndrome by proxy. Malingering is a conscious intent to deceive. There is no masochist syndrome.

7-50 Answer C

Naloxone (Narcan) is the antidote for an overdose of narcotics. It is given at a dose of 0.4–2.0 mg IV and may be repeated every 2–3 minutes. For an acetaminophen overdose, a loading dose of acetylcysteine, 140 mg/kg, followed by 70 mg/kg every 4 hours for 72 hours, is given. Flumazenil (Romazicon) is the antidote for an overdose of benzodiazepines. Activated charcoal is the antidote for phenothiazine overdose.

7-51 Answer D

The most sensitive diagnostic test for identifying an alcoholic client is the γ-glutamyltransferase (GGT) test. GGT is an enzyme produced in the liver after consumption of five or more drinks daily. A GGT of more than 40 units indicates alcoholism. The assay is 70% sensitive and has a similar specificity. The aspartate transaminase, mean corpuscular volume, and alkaline phosphatase levels are all increased in clients who are alcoholics, but the level of sensitivity and specificity is not as impressive as the GGT.

7-52 Answer A

If you suspect that your client abuses alcohol, the most appropriate action would be to confront the client. The first confrontation may be met with one of many responses, but it "keeps the door open" for further conversations. The overall goal of all types of confrontation is to help the client understand the need for abstinence. Then the provider should discuss interventions to assist with attaining this goal. When the client denies alcoholism, one intervention is to have family and friends confront the client at the same time with reflections of how the client's alcohol problem has affected them personally.

7-53 Answer A

In a study on behavioral change related to cigarette smoking, the first stage is the precontemplation phase, during which the client should not be confronted with actually quitting but should be asked the safe question, "What would it take for you to consider quitting?" In the next stage, the contemplation stage, it would be appropriate to ask, "What would it take for you to quit now?" In the preparation stage, one might ask, "What technique do you think will work best for you?" In the action phase, the health-care provider might ask, "What do you think will be your biggest challenge to quitting?" In the maintenance stage, when the client has stopped smoking for more than 6 months, it is appropriate to ask, "What have you learned about people, places, events, and emotions that made you want to smoke?"

7-54 Answer A

The Agency for Health Care Policy and Research recommends in its smoking cessation clinical practice guideline that providers ask and record the tobacco-use status of every client at every visit.

7-55 Answer C

Varenicline (Chantix) has been proved to be more effective than bupropion (Zyban) for smoking cessation. They are both nonnicotine medications. Wellbutrin is the same as Zyban; it is also used for depression. Oxazepam (Serax), clorazepate dipotassium (Tranxene), and alprazolam (Xanax) are all benzodiazepines that are helpful with anxiety.

7-56 Answer D

Marijuana tests positive in the urine for up to 30 days after a person stops smoking the drug.

7-57 Answer A

A hypoactive or weaker-than-normal reflex is scored as 1+. It is present with lower motor neuron involvement, as in a slipped lumbar disk or spinal cord injuries. Hyperactive reflexes, scored as 3+ or 4+, are present with lesions of upper motor neurons, such as a cerebrovascular accident. A normal reflex is scored as 2+.

7-58 Answer A

When the client is supine and you ask him to flex his head to his chest, you are assessing for the Brudzinski sign. Pain, resistance, and flexion of the hips and knees constitute a positive Brudzinski sign and indicate meningeal irritation. A positive Kernig's sign, which also tests for meningeal irritation, occurs when there is excessive pain or resistance assessed when the client lies supine, with hips and knees flexed, and then the knee is straightened. Decorticate and decerebrate posturing are two positions that reflect neurological lesions. In decorticate posturing, the client is rigid with flexed arms, clenched fists, and extended legs. This posturing is characteristic of a lesion at or above the brainstem. In decerebrate posturing, there is rigid extension of the arms and legs, downward pointing of the toes, and backward arching of the head. This posturing is characteristic of a lesion of the midbrain, pons, or diencephalon.

7-59 Answer C

When you move a client's head to the left and the eyes move to the right in relation to the head, the client has doll's eyes. This is the normal response to passive head movement and is an indicator of brainstem function. Doll's eyes are absent when the eyes fail to turn together and eventually remain fixed in the midposition as the head is turned to the side.

7-60 Answer B

A subdural hematoma is the most common of the intracranial hematomas, occurring in 10%–15% of all head injuries. Clients present with headache, drowsiness, agitation, slowed thinking, and confusion. Epidural hematomas occur in 2%–3% of all head injuries. The client usually has a momentary loss of consciousness followed by a lucid period lasting from a few hours to 1–2 days. There is then a rapid deterioration in the level of consciousness. An intracerebral hematoma occurs in 2%–3% of all head injuries. The client presents with a headache, consciousness deteriorating to deep coma, and hemiplegia on the contralateral side. The meninges are the three layers around the brain and spinal cord—the dura mater, arachnoid, and pia mater. A tumor of the nerve tissue is a meningioma.

7-61 Answer C

Clients with eating disorders tend to have low self-esteem. Other factors that appear to increase the risk for an eating disorder include female gender, young age, perfectionist personality, family history of eating disorders, attempts to diet, depression, and living in cultures in which thinness is a standard of beauty.

7-62 Answer D

If you suspect anorexia, the best initial approach is to confront Julie with the fact that you suspect an eating disorder. Clients are usually aware that a problem exists but need the extra "push" that confrontation provides. Once they accept the diagnosis, proven treatments include medical monitoring; nutritional counseling; psychotherapy, including behavioral therapy, family counseling, and stress-reduction techniques; medications; and support group participation.

7-63 Answer B

When a client states, "It's the worst headache I've ever had," it is noteworthy. Other findings suggestive of serious underlying causes of headaches include advanced age, onset with exertion, decreased alertness or cognition, radiation of the pain to between the shoulder blades (suggesting spinal arachnoid irritation), nuchal rigidity, any historical or physical abnormality suggesting infection, and worsening under observation.

7-64 Answer B

The Hallpike maneuver is performed to elicit vertigo. It evaluates the effect of head position on the elicitation of vertigo. The client sits with the head to one side with eyes open. The examiner grasps the head and quickly assists the client to a supine position with the head hanging below the level of the table. After 30 seconds, the client is quickly assisted back to the sitting position, the head is rotated to the other side, and the maneuver repeated. Vertigo will be apparent in clients with a peripheral, but not central, cause of vertigo.

7-65 Answer B

Elisabeth Kübler-Ross' stages of anticipatory grieving are shock, denial, anger, bargaining, depression, and acceptance. Each person goes through each stage at his or her own rate, but the stages vary little from person to person.

7-66 Answer A

The CAGE instrument is a widely used questionnaire that has a high degree of accuracy for identifying clients who abuse alcohol. CAGE is an acronym for four questions: the C stands for "Have you ever felt you should cut down on drinking?"; the A for "Have people annoyed you by criticizing your drinking"; the G for "Have you felt bad or guilty about your drinking"; and the E for "Have you had a drink first thing in the morning (an 'eye opener') to steady your nerves or to get rid of a hangover?"

There are no such measurements as the HEAT instrument or the DRINK tool. The MMSE is the Mini-Mental State Examination, which can help determine the degree of confusion and therefore help to isolate possible causes.

7-67   Answer B

Any medication that is taken more than three times a week for migraines has the potential for creating daily or "rebound" headaches. The worst offender seems to be ergotamine tartrate.

7-68   Answer A

Beta blockers and calcium channel blockers may be used in the treatment of migraine headaches. Beta blockers, by blocking beta receptors, prevent arterial dilation. Propranolol (Inderal) is the most frequently prescribed of the beta blockers. Calcium channel blockers inhibit arterial vasospasm and block the release of serotonin platelets. They also affect cerebral blood flow, neurotransmission, and neuroreceptor blockade to assist in preventing migraines. Verapamil (Calan) is probably the best known of the calcium channel blockers used for this purpose.

7-69   Answer A

Hot showers may exacerbate the symptoms of multiple sclerosis. For the same reason, fevers should be controlled. Teaching points would include avoiding hot showers, controlling fevers, encouraging exercise and plenty of rest, and seeking psychological and emotional support.

7-70   Answer C

The FAQ (Functional Activities Questionnaire) is a measure of functional activities. There are 10 complex, higher-order activities that are appropriate for the initial assessment of Alzheimer's disease. The MMSE (Mini-Mental State Examination) is a test of cognition. The CAGE questionnaire is a screening tool for alcoholism. The Holmes and Rahe Social Readjustment Scale measures major life changes for identifying the impact of stress on an individual.

7-71   Answer C

Bell's palsy, a demyelinating viral inflammatory disease, affects cranial nerve VII (the facial nerve) and results in a unilateral loss of facial expression with difficulty in chewing and diminished taste.

7-72   Answer B

The diagnosis of Guillain-Barré syndrome is confirmed by a rapidly progressive weakness, usually in an ascending pattern from the legs up to the trunk and then to the arms and face. There is no significant sensory loss and the reflexes are usually hyporeflexive or absent.

Guillain-Barré syndrome is a form of peripheral neuropathy. Peripheral neuropathy, which usually involves the distal extremities, does not have the ascending pattern just described. Peripheral neuropathy is also caused by diabetes, alcohol abuse, nutritional deficiencies, trauma, and syphilis. Myasthenia gravis is an autoimmune neuromuscular junction disease in which the client produces antibodies that destroy the acetylcholine receptors on muscle. Radiculopathies are usually caused by mechanical compression and cause neck and low back pain.

7-73   Answer D

Alcoholism is the most common cause of cerebellar disease. Hypothyroidism, use of drugs such as 5-fluorouracil and phenytoin, cerebellar neoplasms, hemorrhages, and infarcts also cause cerebellar disease, but alcoholism is the most frequent offender.

7-74   Answer A

Thrombotic strokes comprise 40% of all strokes, followed by embolic strokes (30%), lacunar strokes (20%), and hemorrhagic strokes (10%). Thrombotic and lacunar strokes usually have a gradual onset, whereas embolic and hemorrhagic strokes usually have a sudden onset.

7-75   Answer B

The leading cause of death after a stroke is pneumonia as a complication. The second and third most common causes of death, respectively, are pulmonary embolus and ischemic heart disease. Pulmonary embolus results from immobilization and ischemic heart disease is present because atherosclerosis affects the coronary arteries, as well as the cerebral vasculature. Septicemia does not usually occur after a stroke.

7-76   Answer A

Generalized absence seizures (petit mal seizures) almost always occur in children. With generalized absence seizures, there is usually no aura or postictal state. The seizure usually lasts just a few seconds and consists of staring, accompanied by an altered mental state.

7-77   Answer D

When you ask a client to walk a straight line placing heel to toe, you are assessing the proprioceptive aspect of the nervous system, which controls posture, balance, and coordination. Assessing dermatomes and the major peripheral nerves tests sensory function. The cerebellum is one of the neural structures involved in proprioception and can be assessed by coordination functions. Cranial nerves are assessed in many ways, but not by walking.

7-78   Answer A

When you place a key in a client's hand while the client's eyes are closed and ask him or her to identify it, you are assessing stereognosis. Stereognosis is the ability to recognize objects by touching and manipulating them. Graphesthesia is the ability to identify letters or numbers written on each palm with a blunt point. Two-point discrimination is the ability to sense whether one or two areas of the skin are being touched at the same time. Position sense (kinesthetic sensation) is the ability to recognize what position parts of the body are in when the eyes are closed; it is tested by actions such as moving a digit.

7-79   Answer A

A grade of 3+ for deep tendon reflexes indicates that the reflexes are brisker than normal, but this is not necessarily indicative of disease. A grade of 4+ is brisk and hyperactive, with clonus of the tendon, and is associated with disease. A grade of 2+ is normal. A grade of 1+ is low normal, indicating a slightly diminished response. A grade of zero indicates that there is no reflex response.

7-80   Answer C

Syncope is a temporary loss of consciousness that is associated with an increased rate of respiration, tachycardia, pallor, perspiration, and coolness of the skin. Lethargy is drowsiness from which the client may be aroused; the client responds appropriately but then may immediately fall asleep again. Delirium is confusion, with disordered perception and a decreased attention span. Delirium may also involve motor and sensory excitement, inappropriate reactions to stimuli, and marked anxiety. A fugue state is a dysfunction of consciousness in which the

individual carries on purposeful activity that he or she does not remember afterward.

7-81   Answer C

A spinal cord injury at the level of C6 allows clients to self-transfer to a wheelchair. Clients can use their shoulders and extend their wrists but have no finger control. An injury at the level of C4 would involve some sensation in the head and neck and some control of the neck and diaphragm, but mobility is restricted. An injury at the level of C5 would allow clients to control their head, neck, and shoulders and flex their elbows, but they would not be able to self-transfer from the wheelchair to the bed. An injury at C7–C8 would allow clients to extend their elbows, flex their wrists, and have some use of their fingers. They would be able to use a manual wheelchair.

7-82   Answer A

The diagnosis of multiple sclerosis (MS) is often difficult given the large variety of symptoms, but it is a strong possibility in this case. Generally, it occurs in clients ages 20–40. For a diagnosis of MS to be made, two or more parts of the CNS must be involved. In addition, there are several patterns that are diagnostic. A pattern of two or more episodes of exacerbations, separated by 1 month or longer and lasting more than 24 hours, with subsequent recovery is one of the patterns exhibited here. The most common symptoms of MS include focal weakness, optic neuritis, focal numbness, cerebellar ataxia, diplopia, nystagmus, and bowel and bladder changes.

7-83   Answer B

Clients with Parkinson's disease may exhibit "cogwheel rigidity," a condition in which there is an increased resistance in muscle tone when the nurse practitioner moves the client's neck, trunk, or limbs. The muscle is stiff and difficult to move. There is a ratchetlike, rhythmic contraction on passive stretching, particularly in the hands.

7-84   Answer B

Fetal alcohol syndrome is most often responsible for developmental delays in children. In descending order, the others are cerebral palsy, Down syndrome, and meningomyelocele.

7-85   Answer C

Bromocriptine and pergolide mimic dopamine. The other mechanisms of antiparkinsonian treatments are as follows: anticholinergics restore acetylcholine-dopamine balance; levodopa restores striatal dopamine; and tolcapone and entacapone reduce systemic degradation of oral dopamine.

7-86   Answer B

A ruptured intervertebral disk at the L5–S1 level affects the first sacral nerve root. The client would have pain in the midgluteal region, as well as the posterior thigh and calf to heel area; paresthesias in the posterior calf and lateral heel, foot, and toes; and difficulty walking on the toes. When the L4–L5 level (fifth lumbar nerve root) is affected, it manifests as pain in the hip, lower back, posterolateral thigh, anterior leg, dorsal surface of the foot, and great toe. In addition, there would be muscle spasms, paresthesia over the lateral leg and web of the great toe, and decreased or absent ankle reflexes. When the C5–C6 level is affected (sixth cervical nerve root), there is pain in the neck, shoulder, anterior upper arm, and radial area of the forearm and thumb; paresthesias of the forearm, thumb, forefinger, and lateral arm; a decreased biceps and supinator reflex; and a triceps reflex that is normal to hyperactive. When the C7–T1 level is affected, there is pain and numbness in the medial two fingers and the ulnar border of the hand and forearm.

7-87   Answer C

A foraminotomy is an enlargement of the opening between the disk and the facet joint to remove bony overgrowth compressing the nerve. A laminectomy is the removal of a part of the vertebral lamina. It relieves pressure on the nerves. A diskectomy is the removal of the nucleus pulposus of an intervertebral disk. Chemonucleolysis is the injection of the enzyme chymopapain into the nucleus pulposus. It hydrolyzes the nucleus pulposus, thus decreasing the size of the protruding herniation.

7-88   Answer B

Sundowning is a common behavioral change in clients with Alzheimer's disease. It is characterized by increased agitation, time disorientation, and wandering behaviors during the afternoon and evening hours. It is frequently worse on overcast days.

7-89   Answer B

It is expected that Marian might be depressed because of her multiple sclerosis (MS). Focusing more on what she has "going for her" rather than the type of MS she has should be the first response. At least partial recovery from acute exacerbations can reasonably be expected, although further relapses can occur. Some disability is likely to result eventually, but usually half of all clients live well without significant disability, even 10 years after the onset of symptoms. There are many different clinical courses of MS. The chronic-relapsing type is only one type; however, it occurs in the highest percentage (40%) of all cases. In the chronic-relapsing clinical type, remissions are fewer and symptoms more disabling and cumulative between exacerbations compared with the exacerbating-remitting form. More symptoms are evident with each exacerbation. The other types of clinical courses, in descending frequency, are exacerbating-remitting (25%), in which attacks are more frequent and begin earlier, remissions are marked by less clearing of manifestations compared with the benign course, and the remissions last longer with stable manifestations between; benign (20%), in which there are minimum deficits from few mild exacerbations to total or nearly total return to the previous functioning; and chronic-progressive (15%) in which the onset is insidious, there are no remissions, and the disabilities become steadily more severe. It is slower in its progression than the chronic-relapsing type.

7-90   Answer B

Plasmapheresis, or plasma exchange, when used with adrenocorticotropic hormone therapy or other pharmacological therapy, has successfully induced remission in some clients with multiple sclerosis. Plasmapheresis is a procedure that removes the plasma component from whole blood, with the goal being to remove inflammatory agents, such as T lymphocytes, through exchanging plasma while suppressing the immune response and inflammation.

7-91   Answer D

Hallucinations are not extrapyramidal symptoms. Extrapyramidal side effects of antipsychotic medications include akathisia (continuous restlessness and fidgeting); dystonia (involuntary muscular movements or spasms of the face, arms, legs, and neck); and parkinsonism (tremors, shuffling gait, drooling, and rigidity, all characteristic of Parkinson's disease).

7-92   Answer C

Methylphenidate (Ritalin) is a central nervous system stimulant commonly used for children with attention deficit-hyperactivity disorder (ADHD). In adults, one of the investigational uses of Ritalin is for depression in the elderly. Drugs used to counteract extrapyramidal side effects include anticholinergic agents, such as benztropine (Cogentin) and trihexyphenidyl (Artane), and dopaminergic agonists, such as amantadine (Symmetrel).

7-93   Answer C

Altered mental status is the most sensitive indicator of increased intracranial pressure and is the first symptom to change as the pressure rises. As the pressure continues to rise, brainstem herniation occurs, along with dilation of the pupil, hyperventilation, and focal neurological signs such as hemiparesis.

7-94   Answer A

Temporal arteritis, also called giant cell arteritis, presents as a systemic illness with generalized symptoms such as fever, myalgia, arthralgia, anemia, and elevated liver function tests. The headache is a new, mild to moderate one with diffuse pain, not necessarily confined to the temples or frontal region of the head. The erythrocyte sedimentation rate, which can be used as a screening tool, is usually very elevated (greater than 100 mm/min) with temporal arteritis, and a temporal artery biopsy shows granulomatous arteritis. A client with meningitis would show signs of irritation of the brain and meninges, such as a stiff neck. The client with subarachnoid and intracerebral hemorrhage would have an altered mental status.

7-95   Answer D

An electroencephalogram (EEG) is not useful in the routine evaluation of George's headache. His headache is most likely a tension headache because it is a weekly occurrence. A CT scan or MRI study is recommended only if the headache pattern is atypical, has changed in pattern, or is accompanied by other symptoms. The nurse practitioner should discuss with George strategies to avoid possible triggers, how to abort an attack, how to obtain relief from pain, and how to decrease the frequency and severity of attacks. The initial focus should be on the use of NSAIDs, cool compresses, and stress reduction techniques.

7-96   Answer D

In the majority of cases of stroke in older adults, hypertension is the body's attempt to maintain

perfusion. More than two-thirds of these clients become normotensive without any intervention within several days after the stroke. If they had been treated, they would have become hypotensive. If the systolic blood pressure is greater than 220 mm Hg in a client with an ischemic stroke, treatment should be considered.

7-97   Answer C

When a diagnosis of encopresis is made, a physical examination should rule out a neurological disorder affecting the lumbosacral spinal cord. Encopresis, repeated involuntary defecation into the clothing, is more common in boys, usually over 4 years of age. Almost half of the children with this condition have abnormal or prolonged external anal sphincter contraction while straining to defecate.

7-98   Answer A

Ticlopidine (Ticlid), an antiplatelet agent, has been shown to be effective in preventing recurrent strokes in clients with transient ischemic attacks (TIAs) or mild strokes. It is a little more effective than aspirin in preventing recurrent strokes in clients with TIAs and those with moderate or large strokes. The benefit of aspirin in women has not been clearly proved. Aspirin also has more side effects than ticlopidine. The desired effect is decreased platelet aggregation rather than anticoagulation, which warfarin would accomplish. Nitroglycerin has no effect on platelets.

7-99   Answer B

A classic migraine (20% of all migraines) is preceded by either a visual aura, a sensory aura, unilateral weakness, or a speech disturbance. Tension headaches are not accompanied by nausea, vomiting, photophobia, or phonophobia. Cluster headaches occur more often in middle-aged men; cause severe unilateral orbital, supraorbital, or temporal pain; and occur in clusters on a seasonal basis, with 3- to 18-month periods of no headaches.

7-100   Answer C

Naproxen sodium (Anaprox DS) is an NSAID that can cause gastrointestinal (GI) distress and must be taken with food. Ergot preparations such as Cafergot may cause nausea and vomiting, but not the GI distress caused by an NSAID. Sumatriptan may cause fatigue and drowsiness, and nadolol may cause hypotension and bradycardia, but neither causes GI distress.

7-101 Answer D

Sixty percent of clients suffer major depression during their first year after a stroke. Other depressive symptoms, as well as major depression, may also occur, although usually less often, with thyroid disorders, Parkinson's disease, heart disease, and dementia.

7-102 Answer D

Direct confrontation should be used when suspecting depression and the possibility of suicide. Fatigue, loss of weight, and insomnia, in combination with the client's history of the death of his spouse, should point in the direction of depression with a suicidal potential. The provider should ask about suicidal ideation and plans, as well as about the availability of companionship and support. Older white men have the highest incidence of suicide among the entire adult population.

7-103 Answer A

The gait of sensory ataxia includes brusqueness of movements of the leg and stamping of the feet. A Parkinsonian gait involves the trunk bent forward, arms slightly flexed, with an unsteady gait, particularly with turning. The legs are stiff and bent at the knees and hips. The client shuffles forward with an accelerating gait known as festination. An antalgic gait occurs with osteoarthritis of the hip, which causes functional shortening of the leg and produces a characteristic limp. A cerebellar gait is unsteady, with a wide-based stride and an irregular swinging of the trunk. It is more prominent when rising from a chair or turning suddenly.

7-104 Answer A

A client's signs and symptoms may lead the practitioner to suspect which part of the brain has been occluded. The basilar artery branches supply the occipital and temporal lobes, the dorsal surface of the thalamus, the upper part of the cerebellum, and the midbrain. Occlusion in these branches would result in the client exhibiting limb paralysis, nystagmus, vertigo, nausea, slurred speech, and cerebellar ataxia. The internal carotid artery supplies the anterior cerebral surfaces, and an occlusion here would result in unilateral sensory and motor disturbances, visual disturbances, and aphasia with a left-sided

lesion. An occlusion of the posterior cerebral surfaces would result in an ipsilateral visual field deficit; contralateral hemiplegia; bilateral motor, sensory, and visual complaints; vertigo; diplopia; and dysphagia. Occlusion of parts of the medulla would result in contralateral impairment of pain and temperature sensation, dysphagia, and vertigo.

7-105 Answer C

Viral encephalitis is the most common type of encephalitis. It is characterized by a progressive altered level of consciousness, seizures, motor weakness, and headache. Herpes simplex virus and microbial encephalitis are other major types of encephalitis. Pneumococcal is a type of meningitis, not encephalitis.

7-106 Answer C

The peripheral facial palsy of Bell's palsy is self-limiting, and complete recovery usually occurs in several weeks or months in the majority of cases. To cope with self-esteem, clients may be encouraged to change their hairstyle, and men may also be encouraged to grow a beard or mustache. There is no suppressive drug therapy. A course of acyclovir may be ordered. Taking prednisone for 10 days has been found to shorten the recovery period and help with symptoms. Long-term therapy is not warranted because the condition is self-limiting.

7-107 Answer D

Middle-aged men who suffer from migraine headaches are 42% more likely to have a myocardial infarction when compared with nonsufferers, according to the Physicians' Health Study involving 20,084 men. Although the exact causation is not known, the president of the American Heart Association believes it is because the blood vessels are very reactive and the cerebral blood flow constricts, resulting in migraine headaches. When occurring systemically, there may be a constriction of coronary vessels, thus potentially leading to a myocardial infarction.

7-108 Answer C

In infants with open spina bifida, the presence of perineal sensation is associated with significantly better long-term outcomes. In several studies, children with perineal sensation as determined by the response to a pinprick in at least one dermatome on one side of the saddle area were continent of urine and feces, never had pressure sores, and were able to walk more than 50 m.

7-109   Answer B

The rates of pain relief and of perceived recovery were faster for clients assigned to early surgery for severe sciatica than those receiving conservative treatment in one large study. Clients are more likely to choose surgery if they are not able to cope with leg pain, find the natural course of recovery from sciatica unacceptably slow, and want to minimize the time to recovery from pain. Clients whose pain is controlled by pain medication may decide to postpone surgery. This does not reduce their chances for complete recovery at 12 months.

7-110   Answer D

Atypical antipsychotics such as risperidone should be avoided in clients with Alzheimer's disease who also have vascular risk factors because they may increase the risk of stroke. All the other medications listed may be ordered for clients with AD.

7-111   Answer D

Occlusion of the basilar artery branches, which supply the occipital and temporal lobes, dorsal surface of the thalamus, upper part of the cerebellum, and the midbrain would result in the following signs and symptoms: limb paralysis, nystagmus, vertigo, nausea, slurred speech, and cerebellar ataxia. Occlusion of the internal carotid artery, which supplies the anterior cerebral surfaces, would result in unilateral sensory and motor disturbances. Occlusion of the branches from the vertebrobasilar system, which supply the posterior cerebral surfaces, would result in ipsilateral visual field deficits, contralateral hemiplegia, vertigo, and dysphagia. Occlusion of the vertebral arteries, which supply parts of the medulla, would result in contralateral impairment of pain and temperature sensation, dysphagia, and vertigo.

7-112   Answer A

Aseptic or viral meningitis is a more benign, self-limited syndrome caused primarily by viruses. Bacterial or purulent meningitis has a rapid onset hours or days after exposure. Chronic or subacute meningitis has symptoms that develop over months and clients are less acutely ill. There is no category titled inflammatory meningitis.

Bibliography

Douglas, D: Perineal sensation in open spina bifida predicts outcome. *Archives of Disabled Children* 92:67–70, 2007.

Dunphy, LM, et al: *Primary Care: The Art and Science of Advanced Practice Nursing,* ed 2. FA Davis, Philadelphia, 2007.

Laino, C: Men's migraines up heart attack risk. From the American Heart Association's Scientific Sessions 2006, Chicago, November 12–15. http://www.medscape.com/viewarticle/547915, accessed 6/4/07.

Lie, D: Early surgery for severe sciatica relieves pain faster than conservative treatment. *New England Journal of Medicine* 356:2239–2243, 2245–2256, 2007.

Reuben, DB, et al: *2007–2008 Geriatrics at Your Fingertips,* ed 9. American Geriatrics Society, New York, 2007.

Rolland, Y: Exercise program for nursing home residents with Alzheimer's disease: A 1-year randomized, controlled trial. *Journal of the American Geriatrics Society* 55(2):158–165, 2007.

Sauer, LR: Primary stroke prevention. *American Journal of Nursing* 106(11):40–49, November 2006.

How well did you do?

85% and above, congratulations! This score shows application of test-taking principles and adequate content knowledge.

75%–85%, keep working! Review test-taking principles and try again.

65%–75%, hang in there! Spend some time reviewing concepts and test-taking principles and then try the test again.

Chapter 8: *Integumentary Problems*

Questions

8-1 *When palpating the skin over the clavicle of James, age 84, you notice tenting, which is*

A. indicative of dehydration.

B. common in thin older adults.

C. a sign of edema.

D. indicative of scleroderma.

8-2 *Thin, spoon-shaped nails are usually seen in*

A. trauma.

B. a fungal infection.

C. anemia.

D. psoriasis.

8-3 *Which lesion results in scales or shedding flakes of greasy, keratinized skin tissue?*

A. Eczema

B. Impetigo

C. Psoriasis

D. Herpes

8-4 *A client with a nutritional deficiency of vitamin C may have*

A. dry skin and loss of skin color.

B. thickened skin that is dry or rough.

C. flaky skin, sores in the mouth, and cracks at the corners of the mouth.

D. bleeding gums and delayed wound healing.

8-5 *Sandra, age 69, is complaining of dry skin. What do you advise her to do?*

A. Bathe every day.

B. Use tepid water and a mild cleansing cream.

C. Use a dehumidifier.

D. Decrease the oral intake of fluids.

8-6 *Why is ultraviolet light therapy used to treat psoriasis?*

A. To dry the lesions

B. To kill the bacteria

C. To decrease the growth rate of epidermal cells

D. To kill the fungi

8-7 *You're teaching Mitch, age 18, about his tinea pedis. You know he doesn't understand your directions when he tells you which of the following?*

A. "I should dry between my toes every day."

B. "I should wash my socks with bleach."

C. "I should use an antifungal powder twice a day."

D. "I should wear rubber shoes in the shower to prevent transmission to others."

8-8 *Abe, age 57, has just been given a diagnosis of herpes zoster. He asks you about exposure to others. You tell him that*

A. once he has been on the medication for a full 24 hours, he is no longer contagious.

B. he should stay away from children and pregnant women who have not had chickenpox.

C. he should wait until the rash is completely gone before going out in crowds.

D. he should be isolated from all persons except his wife.

8-9 *Which form of acne is more common in the middle-aged to older adult and causes changes in skin color, enlarged pores, and thickening of the soft tissues of the nose?*

A. Acne vulgaris

B. Acne rosacea

C. Acne conglobata

D. Nodulocystic acne

8-10 *What is an excessive amount of collagen that develops during scar formation called?*

A. A keloid

B. A skin tag

C. An angioma

D. A keratosis

8-11 *The morphology of which lesion begins as an inflammatory papule that develops within several days into a painless, hemorrhagic, and necrotic abscess, eventually with a dense, black, necrotic eschar forming over the initial lesion?*

A. Furuncle-carbuncle

B. Hidradenitis suppurativa

C. Anthrax

D. Cellulitis

8-12 *What is the initial emergency measure to limit burn severity?*

A. Stabilize the client's condition.

B. Identify the type of burn.

C. Prevent heat loss.

D. Eliminate the heat source.

8-13 *In a burn trauma, which blood measurement rises as a secondary result of hemoconcentration when fluid shifts from the intravascular compartment?*

A. Hemoglobin

B. Sodium

C. Hematocrit

D. Blood urea nitrogen (BUN)

8-14 *In burn trauma, silver sulfadiazine (Silvadene), a sulfonamide, is the most commonly used topical agent. What is its mechanism of action?*

A. It is a synthetic antibiotic that appears to interfere with the metabolism of bacterial cells.

B. It is a bacteriostatic agent that inhibits a wide variety of gram-positive and gram-negative organisms by altering the microbial cell wall and membrane.

C. It is a bactericidal agent that acts on the cell membrane and cell wall of susceptible bacteria and binds to cellular DNA.

D. It is a protective covering that prevents light, air, and invading organisms from penetrating its surface.

8-15 *Tanisha, a 24-year-old African American mother of four young children, presents in the clinic today with varicella. She states that three of her children also have it and that her eruption started less than 24 hours ago. Which action may shorten the course of the disease in Tanisha?*

A. Calamine lotion

B. Cool baths

C. Acyclovir (Zovirax)

D. Corticosteroids

8-16 *Your 24-year-old client, whose varicella rash just erupted yesterday, asks you when she can go back to work. What do you tell her?*

A. "Once all the vesicles are crusted over"

B. "When the rash is entirely gone"

C. "Once you have been on medication for at least 48 hours"

D. "Now, as long as you stay away from children and pregnant women"

8-17 *Jack, age 59, has a nevus on his shoulder that has recently changed from brown to bluish black. You advise him to*

A. have an excisional biopsy.

B. monitor the nevus for a change at the end of 1 month.

C. apply benzoyl peroxide solution.

D. apply hydrocortisone 1% cream.

8-18 *John, age 58, is a farmer. He presents with a painful finger ulcer and a palpable olecranal lymph node. Suspecting an orf skin ulcer, you ask him if he works with*

A. sheep and goats.

B. horses.

C. metals.

D. tile.

8-19 *All of the following are treatments for psoriasis except*

A. topical antifungals.

B. systemic medications.

C. phototherapy.

D. topical corticosteroids.

8-20 *What is the most common rosacea trigger?*

A. Alcohol

B. Cold weather

C. Skin care products

D. Sun exposure

8-21 *The ABCDEs of melanoma identification include which of the following?*

A. Asymmetry: one half does not match the other half

B. Border: the borders are regular; they are not ragged, notched, or blurred

C. Color (pigmentation) is uniform

D. Diameter: the diameter is greater than 10 mm

8-22 *What is the connection between the surface of the skin and an underlying structure called?*

A. An ulcer

B. A sinus

C. An erosion

D. An abscess

8-23 *A Wood's light is especially useful in diagnosing which of the following?*

A. Tinea versicolor

B. Herpes zoster

C. A decubitus ulcer

D. A melanoma

8-24 *A darkfield microscopic examination is used to diagnose*

A. scabies.

B. leprosy.

C. syphilis.

D. *Candida* infections.

8-25 *Jane is the 26-year-old Asian mother of Alysia, age 2 months. She is concerned about the large blue spot covering her infant's entire right lower leg. Jane tells you that Alysia was born with the spot. You tell her that*

A. when the infant reaches her adult height, the macule can be surgically removed.

B. she should take the infant immediately to a plastic surgeon because this is a rare cancerous lesion.

C. this is a mongolian spot. It is common in Asians and blacks and no treatment is necessary because it will fade with age.

D. she should always keep the spot covered because sunlight will aggravate it.

8-26 *Which of the following statements about malignant melanomas is true?*

A. They usually occur in older adult males.

B. The client has no family history of melanoma.

C. They are common in blacks.

D. The prognosis is directly related to the thickness of the lesions.

8-27 *Stephen, age 18, presents with a pruritic rash on his upper trunk and shoulders. You observe flat to slightly elevated brown papules and plaques that scale when they are rubbed. You also note areas of hypopigmentation. What is your initial diagnosis?*

A. Lentigo syndrome

B. Tinea versicolor

C. Localized brown macules

D. Ochronosis

8-28 *A client with a platelet abnormality may present with*

A. red to blue macular plaques.

B. multiple frecklelike macular lesions in sun-exposed areas.

C. numerous small, brown, nonscaly macules that become more prominent with sun exposure.

D. red, flat, nonblanchable petechiae.

8-29 *Which disease usually starts on the cheeks and spreads to the arms and trunk?*

A. Erythema infectiosum (fifth disease)

B. Rocky Mountain spotted fever

C. Rubeola

D. Rubella

8-30 *Debbie, age 29, has a high fever and red, warm, sharply marginated plaques on the right side of her face that are indurated and painful. You diagnose erysipelas. What treatment do you begin?*

A. Systemic steroids

B. Topical steroids

C. Systemic antibiotics

D. NSAIDs

8-31 *What is the "gold standard" used to confirm the suspicion of a true food allergy (IgE reaction) in a young child?*

A. Immediate-reacting IgE skin test

B. Food challenge

C. Double-blind, placebo-controlled food challenge

D. Diagnostic food diet diary and home challenge

8-32 *Janice states that her son is allergic to eggs and she heard that he should not receive the flu vaccine. How do you respond?*

A. "Although measles, mumps, rubella, and influenza vaccines contain a minute amount of egg, most egg-allergic individuals can tolerate these vaccines without any problems."

B. "Most of the allergic reactions are caused by the actual vaccinations; therefore, a skin test should be done first."

C. "You're right. We should not give this vaccination to your son."

D. "He should not have a skin test done if he has this allergy because a serious cellulitis may occur at the testing site."

8-33 *Dry, itchy skin in older adults results from*

A. the reduction of sweat and oil glands.

B. loss of subcutaneous tissue.

C. dermal thinning.

D. decreased elasticity.

8-34 *Marie asks what she can do for Sarah, her 90-year-old mother, who has extremely dry skin. You respond,*

A. "After bathing every day, use a generous supply of moisturizers."

B. "Use a special moisturizing soap every day."

C. "Your mother does not need a bath every day."

D. "Increase your mother's intake of fluids."

8-35 *Clubbing is defined as*

A. elongation of the toes.

B. broadening of each thumb.

C. a birth deformity of the feet.

D. a thickening and broadening of the ends of the fingers.

8-36 *Where is the epitrochlear lymph node located?*

A. In front of the ear

B. Halfway between the angle and the tip of the mandible

C. In the posterior triangle along the edge of the trapezius muscle

D. In the inner condyle of the humerus

8-37 *Gouty pain in the great toe is*

A. toe gout.

B. hyperuricemia of the toe.

C. podagra.

D. tophus.

8-38 *Jerry, age 52, has gout. What do you suggest?*

A. Using salicylates for an acute attack

B. Limiting consumption of purine-rich foods

C. Testing his uric acid level every 6 months

D. Decreasing fluid intake

8-39 *An eczematous skin reaction may result from*

A. penicillin.

B. allopurinol (Zyloprim).

C. an oral contraceptive.

D. phenytoin (Dilantin).

8-40 *Mary just came from visiting her husband, Sam, age 82, who recently had an ileostomy resulting in a stoma. She did not think that Sam's stoma looked "right." You tell her that the color of the stoma should be*

A. pale pink.

B. beefy red.

C. dark red or purple.

D. flesh colored.

8-41 *Lance, age 50, is complaining of an itchy rash that occurred about a half hour after putting on his leather jacket. He recalls a slightly similar rash last year when he wore his jacket. The annular lesions are on his neck and both arms. They are erythematous, sharply circumscribed, and both flat and elevated. His voice seems a little raspy, although he states that his breathing is normal. What is your first action?*

A. Order a short course of systemic corticosteroids.

B. Determine the need for 0.5 mL 1:1000 epinephrine subcutaneously.

C. Start daily antihistamines.

D. Tell Lance to get rid of his leather jacket.

8-42 *Margaret, age 32, comes into the clinic. She has painful joints and a distinctive rash in a butterfly distribution on her face. The rash has red* *papules and plaques with a fine scale. What do you suspect?*

A. Lymphocytoma cutis

B. Relapsing polychondritis

C. Systemic lupus erythematosus

D. None of the above

8-43 *Jennifer, age 32, has genital warts (condylomata) and would like to have them treated. All of the following could be applied except*

A. benzoyl peroxide.

B. podophyllin.

C. trichloroacetic acid.

D. liquid nitrogen.

8-44 *Johnny, age 12, just started taking amoxicillin for otitis media. His mother said that he woke up this morning with a rash on his trunk. What is your first action?*

A. Prescribe systemic antihistamines.

B. Prescribe a short course of systemic steroids.

C. Stop the amoxicillin.

D. Continue the drug; this reaction on the first day is normal.

8-45 *Jim, age 59, presents with recurrent, sharply circumscribed red papules and plaques with a powdery white scale on the extensor aspect of his elbows and knees. What do you suspect?*

A. Actinic keratosis

B. Eczema

C. Psoriasis

D. Seborrheic dermatitis

8-46 *What is a safe and effective treatment for psoriasis?*

A. Coal tar preparations

B. Topical steroids

C. Topical antibiotics

D. Systemic antihistamines

8-47 *A biopsy of a small, yellow-orange papulonodule on the eyelid will probably show*

A. fragmented, calcified elastic tissue.

B. mature sebaceous glands.

C. lipid-laden cells.

D. endothelial swelling and an infiltrate rich in plasma cells.

8-48 *Permethrin (Elimite) applied over the body overnight from the neck down is the preferred treatment for*

A. scabies.

B. eczema.

C. herpes simplex.

D. psoriasis.

8-49 *Elizabeth, age 83, presents with a 3-day history of pain and burning in the left forehead. This morning she noticed a rash with erythematous papules in that site. What do you suspect?*

A. Varicella

B. Herpes zoster

C. Syphilis

D. Rubella

8-50 *A 70-year-old client with herpes zoster has a vesicle on the tip of the nose. This may indicate*

A. ophthalmic zoster.

B. herpes simplex.

C. Kaposi's sarcoma.

D. orf and milker's nodules.

8-51 *What is the most effective treatment for urticaria?*

A. An oral antihistamine

B. Dietary management

C. Avoidance of the offending agent

D. A glucocorticosteroid

8-52 *A linear arrangement along a nerve distribution is a description of which type of skin lesion?*

A. Annular

B. Zosteriform

C. Keratotic

D. Linear

8-53 *Pastia lines are present in which disease?*

A. Toxic shock syndrome

B. Rocky Mountain spotted fever

C. Scarlet fever

D. Meningococcemia

8-54 *The viral exanthem of Koplik's spots is present in*

A. rubeola.

B. rubella.

C. fifth disease.

D. varicella.

8-55 *A darkfield examination is used to cutaneously diagnose which disease?*

A. Syphilis

B. Viral blisters

C. Scabies

D. Candidiasis

8-56 *Which of the following secondary skin lesions usually results from chronic scratching or rubbing?*

A. Crusts

B. Scales

C. Lichenification

D. Atrophy

8-57 *Which skin lesion is morphologically classified as pustular?*

A. A wart

B. Impetigo

C. Herpes simplex

D. Acne rosacea

8-58 *The "herald patch" is present in almost all cases of*

A. pityriasis rosea.

B. psoriasis.

C. impetigo.

D. rubella.

8-59 *The five Ps—purple, polygonal, planar, pruritic papules—are present in*

A. ichthyosis.

B. lichen planus.

C. atopic dermatitis.

D. seborrheic dermatitis.

8-60 *Adverse effects from prolonged or high-potency topical corticosteroid use to an open lesion may include*

A. epidermal proliferation.

B. striae.

C. vitiligo.

D. easy bruisability.

8-61 *Your client had a colostomy several weeks ago and is having difficulty finding a permanent appliance that fits. How long do you tell him to wait for the stoma to shrink before buying a permanent appliance?*

A. 2–4 weeks

B. 4–6 weeks

C. 6–8 weeks

D. Just over 2 months

8-62 *Silas, age 82, comes to your office with a fairly new colostomy. Around the stoma he has a papular rash with satellite lesions. What does this indicate?*

A. A fungal infection, usually *Candida albicans*

B. An allergic reaction to the appliance

C. A normal reaction to fecal drainage

D. A fluid volume deficit

8-63 *Which type of hemangioma in a newborn occurs on the nape of the neck and is usually not noticeable when it becomes covered by hair?*

A. Nevus flammeus (port-wine stain)

B. Stork's beak mark

C. Strawberry hemangioma

D. Cavernous hemangioma

8-64 *Which of the following is a predisposing condition for furunculosis?*

A. Diabetes mellitus

B. Hypertension

C. Peripheral vascular disease

D. Chronic fatigue syndrome

8-65 *What is the treatment for thrush?*

A. Nystatin oral suspension for 2 weeks, 2–3 mL in each side of the mouth, held as long as possible

B. Clotrimazole oral troches (10 mg) two times per day for 7 days

C. Fluconazole (100 mg) twice daily for 1 week

D. Antiseptic mouth rinses after each meal

8-66 *Justin, an obese 42-year-old, cut his right leg 3 days ago while climbing a ladder. Today his right lower leg is warm, reddened, and painful without a sharply demarcated border. What do you suspect?*

A. Diabetic neuropathy

B. Cellulitis

C. Peripheral vascular disease

D. A beginning stasis ulcer

8-67 *Psoriasis may occur after months of using*

A. vitamins.

B. hormone replacement therapy.

C. NSAIDs.

D. antihistamine nasal sprays.

8-68 *What is the drug of choice for acute anaphylaxis?*

A. Diphenhydramine (Benadryl) 25–100 mg PO qid for adults

B. Epinephrine 1:1000 subcutaneously (0.3–0.5 mL) for adults

C. Prednisone (2 mg/kg q 24 hours) PO in one initial daily dose, tapered off over 1 to 2 weeks

D. Amlodipine besylate (Norvasc) 5 mg qid for 4 weeks

8-69 *What is the most important thing a woman can do to have youthful, attractive skin?*

A. Keep well hydrated.

B. Use sunscreen with an SPF of at least 45.

C. Avoid smoking.

D. Use mild defatted or glycerin soaps.

8-70 *The majority of malignant melanomas are*

A. superficially spreading.

B. lentigo maligna.

C. acral-lentiginous.

D. nodular.

8-71 *Large, flaccid bullae with honey-colored crusts around the mouth and nose are characteristic of*

A. a burn.

B. Rocky Mountain spotted fever.

C. measles.

D. impetigo.

8-72 *Balanitis is associated with*

A. diabetes.

B. macular degeneration.

C. *Candida* infection of the penis.

D. measles.

8-73 *Steve, age 29, has a carbuncle on his neck. After an incision and drainage (I&D), an antibiotic is ordered. What is the most common organism involved?*

A. *Streptococcus*

B. *Moraxella catarrhalis*

C. *Staphylococcus aureus*

D. *Klebsiella*

8-74 *A Gram stain of which lesion reveals large, square-ended, gram-positive rods that grow easily on blood agar?*

A. Dermatophyte infection

B. Tuberculosis (scrofuloderma)

C. Sarcoidosis

D. Anthrax

8-75 *Sidney, age 72, has just been diagnosed with temporal arteritis. What do you prescribe?*

A. Systemic corticosteroids

B. Topical corticosteroids

C. Antibiotics

D. Antifungal preparations

8-76 *Jamie, age 6, was bitten by a dog. Her mother asks you if the child needs antirabies treatment. You tell her,*

A. "If the dog was a domestic pet that had been vaccinated, the wound should be cleaned and irrigated."

B. "Antirabies treatment must be started immediately."

C. "Rabies can be contracted only through the bites of wild animals."

D. "Wait until you have observed the animal for 2 weeks to determine if it is rabid."

8-77 *Sophie brings in her husband, Nathan, age 72, who is in a wheelchair. On his sacral area he has a deep crater with full-thickness skin loss involving necrosis of subcutaneous tissue that extends down to the underlying fascia. Which pressure ulcer stage is this?*

A. Stage I

B. Stage II

C. Stage III

D. Stage IV

8-78 *The purpose of a transparent dressing such as Tegaderm applied over a pressure ulcer is to*

A. toughen intact skin and preserve skin integrity.

B. prevent skin breakdown and the entrance of moisture and bacteria but allow permeability of oxygen and moisture vapor.

C. allow necrotic material to soften.

D. use the proteolytic enzymes in the dressing to serve as a debriding agent.

8-79 *Treatment for a stage I pressure ulcer may include*

A. an enzymatic preparation.

B. systemic antibiotics.

C. surgical treatment with muscle flaps.

D. a transparent, semipermeable membrane dressing.

8-80 *Which structure of the skin is responsible for storing melanin?*

A. Epidermis

B. Dermis

C. Sebaceous glands

D. Eccrine sweat glands

8-81 *Buddy, age 12, presents with annular lesions with a scaly border and central clearing on his trunk. What do you suspect?*

A. Psoriasis

B. Erythema multiforme

C. Tinea corporis

D. Syphilis

8-82 *Harry uses a high-potency corticosteroid cream for his dermatoses. You tell him the following:*

A. "You must use this for an extended period of time for it to be effective."

B. "It will work better if you occlude the lesion."

C. "It may exacerbate your concurrent condition of tinea corporis."

D. "Be sure to use it daily."

8-83 *Janine, age 29, has numerous transient lesions that come and go and is diagnosed with urticaria. What do you order?*

A. Aspirin

B. NSAIDs

C. Opioids

D. Antihistamines

8-84 *What is the name of the acquired disorder characterized by complete loss of pigment of the involved skin?*

A. Tinea versicolor

B. Vitiligo

C. Tuberous sclerosis

D. Pityriasis alba

8-85 *Which is the drug of choice for tinea capitis?*

A. A topical corticosteroid

B. Oral griseofulvin (Grisactin)

C. A topical antifungal

D. An antibiotic

8-86 *Which of the following therapeutic modalities is not useful for the management of acute atopic dermatitis?*

A. Emollients

B. Compresses

C. Ultraviolet light

D. Tars

8-87 *A mother complains that her newborn infant lying on his or her side may appear red on the dependent side of the body while appearing pale on the upper side.*

When she picks up the baby, this coloring disappears. You explain to her about

A. a temporary hemangioma.

B. hyperbilirubinemia.

C. harlequin sign.

D. mongolian spots.

8-88 *Suzanne has a 7-year-old daughter who has had two recent infestations of lice. She asks you what she can do to prevent this. You respond,*

A. "After two days of no head lice, her bedding is lice free."

B. "Boys are more susceptible, so watch out for her brother also."

C. "After several infestations, she is now immune and is no longer susceptible."

D. "Don't let her share hats, combs, or brushes with anyone."

8-89 *Which treatment would you order for anogenital pruritus?*

A. Suppositories for pain

B. Antifungal cream for itching

C. A high-fiber diet for constipation

D. Zinc oxide ointment

8-90 *Persons with which skin phototype (SPT) sunburn easily after 30 minutes in the sun but never tan?*

A. SPT I

B. SPT II

C. SPT III

D. SPT IV

8-91 *Nevi arise from*

A. plugged follicles.

B. melanocytes.

C. capillary occlusion.

D. epithelium.

8-92 *Which skin lesions are directly related to chronic sun exposure and photodamage?*

A. Skin tags

B. Seborrheic keratoses

C. Actinic keratoses

D. Angiomas

8-93 *Samantha, age 52, has an acrochordon on her neck. She refers to this as a*

A. nevus.

B. skin tag.

C. lipoma.

D. wart.

8-94 *A basal cell carcinoma is*

A. an epithelial tumor that originates from either the basal layer of the epidermis or cells in the surrounding dermal structures.

B. a malignant tumor of the squamous epithelium of the skin or mucous membranes.

C. an overgrowth and thickening of the cornified epithelium.

D. lined with epithelium and contains fluid or a semisolid material.

8-95 *What is a noninvasive method of treating skin cancer (other than melanoma) that uses liquid nitrogen?*

A. Mohs' micrographic surgery

B. Curettage and electrodesiccation

C. Radiation therapy

D. Cryosurgery

8-96 *Zinc oxide, magnesium silicate, ferric chloride, and kaolin are examples of*

A. chemical sunscreens.

B. physical sunscreens.

C. agents used in tanning booths.

D. emollients.

8-97 *Amy, age 36, is planning to go skiing with her fiancé. He has warned her about frostbite and she is wondering what to do if frostbite should occur. You know she's misunderstood the directions when she tells you which of the following?*

A. "I should remove wet footwear if my feet are frostbitten."

B. "I should rub the area with snow."

C. "I should apply firm pressure with a warm hand to the area."

D. "I should place my hands in my axillae if my hands are frostbitten."

8-98 *Susan states that her fiancé has been frostbitten on the nose while skiing and is fearful that it will happen again. What do you tell her?*

A. "Don't worry—as long as he gets medical help in the first few hours after being frostbitten again, he'll recover."

B. "Once frostbitten, he should not go out skiing again."

C. "If it should happen again, massage the nose with a dry hand."

D. "Infarction and necrosis of the affected tissue can happen with repeated frostbite."

8-99 *The total loss of hair on all parts of the body is referred to as*

A. female pattern alopecia.

B. alopecia areata.

C. alopecia totalis.

D. alopecia universalis.

8-100 *All of the following medications may cause alopecia except*

A. warfarin (Coumadin).

B. minoxidil (Rogaine).

C. levonorgestrel (Norplant).

D. acetylsalicylic acid (aspirin).

8-101 *Susie asks you about the "blackheads" on her face. You tell her these are referred to as*

A. open comedones.

B. closed comedones.

C. papules.

D. pustules.

8-102 *Which of the following warts (HPV) looks like a cauliflower and are usually found in the anogenital region?*

A. Plantar warts

B. Filiform and digitate warts

C. Condyloma acuminata

D. Verruca plana

8-103 *Susan, a new mother, states that when she pushes her index finger on one of her baby's skull bones, it presses in and then returns to normal when she removes*

her finger. She is concerned about this. You tell her that it is common and is called

A. craniotabes.

B. molding.

C. caput succedaneum.

D. cephalhematoma.

8-104 *Candidiasis may occur in many parts of the body. James, age 29, has it in the glans of his penis. What is your diagnosis?*

A. Balanitis

B. Thrush

C. Candidal paronychia

D. Subungual *candida*

8-105 *Shelby has a blister filled with clear fluid on her arm. It is the result of contact with a hot iron. How do you document this?*

A. Bulla

B. Wheal

C. Cyst

D. Pustule

8-106 *You are teaching Harvey about the warts on his hands. What is included in your teaching?*

A. Treatment is usually effective and most warts will not recur afterward.

B. Because warts have roots, it is difficult to remove them surgically.

C. Warts are caused by the human papillomavirus.

D. Shaving the wart may prevent its recurrence.

8-107 *Which treatment is considered the gold standard in tissue-conservative skin cancer removal?*

A. Cryosurgery

B. Simple excision

C. Photodynamic treatment

D. Mohs' micrographic surgery

8-108 *Johnnie, age 52, presents with pruritus with no rash present. He has hypertension, diabetes, and ESRD. One of the differential diagnoses would be*

A. uremia from chronic renal disease.

B. contact dermatitis.

C. lichen planus.

D. psoriasis.

8-109 *Which of the following is a secondary skin lesion?*

A. Acne nodule

B. Neoplasm

C. Seborrheic dermatitis

D. Herpes simplex

8-110 *Client teaching is an integral part of successfully treating pediculosis. Which of the following statements would you incorporate in your teaching plan?*

A. "It's OK to resume sharing combs, headsets, etc. after being lice free for 1 month."

B. "Soak your combs and brushes in rubbing alcohol for 8 hours."

C. "Itching may continue after successful treatment for up to a week."

D. "Spraying of pesticides in the immediate environment is essential to prevent recurrence."

8-111 *Susie, age 6 months, has a candida infection in the diaper area. What do you suggest to the mother?*

A. "Use rubber or plastic pants to contain the infection and prevent it from getting to the thighs."

B. "Keep the area as dry as possible."

C. "Use baby powder with cornstarch."

D. "Keep Susie away from other babies until the infection is cleared up."

8-112 *Tinea unguium is also known as*

A. tinea capitis.

B. pityriasis versicolor.

C. tinea manuum.

D. onychomycosis.

Answers

8-1 Answer B

Tenting, which occurs when pinched skin over the clavicle remains pinched for a few moments before resuming its normal position, is common in thin older adults. Skin turgor is decreased with dehydration and increased with edema and scleroderma.

8-2 Answer C

Thin, spoon-shaped nails are usually seen in anemia. Causes of thick nails include trauma, fungal infections, psoriasis, and decreased peripheral vascular blood supply.

8-3 Answer C

Psoriasis results in scales or shedding flakes of greasy, keratinized skin tissue. The color may be white, gray, or silver, and the texture may vary from fine to thick.

The other lesions—eczema, impetigo, and herpes—result in crusts that are dried blood, serum, or pus left on the skin surface when vesicles or pustules burst. They can be red-brown, orange, or yellow.

8-4 Answer D

A vitamin C deficiency results in bleeding gums and delayed wound healing. A protein deficiency results in dry skin and loss of skin color. A vitamin A deficiency results in thickened skin that is dry or rough. A vitamin B_6 deficiency results in flaky skin, sores in the mouth, and cracks at the corners of the mouth.

8-5 Answer B

If a client is complaining of dry skin, the client should use tepid water and a mild cleansing cream or soap, use a humidifier to humidify the air, and increase the oral intake of fluids to assist in replacing some of the fluids lost from the skin. Advise the client that it is not necessary to take a bath every day because soaps and hot water are drying.

8-6 Answer C

Ultraviolet light therapy is used to treat psoriasis to decrease the growth rate of epidermal cells. This assists in decreasing the hyperkeratosis. Treatments are given daily and last only for seconds.

8-7 Answer D

If a client has tinea pedis, tell the client to dry between the toes every day, wash socks with bleach, and use an antifungal powder twice per day. Rubber- or plastic-soled shoes can harbor the fungus and therefore should not be worn. The shower should be washed with bleach to kill the fungi.

8-8 Answer B

If a client has just been given a diagnosis of herpes zoster, advise the client to stay away from children and pregnant women who have not had chickenpox until crusts have formed over the blistered areas. Herpes zoster is contagious to people who have not had chickenpox.

8-9   Answer B

Acne rosacea is a chronic type of facial acne that occurs in middle-aged to older adults. Over time, the skin changes in color to dark red, pores become enlarged, and the soft tissue of the nose may exhibit rhinophyma, an irregular bullous thickening. Acne vulgaris is the form of acne common in adolescents and young to middle-aged adults. Acne conglobata begins in middle adulthood and causes serious skin lesions such as comedones, papules, pustules, nodules, cysts, and scars, primarily on the back, buttocks, and chest. Severe (nodulocystic) acne consists mostly of nodules and cysts and always results in scar formation.

8-10   Answer A

A keloid is an elevated, irregularly shaped, and progressively enlarging scar that arises from excessive amounts of collagen during scar formation. A skin tag is a soft papule on a pedicle. An angioma is a benign vascular tumor. A keratosis is any skin condition in which there is a benign overgrowth and thickening of the cornified epithelium.

8-11   Answer C

Although cellulitis, furuncle-carbuncles, and hidradenitis suppurativa are all distinctive abscesses, only anthrax has the morphology described. It results in a dense, black, necrotic eschar gradually forming over the initial lesion. A furuncle-carbuncle is a pustular lesion surrounding one or several hair follicles, and a hidradenitis suppurativa lesion results in scarring and fibrotic bands. Cellulitis begins as a tender, warm, erythematous area of the skin and then takes on multiple presentations but not with a dense black necrotic eschar as described here.

8-12   Answer D

The first intervention is to eliminate the heat source. Then, stabilize the client's condition, identify the type of burn, prevent heat loss, reduce wound contamination, and prepare for emergency transportation.

8-13   Answer C

In burn trauma, the hematocrit rises as fluid, not blood, shifts from the intravascular compartment.

The hemoglobin level decreases secondary to hemolysis; the sodium level decreases secondary to massive fluid shifts into the interstitium; and the blood urea nitrogen level increases secondary to dehydration.

8-14   Answer C

Silver sulfadiazine (Silvadene), the most commonly used topical agent for burn trauma, is a bactericidal agent that acts on the cell membrane and cell wall of susceptible bacteria and binds to cellular DNA. It is effective against a wide variety of both gram-negative and gram-positive organisms. Mafenide acetate (Sulfamylon) is a synthetic antibiotic that interferes with the metabolism of bacterial cells. Approximately 3%–5% of clients develop a hypersensitivity to mafenide. Silver nitrate is a bacteriostatic agent that alters the microbial cell wall and membrane. It has limited penetrating ability and is ineffective if used more than 72 hours after a burn injury.

8-15   Answer C

In adolescents and young adults, acyclovir (Zovirax), if started within the first 24–48 hours after the rash appears, may shorten the course of varicella (chickenpox). Acyclovir is not, however, recommended for children. In children, treatment of varicella consists of cool baths with Aveeno for pruritus and calamine lotion to dry the lesions.

8-16   Answer A

A client who has a varicella rash can return to work once all the vesicles are crusted. Varicella is contagious from 48 hours before the onset of the vesicular rash, during the rash formation (usually 4–5 days), and during the several days while the vesicles dry up. The characteristic rash appears 2–3 weeks after exposure. Treatment is effective only if started within the first few days, and then only to shorten the course of the disease. Clients should avoid contact with pregnant women and children who have not been exposed to varicella.

8-17   Answer A

The ABCDEs (asymmetry, border irregularity, color changes, diameter, evolving/elevation) of melanomas should be taught to all clients. A change in the color variation may indicate a melanoma, and an excisional biopsy should be done. Monitoring for a month may enable a melanoma to extend extensively, resulting in death. Benzoyl peroxide and hydrocortisone may be used with folliculitis.

8-18   Answer A

An orf skin ulcer results from a parapoxvirus infection, which causes a common skin disease of sheep and goats. It is occasionally transmitted to humans.

8-19   Answer A

Antifungal agents are ineffective against psoriasis. The most common form of treatment is corticosteroids applied topically. Systemic treatments are used in more severe cases, and phototherapy, from either natural or artificial light, may also be helpful.

8-20   Answer D

Clients with rosacea usually have a long history of flushing in response to sun exposure. Alcohol, cold weather, and skin care products may also be triggers, but not nearly as often. Other triggers may include emotional stress, spicy foods, exercise, wind, hot baths, and hot drinks.

8-21   Answer A

One of the warning signs of cancer is a lesion that does not heal or one that changes in appearance. The ABCDEs of melanoma identification should be taught to all clients. The A is for asymmetry: one half does not match the other half. B is for border irregularity: the edges of a melanoma are ragged, notched, or blurred. The C is for color: pigmentation is not uniform; there may be shades of tan, brown, and black, as well as red, white, and blue. The D is for diameter: greater than 6 mm. E is for an evolving lesion, as well as for elevation.

8-22   Answer B

The connection between the surface of the skin and an underlying structure is called a sinus. An ulcer is a depressed lesion in which the epidermis and part of the dermis have been lost. An erosion is a moist, red, shiny, circumscribed lesion that lacks the upper layer of the skin. An abscess is a circumscribed collection of pus that involves the deeper layers of the skin.

8-23   Answer A

A Wood's light is especially useful in diagnosing tinea versicolor or other fungal infections. A Wood's light produces a "black light" through long-wave ultraviolet rays. It accentuates minor losses of

melanin, which makes it useful in diagnosing tinea versicolor and vitiligo, in which there is hypopigmentation.

8-24   Answer C

A darkfield microscopic examination is used to diagnose syphilis. A darkfield examination, with its special condenser, causes an oblique beam of light to refract off objects too small to be seen by conventional microscopes, such as the narrow organism *Treponema pallidum* that causes syphilis. Application of a special tetracycline solution followed by shining a Wood's light on the skin may accentuate the burrow of scabietic mites, thus helping to diagnose scabies. A direct acid-fast stain is used to diagnose leprosy, and a potassium hydroxide (KOH) stain helps diagnose *candida* infections.

8-25   Answer C

Mongolian spots (congenital dermal melanocytosis) are poorly defined, blue to blue-black flat lesions that usually occur on the trunk and buttocks but may occur anywhere. They are present at birth and are asymptomatic. No treatment is necessary because the spots fade with age.

8-26   Answer D

Prognosis is directly related to the thickness of the lesion. Malignant melanomas usually occur in middle-aged adults of both sexes. The client usually has a family history of melanoma. Melanomas occur rarely in blacks; when they do, the lesions usually develop on the palms and soles and under the nails.

8-27   Answer B

If a client presents with a pruritic rash on his upper trunk and shoulders and you observe areas of hypopigmentation and flat to slightly elevated brown papules and plaques that scale when they are rubbed, suspect tinea versicolor. Lentigines are macular tan to black lesions, ranging from 1 mm to 1 cm in size. They do not increase in color with exposure to the sun. One or more lentigines are seen in normal individuals. Multiple ones need to be further assessed. Localized brown macules are freckles. Ochronosis is a condition with poorly circumscribed, blue-black macules.

8-28   Answer D

A client with a platelet abnormality may present with red, flat, nonblanchable petechiae. Red to blue macular plaques describe ecchymoses; multiple frecklelike macular lesions in sun-exposed areas indicate xeroderma pigmentosum; and numerous small, brown, nonscaly macules that become more prominent with sun exposure are freckles.

8-29   Answer A

Erythema infectiosum (fifth disease) usually starts on the cheeks and spreads to the arms and trunk. Rocky Mountain spotted fever, which is associated with a history of tick bites, starts as a maculopapular rash with erythematous borders appearing first on the wrists, ankles, palms, soles, and forearms. Rubeola (measles) starts as a brownish-pink maculopapular rash around the ears, face, and neck and then progresses over the trunk and limbs. Rubella (German measles) starts as a fine, pinkish, macular rash that becomes confluent and pinpoint after 24 hours.

8-30   Answer C

Erysipelas is caused by *Streptococcus hemolyticus* and must be treated with appropriate antibiotics. A 7-day course of therapy is recommended: penicillin VK 250 mg, dicloxacillin 250 mg, or a first-generation cephalosporin 250 mg PO qid. In penicillin-allergic clients, either erythromycin 250 mg qid for 7–14 days or clarithromycin 250 mg bid for 7–14 days is a good choice.

8-31   Answer C

The "gold standard" used to confirm the suspicion of a true food allergy (IgE reaction) in a young child is the double-blind, placebo-controlled food challenge. It is necessary in research studies and in all unclear clinical situations to confirm the suspicion of a true allergy. An immediate-reacting IgE skin test is a good screening test that can virtually rule out the allergy. A positive result indicates likelihood of an allergy. A food challenge is the only method to confirm the suspicion of a food reaction regardless of the mechanism (allergy or otherwise). A diagnostic food diet diary and home challenge are possibly helpful when the reactions are not life threatening.

8-32   Answer A

If a client is allergic to eggs and does not think that he or she should receive the flu vaccine, advise the client that, although measles, mumps, rubella, and influenza vaccines contain a minute amount of egg, most individuals who are allergic to eggs can tolerate these vaccines without any problems; that some of the allergic reactions are caused by the gelatins in the vaccinations and not the actual vaccinations; and that if the client can eat a whole egg with no reaction, he or she should have no problem with the vaccination. If the history of the allergy is questionable, it is safest to perform a skin test using the vaccine in dilute amounts and then administer the vaccine under strict observation, allowing a 2-hour wait to observe for any reaction.

8-33   Answer A

Dry, itchy skin in older adults results from the reduction of sweat and oil glands. Loss of subcutaneous tissue, dermal thinning, and decreased elasticity are normal changes associated with aging, and they may cause wrinkles and sagging of the skin.

8-34   Answer C

Although increasing fluids and a moisturizing cream will help the general problem, Sarah does not need a bath every day because that will exacerbate the dryness of her skin. Plain water should be used rather than special soap.

8-35   Answer D

Clubbing is defined as a thickening and broadening of the ends of the fingers. Clubbing is a bulbous appearance and swelling of the terminal phalanges, increasing the normal 160° angle between the nailbed and the digit to 180°. In adults, it is usually caused by pulmonary disease and the resultant hypoxia.

8-36   Answer D

The epitrochlear lymph node is located in the inner condyle of the humerus. The preauricular lymph node is located in front of the ear; the submaxillary (submandibular) lymph node is halfway between the angle and the tip of the mandible; and the posterior cervical lymph node is in the posterior triangle along the edge of the trapezius muscle.

8-37   Answer C

Podagra is gouty pain in the great toe. Hyperuricemia results in the deposition of uric acid crystals in the joints.

8-38   Answer B

For the client with gout, the consumption of purine-rich foods, such as organ meats, should be limited to prevent uric acid buildup. Alcohol should also be limited and fluids increased to 2 L per day. Salicylates should be avoided because they block renal excretion of uric acid. An annual testing of the serum uric acid level is sufficient.

8-39 Answer A

Penicillin, neomycin, phenothiazines, and local anesthetics may cause an eczematous type of skin reaction. Allopurinol (Zyloprim) and sulfonamides may cause exfoliative dermatitis, oral contraceptives may cause erythema nodosum, and phenytoin (Dilantin) and procainamide (Pronestyl) may cause drug-related systemic lupus erythematosus.

8-40 Answer B

A normal stoma is moist and beefy red. A pale pink color may indicate a low hemoglobin level. A dark-red or purple stoma may indicate early ischemia. A black stoma is the result of necrosis. Stomas are never flesh colored.

8-41 Answer B

Lance has hives. Although all the actions are appropriate, the first step is to determine the need for 0.5 mL 1:1000 epinephrine subcutaneously (SQ). With Lance's neck involvement, it is most important to determine if respiratory distress is imminent, in which case the epinephrine must be administered.

8-42 Answer C

If a client comes into the clinic complaining of painful joints and has a distinctive rash in a butterfly distribution on the face that has red papules and plaques with a fine scale, suspect systemic lupus erythematosus. Acute lupus erythematosus occurs most often in young adult women and has a classic presentation of a rash in a butterfly distribution. The lesions are red papules and plaques with a fine scale. In the acute phase, the client is febrile and ill. The presence of these skin lesions in a client with neurological disease, arthritis, renal disease, or neuropsychiatric disturbances also supports the diagnosis. Lymphocytoma cutis is also most common on the face and neck. It occurs in both sexes and has smooth, red to yellow-brown papules up to 5 cm in diameter. Relapsing polychondritis occurs in adults with a history of arthritis. It appears as a macular erythema, tenderness, and swelling over the cartilaginous portions of the ear.

8-43 Answer A

Genital warts (condylomata) may be treated using podophyllin (contraindicated in pregnant clients), trichloroacetic acid, or liquid nitrogen. Benzoyl peroxide is used for acne.

8-44 Answer C

If you suspect a drug reaction to amoxicillin, stop the amoxicillin. Symptomatic relief may be obtained by systemic antihistamines and steroids. Systemic steroids may be necessary with severely symptomatic clients, although topical steroids may help clients with the pruritus.

8-45 Answer C

If a client presents with recurrent, sharply circumscribed red papules and plaques with a powdery white scale on the extensor aspect of his elbows and knees, suspect psoriasis. This is a classic presentation of psoriasis. Besides the extensor aspect of the elbows and knees, it occurs frequently in the presacral area and scalp, although lesions may occur anywhere. Actinic keratosis is distributed on sun-exposed areas such as the face, head, neck, and dorsum of the hand and appears as poorly circumscribed, pink to red, slightly scaly lesions. Eczema presents as a group of pinpoint pruritic vesicles and papules on a coin-shaped erythematous base that usually worsens in winter. Seborrheic dermatitis has a symmetric appearance of raised, scaly, red, greasy papules and plaques that may be sharply or poorly circumscribed.

8-46 Answer A

A safe and effective treatment for psoriasis is the use of coal tar preparations. The concentration is increased every few days from 0.5% to a maximum of 10%. A contact period of several hours is required and the odor is unpleasant. Topical steroids are used in the treatment of atopic dermatitis; topical antibiotics are indicated for acne rosacea; and systemic antihistamines are indicated for pityriasis rosea. Some of the chemicals in coal tar may cause cancer but only in very high concentrations as in coal tar used for industrial paving. Any client using coal tar regularly should be aware of the signs and symptoms and have a skin cancer checkup annually. Ongoing treatment for psoriasis may include topical creams and ointments, such as vitamin D compounds like calcipotriene, corticosteroids, retinoids such as tazarotene, and anthralin. These may be used in combination with sunlight (phototherapy). For severe psoriasis, systemic therapy may be required; this includes the use of such medications as retinoids, methotrexate, and cyclosporine, usually in addition to continued topical treatments and exposure to ultraviolet light.

8-47 Answer C

A biopsy of a small, yellow-orange papulonodule on the eyelid will probably show lipid-laden cells. This is a description of a noneruptive xanthoma of the eyelid (xanthelasma). Fragmented, calcified elastic tissue is diagnostic of pseudoxanthoma elasticum. A biopsy of sebaceous hyperplasia will show large, mature sebaceous glands. A biopsy revealing endothelial swelling and perivascular round-cell infiltrate that is rich in plasma cells is diagnostic of syphilis.

8-48 Answer A

Permethrin (Elimite) applied over the body overnight from the neck down is the preferred treatment for scabies. Lindane (Kwell) is also often effective. Topical corticosteroids or systemic antihistamines are indicated for eczema. Acyclovir (Zovirax) is the treatment for herpes simplex, and coal tar preparations are used to treat psoriasis.

8-49 Answer B

The rash of herpes zoster is characteristic in that it appears on only one side of the body. Herpes zoster begins in a dermatomal distribution, most commonly in the thoracic, cervical, and lumbosacral areas, although it also occurs on the face. Although herpes zoster is caused by the reactivation of latent varicella virus in the distribution of the affected nerve, varicella (chickenpox) presents with a scattered rash on both sides of the body. A client with syphilis would present with sharply circumscribed, ham-colored papules with a slight scale and lesions over the entire body, especially on the palms and soles. Rubella (German measles) occurs in childhood. It begins on the face and rapidly (in hours) spreads down to the trunk.

8-50 Answer A

Ophthalmic zoster (herpes zoster ophthalmica) involves the ciliary body and may appear clinically as vesicles on the tip of the nose. The client with a herpetic lesion on the nose indicating ophthalmic zoster needs to be referred to an ophthalmologist to preserve the eyesight. Herpes simplex primarily occurs on the perioral, labial, and genital areas of the body. Kaposi's sarcoma in the older adult usually occurs in the lower extremities. Orf and milker's nodules almost always appear on the hands.

8-51 Answer C

The most effective treatment for urticaria (hives) is avoidance of the offending agent. Usually the offending antigen is identifiable and exposure is self-limited. Treatment with oral antihistamines is usually effective for symptomatic relief of itching, swelling, and nasal symptoms. Dietary management may sometimes be helpful if the cause of the problem is a known food, such as shellfish, nuts, fish, eggs, chocolate, or cheese. Glucocorticoids have a minimal role in treating urticaria; a brief trial may be indicated for temporary relief in a difficult case.

8-52 Answer B

A zosteriform lesion is a linear arrangement along a nerve distribution and typifies herpes zoster. An annular lesion is ring shaped. Linear simply implies that the lesion appears in lines. A keratotic lesion has horny thickenings.

8-53 Answer C

Pastia lines are present in scarlet fever. All of the diseases listed are caused by bacteria. In scarlet fever, there is diffuse erythema with a sandpaper texture and gooseflesh appearance, with accentuation of erythema in the flexural creases referred to as Pastia lines. In toxic shock syndrome, there is a diffuse sunburnlike erythroderma. In Rocky Mountain spotted fever, there is an early maculopapular rash and then petechial or, rarely, purpuric lesions present on the extremities. In meningococcemia, there are erythematous, nonconfluent, discrete papules early in the disease.

8-54 Answer A

The viral exanthem of Koplik's spots is present in rubeola (measles). Koplik's spots are observed on the buccal mucosa before the rash appears. In rubella (German measles), there are variable erythematous macules on the soft palate, and in fifth disease (erythema infectiosum), there is no exanthem. In varicella (chickenpox), there may be sparse lesions on the mucosal surfaces, especially the hard palate.

8-55   Answer A

A darkfield examination is used to diagnose syphilis cutaneously. Viral blisters can be diagnosed cutaneously by the Tzanck smear; a scraping can be done to look for scabies; and a potassium hydroxide preparation and culture are used to diagnose candidiasis.

8-56   Answer C

Lichenification is a thickening of the skin that usually results from chronic scratching or rubbing. Crusts represent dried serum, blood, pus, or exudate. Scales are yellow, white, or brownish flakes on the surface of the skin that represent desquamation of stratum corneum. Atrophy represents loss of substance of the skin.

8-57   Answer D

Acne rosacea, acne vulgaris, folliculitis, candidiasis, and miliaria are classified as pustular lesions. Papular lesions include warts, corns, Kaposi's sarcoma, basal cell carcinoma, and scabies. Vesicular lesions include herpes simplex, varicella, and herpes zoster. Erosive lesions include impetigo, lichen planus, and erythema multiforme.

8-58   Answer A

The "herald patch" is present in almost all cases of pityriasis rosea. Pityriasis rosea is a common, acute, viral, self-limited eruption that usually begins with a solitary oval, pink, scaly plaque, approximately 3–5 cm in diameter, on the trunk or proximal extremities. It is referred to as the herald patch because it has an elevated red border and a central clearing.

8-59   Answer B

The five Ps—purple, polygonal, planar, pruritic papules—are present in lichen planus. Lichen planus occurs in clients of all ages but is more common in adults. It has a primary skin lesion with the five Ps that looks like a shiny, violaceous, flat-topped papule that is very pruritic. Ichthyosis vulgaris lesions are fine, small, flaky white scales with minimal underlying erythema that can be found anywhere but are more prominent on the extensor aspects of the extremities. Atopic dermatitis (eczema) presents differently at different ages and in persons of different races, but it usually starts as red, weepy, shiny patches. Seborrheic dermatitis presents as dry scales with underlying erythema.

8-60   Answer D

Adverse effects from prolonged or high-potency topical corticosteroid use may include cutaneous atrophy, telangiectases, and easy bruisability, as well as systemic absorption, which may include growth retardation, electrolyte abnormalities, hyperglycemia, hypertension, and increased susceptibility to infection. Vitiligo is caused by loss of melanin. Striae may occur after use of oral corticosteroids or occlusive topical corticosteroid therapy.

8-61   Answer C

Stomas shrink within 6–8 weeks after surgery. At that time, it is safe to buy a permanent appliance. Before that, the stoma needs to be measured weekly to find a well-fitting appliance.

8-62   Answer A

A papular rash with satellite lesions around a stoma indicates a fungal infection. It may be a consequence of persistent skin moisture or an adverse effect of antibiotic therapy. If Silas were having an allergic reaction to the appliance, he would have an erythematous vesicular rash limited to the site of the faceplate of the appliance. If the appliance fits properly, fecal drainage should not come in contact with the skin. Fluid and electrolyte imbalances may occur, but the signs and symptoms would be systemic in nature.

8-63   Answer B

A stork's beak mark usually occurs on the nape of the neck and blanches on pressure. Although it does not fade, when it is covered by hair it is usually not noticeable. A nevus flammeus (port-wine stain) is deep red to purple, does not blanch on pressure, and does not fade with age. A strawberry hemangioma is the result of dilated capillaries in the entire dermal and subdermal layers of the skin. Although it continues to enlarge after birth, it usually disappears by 10 years of age. A cavernous hemangioma is the result of a communicating network of venules in the subcutaneous tissue and does not fade with age.

8-64   Answer A

Predisposing conditions for furunculosis or carbuncles include diabetes mellitus, human immunodeficiency virus (HIV) disease, and injection drug use. Furunculosis (boils) and carbuncles are very painful inflammatory swellings of a hair follicle that result in an abscess, caused by coagulase-positive *Staphylococcus aureus*.

8-65   Answer A

One treatment for thrush includes nystatin oral suspension for 2 weeks, 2–3 mL in each side of the mouth, held as long as possible. When clotrimazole oral troches (10 mg) are used, they should be used five times per day for 14 days (not two times per day for 7 days). Fluconazole 100 mg may be given as a single dose (not twice per day for 1 week). Antiseptic mouthwashes are not effective for thrush.

8-66   Answer B

Cellulitis is a spreading infection of the epidermis and subcutaneous tissue that usually begins after a break in the skin. The skin is warm, red, and painful. Although Justin may have diabetic neuropathy, peripheral vascular disease, or a stasis ulcer, the information is not complete enough for you to suspect those conditions. The information and assessment data given fully support a diagnosis of cellulitis.

8-67   Answer C

Psoriasis may occur after extended therapy with many medications, including beta blockers, lithium, NSAIDs, gold, antimalarials, and angiotensin-converting enzyme (ACE) inhibitors, and after heavy alcohol intake.

8-68   Answer B

The drug of choice for acute anaphylaxis is epinephrine 1:1000 subcutaneously (0.3–0.5 mL) for adults. Diphenhydramine IV (Benadryl) is a second-line emergency drug; the oral form would work well as an antihistamine. Prednisone is beneficial in severe or refractory urticaria. Calcium channel blockers, such as amlodipine besylate (Norvasc), may be of value in clients with chronic urticaria unresponsive to antihistamines when used for at least 4 weeks.

8-69   Answer C

The most important thing a woman can do to have youthful, attractive skin is not smoke. Smokers develop more wrinkles and have elastosis, decreased tissue perfusion and oxygenation, and an adverse exposure to free radicals on elastic tissue. Other important things to promote the health of the skin are use of a sunscreen with a sun protective factor of at least 15 and keeping the skin well hydrated. Although keeping the skin well hydrated promotes skin health, it does not prevent wrinkles. Using mild defatted glycerin soaps maintains texture and hydration but does not help prevent wrinkles.

8-70   Answer A

The majority (70%) of malignant melanomas are superficially spreading. These have a good prognosis because they tend to spread superficially before invading the tissues. The next most common type (10%) presents as a black nodule; 5% of melanomas present as lentigo maligna, which arise from precursor lesions, and another 5% are acral-lentiginous. These arise on the hands or feet and are the most common type seen in Asians and African Americans.

8-71   Answer D

Large, flaccid bullae with honey-colored crusts around the mouth and nose are characteristic of impetigo. These weeping erosions can appear anywhere but usually appear on the face and nose and around the mouth. Hemorrhagic blisters may be present with a burn. Rocky Mountain spotted fever presents with petechiae beginning at the wrist and ankles and going to the palms and soles, then centrally to the face. Measles begins with red macules on the back of the neck, then spreads over the face and upper trunk. The lesions then become papular and may be confluent over the face.

8-72   Answer C

Balanitis is associated with *candida* infection of the penis. Candidiasis (moniliasis) may affect the mouth (thrush), penis (balanitis), or vagina (vaginitis).

8-73   Answer C

Treatment for a furuncle (boil) or carbuncle (cluster of boils) may involve systemic antibiotics. The most common offending organism is *Staphylococcus aureus*. *Streptococcus*, *Klebsiella*, and *Moraxella catarrhalis*, as well as *Staphylococcus aureus*, are all causative organisms of pneumonia.

8-74   Answer D

Anthrax is diagnosed with a Gram stain of the lesion, which reveals large, square-ended gram-positive rods that grow easily on blood agar. A dermatophyte infection is diagnosed with a potassium hydroxide preparation revealing hyphae and spores. In addition, fungal cultures demonstrate different fungi. Tuberculosis (scrofuloderma) is diagnosed with a histologic examination that reveals caseation necrosis and acid-fast bacilli. Sarcoidosis is diagnosed with a biopsy revealing noncaseating granulomas.

8-75   Answer A

Treatment for temporal arteritis involves systemic corticosteroids and immunosuppressives. The erythrocyte sedimentation rate is frequently elevated and a biopsy reveals granulomas and giant cells. Antibiotics and antifungal preparations are not indicated.

8-76   Answer A

Dogs are responsible for 80%–90% of animal bites to humans. Annually, 10–20 deaths occur from dog bites. Most of these deaths result from the exsanguination associated with head and neck bites in children younger than age 4. The wound should be washed thoroughly with soap and water and then treated like any other wound. Because rabies may be contracted from domestic dogs and cats that have not been vaccinated, the animal should be confined for observation. A rabid animal has an initial anxiety stage, followed by a furious stage. Preventive treatment of suspected rabies is based on immunization through a series of vaccine and immune serum injections. Domestic pets that do not appear rabid are assumed to have been vaccinated against rabies; this needs to be confirmed by the owner. Biting animals with an unknown vaccination record that appear healthy should be kept under observation for 7–10 days. Sick or dead animals should be examined for rabies. Because rabies is almost always fatal, when in doubt, treat. The type of immunization determines the timing of the treatment. If immune globulin is given, half of it is infiltrated around the wound and the remainder is administered intramuscularly. Inactivated human diploid cell rabies vaccine (HDCV) is given as a series of five injections beginning immediately and ending on day 28.

8-77   Answer C

A stage III pressure ulcer is one that has a deep crater with full-thickness skin loss involving necrosis of subcutaneous tissue extending down to the underlying fascia. Stage I is nonblanchable erythema of intact skin. Stage II is partial-thickness skin loss involving the epidermis and/or dermis. It may appear as an abrasion, blister, or shallow ulcer. Stage IV involves full-thickness skin loss with

extensive destruction; tissue necrosis; or damage to muscle, bone, or supporting structures.

8-78   Answer B

A transparent dressing is applied over a pressure ulcer to prevent skin breakdown and the entrance of moisture and bacteria but allow permeability of oxygen and moisture vapor. A liquid preparation such as benzoin is used to toughen intact skin and preserve skin integrity. Wet-to-dry gauze dressings allow necrotic material to soften. They adhere to the gauze, so the wound is debrided. A proteolytic enzyme such as Elase may serve as a debriding agent in inflamed and infected lesions.

8-79   Answer D

Treatment for a stage I pressure ulcer may include a hydrocolloid or transparent semipermeable membrane. An enzymatic preparation is used for a stage IV ulcer, and surgery may possibly be necessary. The use of antibiotics is recommended only for clients with clinical signs of sepsis. Antibiotics are not indicated when signs of infection are localized.

8-80   Answer A

The epidermis stores melanin, which protects tissues from the harmful effects of ultraviolet radiation in sunlight. The epidermis also protects tissues from physical, chemical, and biological damage; prevents water loss; converts cholesterol molecules to vitamin D when exposed to sunlight; and contains phagocytes that prevent bacteria from penetrating the skin. The dermis is the second layer of the skin. Its fibrous connective tissue gives the skin its strength and elasticity. The sebaceous glands are sebum-producing glands that assist in retarding evaporation and water loss from the epidermal cells. The eccrine sweat glands open directly onto the skin's surface and are widely distributed throughout the body in the subcutaneous tissue.

8-81   Answer C

Psoriasis, erythema multiforme, tinea corporis, and syphilis all have lesions with annular configurations. Tinea corporis (ringworm) has ring-shaped lesions with a scaly border and central clearing or scaly patches with a distinct border on exposed skin surfaces or on the trunk. Psoriasis has annular lesions on the elbows, knees, scalp, and nails. Erythema multiforme has annular lesions that are mostly acral in distribution and are often associated with a recent herpes simplex infection. Secondary syphilis lesions are usually on the palmar, plantar, and mucous membrane surfaces.

8-82   Answer C

If a client uses a high-potency corticosteroid cream for a dermatosis, tell the client that it may exacerbate concurrent conditions such as tinea corporis and acne. Topical corticosteroids should not be used indiscriminately on all cutaneous eruptions. They should not be used for an extended period of time, and the lesion should not be occluded. Intermittent therapy with high-potency agents, such as every other day, or 3–4 consecutive days per week, may be more effective and cause fewer adverse effects than continuous regimens. This is also true of lower-potency corticosteroids.

8-83   Answer D

Transient urticaria requires antihistamines on a regular basis. Aspirin, NSAIDs, and opioids are to be avoided.

8-84   Answer B

Vitiligo, which usually appears in childhood, is an acquired disorder characterized by complete loss of pigment of the involved skin. Although tinea versicolor does have areas of hypopigmentation, they are scattered and do not have complete loss of pigment. In tuberous sclerosis, ash-leaf spots, which are hypopigmented macules, about 2–3 cm in size, are present at birth. Pityriasis alba is also an acquired disorder of hypopigmentation characterized by poorly demarcated, slightly scaly, oval hypopigmented macules that vary from 1.5–2 cm in size.

8-85   Answer B

The drug of choice for tinea capitis is oral griseofulvin (Grisactin), taken for 6–8 weeks. It should be administered with fat-containing foods because fat is required for optimal absorption. Although topical antifungal agents are effective, they take an extremely long time to work. Topical corticosteroids and antibiotics are not effective for fungal lesions.

8-86   Answer D

Therapeutic modalities useful for the management of acute atopic dermatitis include emollients, compresses, and ultraviolet light. Although tars are useful for chronic, dry, lichenified lesions, they are not helpful for acute dermatitis. Emollients are best applied and most helpful if used immediately after bathing or showering. Compresses are indicated for acute weeping lesions to help cool and dry the skin, which reduces inflammation. Ultraviolet light is useful for severe, uncontrollable atopic dermatitis.

8-87   Answer C

The harlequin sign is a transient phenomenon in a newborn who has been lying on his or her side. The dependent side is red while the upper side is pale, as if a line has been drawn down the middle of the body. This disappears when the infant's position is changed. Hyperbilirubinemia results in jaundice. Hemangiomas and mongolian spots are birthmarks.

8-88   Answer D

Head lice may be transmitted by sharing hats, combs, or brushes, so these practices should be discouraged. The louse can survive for more than 2 days off the scalp, so it can still survive in the bed linen. Girls are more susceptible than boys, and lice occur more often in whites. Immunity against head lice is never acquired.

8-89   Answer C

Treating constipation, preferably with a high-fiber diet, may help anogenital pruritus. Most cases of anogenital pruritus have no obvious cause and chiefly cause nocturnal itching without pain. Although the condition is benign, it may be persistent and recurrent. Hydrocortisone-pramoxine (Pramosone) 1% or 2.5% cream, lotion, or ointment helps with pruritus. Suppositories are not necessary. Anogenital hygiene needs to be stressed. Potent fluorinated topical corticosteroids and antifungals may lead to atrophy and striae after several days and should be avoided.

8-90   Answer A

Skin phototyping (SPT) is a risk classification system designed to estimate one's risk for sun damage. SPT ranges from I to VI. A person with SPT I sunburns easily but never tans. Persons with black skin are termed SPT VI. Persons in the middle types tan easily with minimal sunburn.

8-91   Answer B

Nevi, commonly called moles, are flat or raised macules or papules that arise from melanocytes during early childhood. A nevus flammeus (port-wine stain) is an angioma, a congenital vascular lesion that involves the capillaries.

8-92   Answer C

Actinic keratoses, also called senile or solar keratoses, are epidermal skin lesions that are directly related to chronic sun exposure and photodamage. Skin tags occur in middle-aged adults of both genders and may be associated with acromegaly or acanthosis nigricans. Seborrheic keratoses are lesions most often seen in older adults and do not appear to be related to damage from sun exposure. Angiomas are common, small, red to purple papules unrelated to sun exposure.

8-93   Answer B

Skin tags (acrochordons) are benign overgrowths of skin, commonly seen after middle age and usually found on the neck, axilla, groin, upper trunk, and eyelid. A nevus is a mole, and a lipoma is a benign subcutaneous tumor that consists of adipose tissue. A wart is a circumscribed elevation due to hypertrophy of the papillae and epidermis.

8-94   Answer A

A basal cell carcinoma is an epithelial tumor that originates from either the basal layer of the epidermis or cells in the surrounding dermal structures. A squamous cell carcinoma is malignant and originates in the squamous epithelium. An overgrowth and thickening of the cornified epithelium is a keratosis. A cyst is a benign closed sac in or under the skin surface that is lined with epithelium and contains fluid or a semisolid material.

8-95   Answer D

Cryosurgery is a noninvasive method of treating skin cancer other than melanoma in which liquid nitrogen is used to freeze and destroy the tumor tissue. Mohs' micrographic surgery involves shaving thin layers of the tumor tissue horizontally, then taking a frozen section to determine tumor margins. Curettage and electrodesiccation are used to treat basal cell cancers less than 2 cm in diameter and primary squamous cell cancers that are less than 1 cm in diameter. Radiation therapy is used for lesions that are inoperable because of their location.

8-96   Answer B

Zinc oxide, magnesium silicate, ferric chloride, and kaolin are examples of physical sunscreens that reflect and scatter ultraviolet light. Chemical sunscreens such as PABA, benzophenones, and salicylates absorb ultraviolet light and act as a radiation filter. Tanning booths should be avoided because ultraviolet (UVA) radiation emitted by tanning booths damages the deep skin layers.

8-97   Answer B

Rubbing or massaging the frostbitten areas, especially with snow, may cause permanent tissue damage. Advise the client to remove wet footwear if the feet are frostbitten; apply firm pressure with a warm hand to the area; and place the hands in the axillae if the hands are frostbitten.

8-98   Answer D

Permanent tissue damage can occur with a second episode of frostbite on the same skin surface. Susan's fiancé should be extremely careful and wear a warm knit mask covering the entire face with only small holes for his orifices if he insists on skiing. With continued exposure, vasoconstriction and increased viscosity of the blood can cause infarction and necrosis of the nose. Massaging a frostbitten nose may cause tissue damage.

8-99   Answer D

Alopecia universalis is the loss of hair on all parts of the body. Female pattern alopecia is progressive thinning and loss of hair over the central part of the scalp. Alopecia areata appears as round or oval bald patches on the scalp and other hairy parts of the body. Alopecia totalis is the loss of all hair on the scalp.

8-100   Answer B

Minoxidil (Rogaine) is a vasodilator and may stimulate vertex hair growth. Anticoagulants (e.g., warfarin), oral contraceptives, and salicylates (aspirin) may cause alopecia. Other drugs that may also cause alopecia include antithyroid drugs, allopurinol, propranolol, amphetamines, and levodopa.

8-101   Answer A

Open comedones are known as blackheads. A person with acne vulgaris may have open comedones, closed comedones (whiteheads), papules, pustules, cysts, and even scars.

8-102   Answer C

Condyloma acuminata is a cauliflower-like wart usually found in anogenital regions and is usually sexually transmitted. Plantar warts appear at maximum points of pressure such as the heads of metatarsal bones or heels; filiform or digitate warts are fingerlike, flesh-colored projections emanating from a narrow or broad base, usually in the facial region; and verruca plana are flat warts that are pink, light brown, or yellow with slightly elevated papules that may undergo spontaneous remission.

8-103   Answer A

Craniotabes is localized softening of the cranial bones that are so soft that they may be indented by the pressure of a finger. When the pressure is removed, the bone returns to its normal position. This condition corrects itself in a matter of months without treatment. Molding is when the vertex of the head is molded to fit the cervix contours during delivery. The head usually returns to its normal shape within a few days. Caput succedaneum is edema of the scalp that is usually absorbed and disappears by the third day of life without treatment. A cephalhematoma is a collection of blood on the skull bone caused by rupture of a periosteum capillary due to the pressure of birth and usually occurs 24 hours after birth and may take weeks to be absorbed.

8-104   Answer A

Candidiasis of the glans of the penis is balanitis. Thrush is oral candidiasis; candidal paronychia involves the tissue surrounding the nail; and subungual *candida* is candidiasis under the nail.

8-105   Answer A

A bulla is a primary skin lesion filled with fluid that is larger than 1 cm in diameter. It is also known as a vesicle. A wheal is also a primary skin lesion larger than 1 cm in diameter that is transient, elevated, and hivelike, with local edema and inflammation. A cyst is filled with fluid and may occur in a variety of sizes. A pustule is a superficial, elevated lesion filled with purulent fluid.

8-106   Answer C

Warts are caused by the human papillomavirus. One in four people is infected with this virus and, despite treatment, most warts recur. Broken or abraded skin can spread the transport of the virus as well as vigorous rubbing, shaving, nail biting, and sexual intercourse. Warts do not have roots, contrary to popular opinion. The underside of a wart is smooth and round.

8-107   Answer D

Mohs' micrographic surgery (MMS) is considered the gold standard in tissue-conservative skin cancer removal. MMS is a specialized type of surgery consisting of the removal of the entire tumor with the smallest possible margin of normal skin. Cryosurgery involves using liquid nitrogen to burn off the lesions. Simple excision uses a scalpel to excise the lesion. Photodynamic therapy may be used with acne.

8-108   Answer A

All of the conditions listed result in pruritus. Only uremia from chronic renal disease, however, results in pruritus with no rash present. The other conditions—contact dermatitis, lichen planus, and psoriasis—all have a rash present.

8-109   Answer C

Primary skin lesions are original lesions arising from previously normal skin. Secondary lesions can originate from primary lesions. Seborrheic dermatitis is a scale and the only secondary lesion listed. The others—acne nodule, tumor (neoplasm), and a vesicle—are primary lesions.

8-110   Answer C

Client education is essential when treating pediculosis. Clients should be informed that itching may continue after successful treatment for up to a week because of the slow resolution of the inflammatory reaction caused by the lice infestation. Clients and parents should be instructed not to share hats, combs, scarves, headsets, towels, and bedding. Combs and brushes can be soaked in rubbing alcohol for 1 hour. Excessive decontamination of the environment is not necessary. Environmental spraying of pesticides is not effective and therefore is not recommended. Bedclothes and clothing should be washed in hot, soapy water.

8-111   Answer B

Clients must be taught to decrease favorable environmental conditions for *candida* such as moisture, warmth, and poor air circulation. To prevent diaper rash, the infant should be kept dry as much as possible and the use of rubber or plastic pants should be discouraged. Baby powder with cornstarch should not be used because it will worsen the infection (*candida* can utilize the cornstarch as food).

8-112   Answer D

Tinea unguium is tinea of the nails, also known as onychomycosis. Tinea capitis is tinea of the scalp; pityriasis versicolor is tinea versicolor; and tinea manuum is tinea of the hands.

Bibliography

Naldi, L. Traditional Therapies in the Management of Moderate to Severe Chronic Plaque Psoriasis: An Assessment of the Benefits and Risks. *British Journal of Dermatology* 2005: 152(4): 597-615l http://www.medscape.com/viewarticle/503441 accessed 6/5/2007.

Nouri, K.; Rivas, P. *A Primer of Mohs Micrographic Surgery: Common Indications. Skinmed* 3(4): 191-196, 2004.

Winland-Brown, JW; Porter, BO; Leik, M: Skin problems. Chap. 6 in Dunphy, L. et al. *Primary Care: The Art and Science of Advanced Practice Nursing.* FA Davis, Philadelphia, 2007.

How well did you do?

85% and above, congratulations! This score shows application of test-taking principles and adequate content knowledge.

75%–85%, keep working! Review test-taking principles and try again.

65%–75%, hang in there! Spend some time reviewing concepts and test-taking principles and then try the test again.

Chapter 9: *Head and Neck Problems*

DIANE GERZEVITZ
JILL E. WINLAND-BROWN
LYNNE M. DUNPHY

Questions

9-1 *When assessing Lenore, age 59, who has a sore throat, you note that she has a positive history of diabetes and rheumatic fever. These facts increase the likelihood that which of the following agents caused her sore throat?*

A. *Neisseria gonorrhoeae*

B. Epstein-Barr virus

C. *Haemophilus influenzae*

D. Group A beta-hemolytic streptococcus

9-2 *The first-line antibiotic therapy for an adult with no known allergies and suspected group A beta-hemolytic streptococcal pharyngitis is*

A. penicillin.

B. erythromycin (E-Mycin).

C. azithromycin (Zithromax).

D. cephalexin (Keflex).

9-3 *Tee, age 64, presents with a sore throat. Your assessment reveals tonsillar exudate, anterior cervical adenopathy, presence of a fever, and absence of a cough. There is a high probability of which causative agent?*

A. *Haemophilus influenzae*

B. Group A beta-hemolytic streptococcus

C. Epstein-Barr virus

D. Rhinovirus

9-4 *Which of the following symptom(s) is (are) most indicative of mononucleosis (Epstein-Barr virus)?*

A. Rapid onset of anterior cervical adenopathy, fatigue, malaise, and headache

B. Gradual onset of fatigue, posterior cervical adenopathy, fever, and sore throat

C. Gradual and seasonal onset of pharyngeal erythema

D. Rapid onset of cough, congestion, and headache

9-5 *Which method can be safely used to remove cerumen in a 12-month-old child's ear?*

A. A size 2 ear curette

B. Irrigation using hot water from a 3-cc syringe

C. A commercial jet tooth cleanser

D. Cerumen should not be removed from a child this young.

9-6 *Mark, age 18, has a persistent sore throat, fever, and malaise not relieved with penicillin therapy. What would you order next?*

A. A throat culture

B. A monospot test

C. A rapid antigen test

D. A Thayer-Martin plate test

9-7 *A sexual history of oral-genital contact in a client presenting with pharyngitis is significant when which of the following organisms is suspected?*

A. *Escherichia coli*

B. *Haemophilus influenzae*

C. *Neisseria gonorrhoeae*

D. *Streptococcus pneumoniae*

9-8 *When a practitioner places a vibrating tuning fork in the midline of a client's skull and asks if the tone sounds the same in both ears or is better in one, the examiner is performing*

A. the Rinne test.

B. the Weber test.

C. the caloric test.

D. a hearing acuity test.

9-9 *Sharon, age 29, is pregnant for the first time. She complains of nasal stuffiness and occasional epistaxis. What do you do?*

A. Order lab tests, such as a complete blood count with differential, hemoglobin, and hematocrit.

B. Prescribe an antihistamine.

C. You do nothing except for client teaching.

D. Refer the client to an ear, nose, and throat specialist.

9-10   *You note a completely split uvula in Noi, a 42-year-old Asian. What is your next course of action?*

A. Do nothing.

B. Refer Noi to a specialist.

C. Perform a throat culture.

D. Order a complete blood count.

9-11   *The most common cause of a white pupil (leukokoria or leukocoria) in a newborn is*

A. a cataract.

B. retinoblastoma.

C. persistent hyperplastic primary vitreous.

D. retinal detachment.

9-12   *Natasha, age 4, has amblyopia. How do you respond when her mother asks about treatment?*

A. "We'll wait until she's 7 years old before starting treatment."

B. "Treatment needs to be started now. We'll cover her 'bad' eye."

C. "Treatment needs to be started now. We'll cover her 'good' eye."

D. "No treatment is necessary. She'll outgrow this."

9-13   *How do you respond when Diane, age 29, asks why she gets sores on her lips every time she sits out in the sun for an extended period of time?*

A. "You are allergic to the sun and must wear sunblock on your lips."

B. "Your lips are dry to begin with and you must keep them moist at all times."

C. "You have herpes simplex that recurs with sunlight exposure."

D. "You're probably allergic to your lip balm."

9-14   *Mavis has persistent pruritus of the external auditory canal. External otitis and dermatological conditions such as seborrheic dermatitis and psoriasis have been ruled out. What can you advise her to do?*

A. Use a cotton-tipped applicator daily to remove all moisture and potential bacteria.

B. Wash daily with soap and water.

C. Apply mineral oil to counteract dryness.

D. Avoid topical corticosteroids.

9-15   *How do you test for near vision?*

A. By using the Snellen eye chart

B. By using the Rosenbaum chart

C. By asking the client to read from a magazine or newspaper

D. By testing the cardinal fields

9-16   *When you are assessing the corneal light reflex, an abnormal finding indicates*

A. possible use of eye medications.

B. a neurological problem.

C. improper alignment of the eyes.

D. strabismus.

9-17   *When you are assessing the internal structure of the eye, absence of a red reflex may indicate*

A. a cataract or a hemorrhage into the vitreous humor.

B. acute iritis.

C. nothing; this is a normal finding in older adults.

D. diabetes or long-standing hypertension.

9-18   *Mavis is 70 years old and wonders if she can donate her corneas when she dies. How do you respond?*

A. "As long as you don't have any chronic illness, your corneas may be harvested."

B. "They will use corneas only from persons younger than age 65."

C. "What makes you feel like you are dying?"

D. "Don't think about such terrible things now."

9-19   *Tara was born with a cleft lip and palate. When should treatment begin for this condition?*

A. Immediately after birth

B. At age 3 months

C. At age 6 months

D. When Tara is ready to drink from a cup

9-20   *The trachea deviates toward the unaffected side in all of the following conditions except*

A. aortic aneurysm.

B. unilateral thyroid lobe enlargement.

C. large atelectasis.

D. pneumothorax.

9-21 *A child's head circumference is routinely measured at each well-child visit until age*

A. 12 months.

B. 18 months.

C. 2 years.

D. 5 years.

9-22 *Jim, age 49, comes to the office with a rapid-onset complete paralysis of one-half of his face. He is unable to raise his eyebrow, close his eye, whistle, or show his teeth. You suspect a lower motor neuron lesion resulting in cranial nerve VII paralysis. What is your working diagnosis?*

A. Cerebrovascular accident

B. Trigeminal neuralgia

C. Bell's palsy

D. Tic douloureux

9-23 *A child's central visual acuity is 20/30 by age*

A. 18 months.

B. 2 years.

C. 3 years.

D. 4 years.

9-24 *When Judith, age 15, asks you to explain the 20/50 vision in her right eye, you respond,*

A. "You can see at 20 ft with your left eye what the normal person can see at 50 ft."

B. "You can see at 20 ft with your right eye what the normal person can see at 50 ft."

C. "You can see at 50 ft with your right eye what the normal person can see at 20 ft."

D. "You can see at 50 ft with the left eye what the normal person can see at 20 ft."

9-25 *Which assessment test is a gross measurement of peripheral vision?*

A. The cover test

B. The corneal light reflex test

C. The confrontation test

D. The Snellen eye-chart test

9-26 *The normal ratio of the artery-to-vein width in the retina as viewed through the ophthalmoscope is*

A. 2:3.

B. 3:2.

C. 1:3.

D. 3:1.

9-27 *You observe a mother showing her infant a toy. You note that the infant can fixate on, briefly follow, and then reach for the toy. You suspect that the infant is*

A. 2 months old.

B. 4 months old.

C. 6 months old.

D. 8 months old.

9-28 *You have made a diagnosis of acute sinusitis based on Martha's history and the fact that she complains of pain behind her eye. Which sinuses are affected?*

A. Maxillary

B. Ethmoid

C. Frontal

D. Sphenoid

9-29 *You diagnose acute epiglottitis in Sally, age 5, and immediately send her to the local emergency room. Which of the following symptoms would indicate that an airway obstruction is imminent?*

A. Reddened face

B. Screaming

C. Grabbing her throat

D. Stridor

9-30 *Darren, age 26, has AIDS and presents with a painful tongue covered with what looks like creamy-white, curdlike patches overlying erythematous mucosa. You are able to scrape off these "curds" with a tongue depressor, which assists you in making which of the following diagnoses?*

A. Leukoplakia

B. Lichen planus

C. Oral candidiasis

D. Oral cancer

9-31 *What is the easiest way to differentiate between otitis externa and otitis media?*

A. With otitis media, tender swelling is usually visible.

B. With otitis media, there is usually bilateral pain in the ears.

C. With otitis media, there is usually tenderness on palpation over the mastoid process.

D. With otitis externa, movement or pressure on the pinna is extremely painful.

9-32 *Which of the following refractive errors in vision is a result of the natural loss of accommodative capacity with age?*

A. Presbyopia

B. Hyperopia

C. Myopia

D. Astigmatism

9-33 *The most frequent cause of laryngeal obstruction in an adult is*

A. a piece of meat.

B. a tumor.

C. mucosal swelling from an allergic reaction.

D. inhalation of a carcinogen.

9-34 *Marnie, who has asthma, has been told that she has nasal polyps. What do you tell her about them?*

A. Nasal polyps are usually precancerous.

B. Nasal polyps are benign growths.

C. The majority of nasal polyps are neoplastic.

D. They are probably inflamed turbinates, not polyps, because polyps are infrequent in clients with asthma.

9-35 *Mary, age 82, presents with several eye problems. She states that her eyes are always dry and look "sunken in." What do you suspect?*

A. Hypothyroidism

B. Normal age-related changes

C. Cushing's syndrome

D. A detached retina

9-36 *Marian, age 79, is at a higher risk than a middle-aged client for developing an eye infection because of which age-related change?*

A. Increased eyestrain

B. Loss of subcutaneous tissue

C. Change in pupil size

D. A decrease in tear production

9-37 *Marty has a hordeolum in his right eye. You suspect that the offending organism is*

A. herpes simplex virus.

B. *Staphylococcus.*

C. *Candida albicans.*

D. *Escherichia coli.*

9-38 *June, age 50, presents with soft, raised, yellow plaques on her eyelids at the inner canthus. She is concerned that they may be cancerous skin lesions. You tell her that they are probably*

A. xanthelasmas.

B. pingueculae.

C. the result of arcus senilis.

D. actinic keratoses.

9-39 *Which cranial nerve (CN) is affected in sensorineural or perceptive hearing loss?*

A. CN II

B. CN IV

C. CN VIII

D. CN XI

9-40 *Regular ocular pressure testing is indicated for older adults taking*

A. high-dose inhaled glucocorticoids.

B. NSAIDs.

C. angiotensin-converting enzyme (ACE) inhibitors.

D. insulin.

9-41 *What condition occurs in almost all persons beginning around age 42–46?*

A. Arcus senilis

B. Presbyopia

C. Cataracts

D. Glaucoma

9-42 *In older adults, the most common cause of decreased visual functioning is*

A. cataract formation.

B. glaucoma.

C. macular degeneration.

D. arcus senilis.

9-43   *How should Tommy, age 2½, have his vision screened?*

A. Using a Snellen letter chart

B. Using the Allen test

C. Using a Snellen E chart

D. Using a Rosenbaum chart

9-44   *Leah, 4 months old, has both eyes turning inward. What is this called?*

A. Pseudostrabismus

B. Strabismus

C. Esotropia

D. Exotropia

9-45   *Maury, age 52, has throbbing pain in the left eye, an irregular pupil shape, marked photophobia, and redness around the iris. What is your initial diagnosis?*

A. Conjunctivitis

B. Iritis

C. Subconjunctival hemorrhage

D. Acute glaucoma

9-46   *Purulent matter in the anterior chamber of the eye is called*

A. hyphema.

B. hypopyon.

C. anisocoria.

D. pterygium.

9-47   *A common cause of conductive hearing loss in adults ages 20–40 is*

A. trauma.

B. otitis media.

C. presbycusis.

D. otosclerosis.

9-48   *If a client presents with a deep aching, red eye and there is no discharge, you should suspect*

A. bacterial conjunctivitis.

B. viral conjunctivitis.

C. allergic conjunctivitis.

D. iritis.

9-49   *Acute otitis media is diagnosed when there is*

A. fluid in the middle ear without signs or symptoms of an ear infection.

B. a diagnosis of three or more episodes of otitis media within 1 year.

C. fluid in the middle ear accompanied by otalgia and fever.

D. fluid within the middle ear for at least 3 months.

9-50   *Judy, age 67, complains of a sudden onset of impaired vision, severe eye pain, vomiting, and a headache. You diagnose the following condition and refer for urgent treatment.*

A. Cataracts

B. Macular degeneration

C. Presbyopia

D. Acute glaucoma

9-51   *Clonazepam (Klonopin) is occasionally ordered for temporal mandibular joint (TMJ) disease. Which of the following statements applies to this medicine?*

A. It is ordered for inflammatory pain.

B. It is ordered for neuropathic pain.

C. It is ordered for a short course of therapy for 1–2 weeks only.

D. It is ordered for muscle relaxation.

9-52   *The antibiotic of choice for beta-lactamase coverage of otitis media is*

A. amoxicillin (Amoxil).

B. amoxicillin and potassium clavulanate (Augmentin).

C. azithromycin (Zithromax).

D. prednisone (Deltasone).

9-53   *Sam, age 4, is brought into the clinic by his father. His tympanic membrane is perforated from otitis media. His father asks about repair of the eardrum. How do you respond?*

A. "The eardrum, in most cases, heals within several weeks."

B. "We need to schedule Sam for a surgical repair."

C. "He must absolutely stay out of the water for 3–6 months."

D. "If the eardrum is not healed in several months, it can be surgically repaired."

9-54 *What significant finding(s) in a child with otitis media with effusion would prompt more aggressive treatment?*

A. There is a change in the child's hearing threshold to less than or equal to 20 decibels (dB).

B. The child becomes a fussy eater.

C. The child's speech and language skills seem slightly delayed.

D. Persistent rhinitis is present.

9-55 *The immediate goal of myringotomy and tube placement in a child with recurrent episodes of otitis media is to*

A. prevent future infections.

B. have an open access to the middle ear for irrigation and instillation of antibiotics.

C. allow removal of suppurative or mucoid material.

D. relieve pain.

9-56 *Marcia, age 4, is brought into the office by her mother. She has a sore throat, difficulty swallowing, copious oral secretions, respiratory difficulty, stridor, and a temperature of 102°F but no pharyngeal erythema or cough. What do you suspect?*

A. Epiglottitis

B. Group A beta-hemolytic streptococcal infection pharyngitis

C. Tonsillitis

D. Diphtheria

9-57 *John, age 19, has just been given a diagnosis of mononucleosis. Which of the following statements is true?*

A. The offending organism is bacteria and should be treated with antibiotics.

B. Convalescence is usually only a few days and John should be back to normal in a week.

C. Mono is rarely contagious.

D. John should avoid contact sports and heavy lifting.

9-58 *Barbara, age 72, states that she was told she had atrophic macular degeneration and asks you if there is any treatment. How do you respond?*

A. "No, but 5 years from the time of the first symptoms, the process usually stops."

B. "Yes, there is a surgical procedure that will cure this."

C. "If we start medications now, they may prevent any further damage."

D. "Unfortunately, there is no effective treatment, but I can refer you to a rehabilitation agency that can help you adjust to the visual loss."

9-59 *Nathan, age 19, is a college swimmer. He frequently gets swimmer's ear and asks if there is anything he can do to help prevent it other than wearing earplugs, which don't really work for him. What do you suggest?*

A. Use a cotton-tipped applicator to dry the ears after swimming.

B. Use eardrops made of a solution of equal parts of alcohol and vinegar in each ear after swimming.

C. Use a hair dryer on the highest setting to dry the ears.

D. Tell Nathan he must change his sport.

9-60 *Harry, age 69, has had Ménière's disease for several years. He has some hearing loss but now has persistent vertigo. What treatment might be instituted to relieve the vertigo?*

A. A labyrinthectomy

B. Pharmacological therapy

C. A vestibular neurectomy

D. Wearing an earplug in the ear with the most hearing loss

9-61 *Marvin has sudden eye redness that occurred after a strenuous coughing episode. You diagnose a subconjunctival hemorrhage. Your next step is to*

A. refer him to an ophthalmologist.

B. order antibiotics.

C. do nothing other than provide reassurance.

D. consult with your collaborating physician.

9-62 *The leading cause of blindness in persons ages 20–60 in the United States is*

A. macular degeneration.

B. glaucoma.

C. diabetic retinopathy.

D. trauma.

9-63 *Samantha, age 12, appears with ear pain. When you begin to assess her ear, you tug on her* *normal-appearing auricle, eliciting severe pain. This leads you to suspect*

A. otitis media.

B. otitis media with effusion.

C. otitis externa.

D. primary otalgia.

9-64 *David, age 32, states that he thinks he has an ear infection because he just flew back from a business trip and feels unusual pressure in his ear. You diagnose barotrauma. What is your next action?*

A. Prescribe nasal steroids and oral decongestants.

B. Prescribe antibiotic eardrops.

C. Prescribe systemic antibiotics.

D. Refer David to an ear, nose, and throat specialist.

9-65 *Jill states that her 5-year-old daughter continually grinds her teeth at night. You document this as*

A. temporal mandibular joint malocclusion.

B. bruxism.

C. a psychosis.

D. an oropharyngeal lesion.

9-66 *The most common cause of sensorineural hearing loss is*

A. trauma.

B. tympanic membrane sclerosis and scarring.

C. otosclerosis.

D. presbycusis.

9-67 *In a young child, unilateral purulent rhinitis is most often caused by*

A. a foreign body.

B. a viral infection.

C. a bacterial infection.

D. an allergic reaction.

9-68 *Henry is having difficulty getting rid of a corneal infection. He asks you why. How do you respond?*

A. "We can't determine the causative agent."

B. "Antibiotics have difficulty getting to that area."

C. "Because the infection was painless, it was not treated early enough."

D. "Because the cornea doesn't have a blood supply, an infection can't be fought off as usual."

9-69 *Sylvia has glaucoma and has started taking a medication that acts as a diuretic to reduce the intraocular pressure. Which medication is she taking?*

A. A carbonic anhydrase inhibitor

B. A beta-adrenergic receptor blocker

C. A miotic

D. A mydriatic

9-70 *Cydney, age 7, is complaining that she feels as though something is stuck in her ear. What action is contraindicated?*

A. Inspecting the ear canal with an otoscope

B. Using a small suction device to try to remove the object

C. Flushing the ear with water

D. Instilling several drops of mineral oil in the ear

9-71 *Ty, age 68, has a hearing problem. He tells you he is ready for a drastic solution to the problem because he likes to play bingo but cannot hear the calls. What can you do for him?*

A. Refer him to a hearing aid specialist.

B. Refer him for further testing.

C. Perform a gross hearing test in the office, then repeat it in 6 months to determine if there is any further loss.

D. Nothing. Tell him that a gradual hearing loss is to be expected with aging.

9-72 *How would you describe the cervical lymphadenopathy associated with asymptomatic HIV infection?*

A. Movable, discrete, soft, and nontender lymph nodes

B. Enlarged, warm, tender, firm, but freely movable lymph nodes

C. Hard, unilateral, nontender, and fixed lymph nodes

D. Firm but not hard, nontender, and mobile lymph nodes

9-73 *Microtia refers to the size of the*

A. ears.

B. skull.

C. pupils.

D. eyes.

9-74 *With a chronic allergy, a client's nasal mucosa appear*

A. swollen and red.

B. swollen, boggy, pale, and gray.

C. hard, pale, and inflamed.

D. bright pink and inflamed.

9-75 *Which manifestation is noted with carbon monoxide poisoning?*

A. Circumoral pallor of the lips

B. Cherry-red lips

C. Cyanosis of the lips

D. Pale pink lips

9-76 *Which manifestation of the buccal mucosa is present in a client with mumps?*

A. Pink, smooth, moist appearance with some patchy hyperpigmentation

B. Dappled brown patches

C. The orifice of Stensen's duct appearing red

D. Koplik's spots

9-77 *How would you grade tonsils that touch the uvula?*

A. Grade 1+

B. Grade 2+

C. Grade 3+

D. Grade 4+

9-78 *Claude, age 78, is being treated with timolol maleate (Timoptic) drops for his chronic open-angle glaucoma. While performing a new client history and physical, you note that he is taking other medications. Which medication would you be most concerned about?*

A. Aspirin therapy as prophylaxis for heart attack

B. Ranitidine (Zantac) for gastroesophageal reflux disease

C. Alprazolam (Xanax), an anxiolytic for anxiety

D. Atenolol (Tenormin), a beta blocker for high blood pressure

9-79 *Manny, age 16, was hit in the eye with a baseball. He developed pain in the eye, decreased visual acuity, and injection of the globe. You confirm the diagnosis of hyphema by finding blood in the anterior chamber. What*

treatment would you recommend while Manny is waiting to see the ophthalmologist?

A. Apply bilateral eye patches.

B. Have Manny lie flat.

C. Refer him to an ophthalmologist within a week.

D. Make sure Manny is able to be awakened every 30 minutes.

9-80 *Jill presents with symptoms of hay fever and you assess the nasal mucosa of her turbinates to be pale. What diagnosis do you suspect?*

A. Allergic rhinitis

B. Viral rhinitis

C. Nasal polyps

D. Nasal vestibulitis from folliculitis

9-81 *Joy, age 36, has a sudden onset of shivering, sweating, headache, aching in the orbits, and general malaise and misery. Her temperature is 102°F. You diagnose influenza (flu). What is your next course of action?*

A. Order amoxicillin (Amoxil) 500 mg every 12 hours for 7 days.

B. Prescribe rest, fluids, acetaminophen (Tylenol), and possibly a decongestant and an antitussive.

C. Order a complete blood count.

D. Consult with your collaborating physician.

9-82 *Mandy was given a diagnosis of flu 2 days ago and wants to start on the "new flu medicine" right away. What do you tell her?*

A. "The medication is effective only if started within the first 48 hours after symptoms begin."

B. "If you treat a cold, it goes away in 7 days; if you don't treat it, it goes away in 1 week."

C. "The medicine has not proven its effectiveness."

D. "I'll start you on zanamivir today. It may shorten the course of the disease and perhaps lessen the severity of your symptoms."

9-83 *Matthew, age 52, has allergic rhinitis and would like some medicine to relieve his symptoms. He is taking cimetidine (Tagamet) for gastroesophageal reflux disease. Which medication would you not order?*

A. A first-generation antihistamine

B. A second-generation antihistamine

C. A decongestant

D. A topical nasal corticosteroid

9-84   Sara, age 29, states that she has painless, white, slightly raised patches in her mouth. They are probably caused by

A. herpes simplex.

B. aphthous ulcers.

C. candidiasis.

D. oral cancer.

9-85   Mycostatin (Nystatin) is ordered for Michael, who has an oral fungal infection. What instructions do you give Michael for taking the medication?

A. "Don't swallow the medication because it's irritating to the gastric mucosa."

B. "Take the medication with meals so that it's absorbed better."

C. "Swish and swallow the medication."

D. "Apply the medication only to the lesions."

9-86   Risk factors for oral cancers include

A. a family history, poor dental habits, and use of alcohol.

B. obesity, sedentary lifestyle, and chewing tobacco.

C. a history of diabetes, smoking, and a high fat intake.

D. smoking, use of alcohol, and chewing tobacco.

9-87   Your neighbor calls you because her son, age 9, fell on the sidewalk while playing outside and a tooth fell out. She wants to know what she should put the tooth in to transport it to the dentist. You tell her that the best solution to put it in is

A. salt water.

B. saliva.

C. milk.

D. water.

9-88   Monique brings her 4-week-old infant into the office because she noticed small, yellow-white, glistening bumps on her infant's gums. She says they look like teeth, but she is worried that they may be cancer. You diagnose these bumps as

A. Bednar's aphthae.

B. Epstein's pearls.

C. buccal tumors.

D. exostosis.

9-89   Mattie says she has heard that it is not good to let a baby go to bed with a bottle. She says that she has always done this with her other children and wonders why it is not recommended. How do you respond?

A. "A bottle in the baby's mouth forces the baby to breathe through the nose. If the nose is clogged, the baby will not get enough oxygen."

B. "A nipple, when placed in the mouth for long periods of time, can cause tooth displacement. This will also affect the adult teeth not grown in yet and will necessitate braces in the teen years."

C. "Normal mouth bacteria act on the sugar in the bottle contents to form acids, which will break down the tooth enamel and destroy the teeth even before they come in."

D. "This encourages the baby to continually want to drink at night. When the child is older, it will become a habit, and the child will end up wearing diapers into the preschool years."

9-90   When the Weber test is performed with a tuning fork to assess hearing and there is no lateralization, this indicates

A. conductive deafness.

B. perceptive deafness.

C. a normal finding.

D. nerve damage.

9-91   A smooth tongue may indicate

A. a normal finding.

B. alcohol abuse.

C. a vitamin deficiency.

D. nicotine addiction.

9-92   Signs and symptoms of acute angle-closure glaucoma include

A. painless redness of the eyes.

B. loss of peripheral vision.

C. translucent corneas.

D. halos around lights.

9-93   Greg, age 72, is brought to the office by his son, who states that his father has been unable to see clearly since last night. Greg reports that his vision is "like looking through a veil." He also sees floaters and flashing lights but is not having any pain. What do you suspect?

A. Cataracts

B. Glaucoma

C. Retinal detachment

D. Iritis

9-94 *The most common offending allergens causing allergic rhinitis are*

A. pollens of grasses, trees, and weeds.

B. fungi.

C. animal allergens.

D. food sensitivity.

9-95 *Shelley, age 47, is complaining of a red eye. You are trying to decide between a diagnosis of conjunctivitis and iritis. One distinguishing characteristic between the two is*

A. eye discomfort.

B. slow progression.

C. a ciliary flush.

D. no change in or slightly blurred vision.

9-96 *Clients with allergic conjunctivitis have which type of discharge?*

A. Purulent

B. Serous or clear

C. Stringy and white

D. Profuse mucoid or mucopurulent

9-97 *Which is the most common localized infection of one of the glands of the eyelids?*

A. Hordeolum

B. Chalazion

C. Bacterial conjunctivitis

D. Herpes simplex

9-98 *Sara, age 92, presents with dry eyes, redness, and a scratchy feeling. You note that this is one of the most common disorders, particularly in older women, and diagnose this as*

A. viral conjunctivitis.

B. keratoconjunctivitis sicca.

C. allergic eye disease.

D. corneal ulcer.

9-99 *Mattie, age 64, presents with blurred vision in one eye and states that it felt like "a curtain came down over my eye." She doesn't have any pain or redness. What do you suspect?*

A. Retinal detachment

B. Acute angle-closure glaucoma

C. Open-angle glaucoma

D. Cataract

9-100 *Martin, age 24, presents with an erythematous ear canal, pain, and a recent history of swimming. What do you suspect?*

A. Acute otitis media

B. Chronic otitis media

C. External otitis

D. Temporomandibular joint syndrome

9-101 *What therapy has proved beneficial for long-term symptom relief of tinnitus?*

A. Aspirin

B. Lidocaine

C. Cognitive behavioral therapy

D. Corticosporin otic gtts prn

9-102 *Sally, age 19, presents with pain and pressure over her cheeks and discolored nasal discharge. You cannot transilluminate the sinuses. You suspect which common sinus to be affected?*

A. Maxillary sinus

B. Ethmoid sinus

C. Temporal sinus

D. Frontal sinus

9-103 *While doing a face, head, and neck examination, you note that the palpebral fissures are abnormally narrow. What are you examining?*

A. Nasolabial folds

B. The openings between the margins of the upper and lower eyelids

C. The thyroid gland in relation to the trachea

D. The distance between the trigeminal nerve branches

9-104 *A 42-year-old stockbroker comes to your office for evaluation of a pulsating headache over the left temporal region and he rates the pain as an 8 on a scale of 1–10. The pain has been constant for the past several hours and is accompanied by nausea and sensitivity to light. He has had frequent headaches for many years but not as severe and they are usually relieved by over-the-counter medicines. He is unclear as to a precipitating event but notes that he has had visual disturbances before each headache and he has been under a lot of stress in his* job. Based on this description, what is the most likely diagnosis of this type of headache?

A. Tension

B. Migraine

C. Cluster

D. Temporal arteritis

9-105 Maggie, a 56-year-old woman, comes to the office requesting a test for thyroid disease. She has had some weight gain since menopause and she read on the Internet that all women should have a thyroid test. Based on the recommendations from the U.S. Preventive Services Task Force, which one of the following statements should be considered in this woman's care?

A. All adults should be screened for thyroid disease.

B. Evidence is insufficient for or against routine screening for thyroid disease in asymptomatic adults.

C. All adults older than 50 should be screened for thyroid disease.

D. All perimenopausal women should be screened for thyroid disease.

9-106 A 62-year-old obese woman comes in today complaining of difficulty swallowing for the past 3 weeks. She states that "some foods get stuck" and she has been having "heartburn" at night when she lies down, especially if she has had a heavy meal. Occasionally she will awake at night coughing. She denies weight gain and/or weight loss, vomiting, or change in bowel movements. She does not drink or smoke. There is no pertinent family history or findings on review of systems (ROS). Physical examination is normal with no abdominal tenderness, and the stool is OB negative. What is the most likely diagnosis?

A. Esophageal varices

B. Esophageal cancer

C. Gastroesophageal reflux disease (GERD)

D. Peptic ulcer disease (PUD)

9-107 Jessica, an 8-year-old third-grader is brought to the office by her grandmother, who is the child's babysitter. She has complained of fever and sore throat for the past 2 days. Five other children in her class have been sick with sore throats. She denies difficulty swallowing and has been drinking fluids but she has no appetite. ROS reveals that she has clear nasal drainage, hoarseness, and a nonproductive cough. She denies vomiting but has had mild diarrhea. On examination she has a temperature of

101.5°F; 3+ erythematous tonsils; and palpable, tender cervical lymph nodes. Based on these findings, what is the most likely diagnosis?

A. Mono

B. Sinusitis

C. Strep pharyngitis

D. Viral pharyngitis

9-108 Which of the following conditions produces sharp, piercing facial pain that lasts for seconds to minutes?

A. Trigeminal neuralgia

B. TMJ

C. Goiter

D. Preauricular adenitis

9-109 A client comes in complaining of 1 week of pain in the posterior neck with difficulty turning the head to the right. What additional history is needed?

A. Recent trauma

B. Difficulty swallowing

C. Stiffness in the right shoulder

D. Change in sleeping habits

9-110 A client complains of frequent bouts of severe, intense, disabling left-sided facial pain accompanied by excessive left eye lacrimation (tearing) and worsening anxiety. The pain wakes him at night and he has even contemplated harming himself during these episodes due to the intensity and unrelenting nature of the pain. What kind of headache is he describing?

A. Classic migraine

B. Tension headache

C. Sinus headache

D. Cluster headache

9-111 A 65-year-old man presents complaining of left-sided, deep, throbbing headache along with mild fatigue. On examination the client has a tender, tortuous temporal artery. You suspect temporal arteritis. How do you confirm your diagnosis?

A. MRI of the head

B. Erythrocyte sedimentation rate (ESR)

C. EEG

D. Otoscopy

9-112 *An 80-year-old woman comes in today with complaints of a rash on the left side of her face that is blistered and painful and accompanied by left-sided eye pain. The rash broke out 2 days ago, and she remembers being very tired and feeling feverish for a week before the rash appeared. On examination the rash follows the trigeminal nerve on the left and she has some scleral injection and tearing. You suspect herpes zoster ophthalmicus. Based on what you know to be complications of this disease, you explain to her that she needs*

A. antibiotics.

B. a biopsy of the rash.

C. immediate hospitalization.

D. ophthalmological consultation.

9-113 *When you examine the tympanic membrane, which of these structures is visible?*

A. Stapes

B. Cochlea

C. Pars flaccida

D. Round window

9-114 *A 22-year-old client who plays in a rock band complains that he finds it difficult to understand his fellow musicians at the end of a night of performing, a problem that is compounded by the noisy environment of the "club." These symptoms are most characteristic of which of the following?*

A. Sensorineural loss

B. Conductive loss

C. Tinnitus

D. Vertigo

9-115 *Which of the following signs of thyroid dysfunction is a sign of hyperthyroidism?*

A. Slow pulse

B. Decreased systolic BP

C. Exophthalmos

D. Dry, coarse, cool skin

9-116 *Your client is unable to differentiate between sharp and dull stimulation on both sides of her face. You suspect*

A. Bell's palsy.

B. a lesion affecting the trigeminal nerve.

C. a stroke.

D. shingles.

Answers

9-1   Answer D

If a client has a sore throat and a history of diabetes or rheumatic fever, it is very likely that the infection is a result of group A beta-hemolytic streptococcus.

9-2   Answer A

The first-line antibiotic therapy for an adult with no known allergies and suspected group A beta-hemolytic streptococcus pharyngitis is penicillin.

9-3   Answer B

When the following four symptoms present as a cluster, there is a high probability (43%) that the infection is caused by group A beta-hemolytic streptococcus: throat pain with tonsillar exudate, anterior cervical adenopathy, presence of fever, and absence of cough.

9-4   Answer B

Symptoms most indicative of mononucleosis (Epstein-Barr virus) are gradual onset of fatigue, sore throat, fever, posterior cervical adenopathy, palatine petechiae, and hepatosplenomegaly.

9-5   Answer C

Irrigation with a soft bulb syringe or a commercial jet tooth cleanser may be used to remove cerumen. Irrigation using lukewarm water should be done when the cerumen is dry and hard but not if the tympanic membrane might be perforated. Cerumen can be safely removed from an infant's ear by the practitioner for adequate visualization of the tympanic membrane by using an ear curette through an operating otoscope, or if an operating otoscope is not available, by using a size 00 ear curette through a size 3-mm speculum.

9-6   Answer B

If a client has a persistent sore throat, fever, and malaise not relieved with penicillin therapy, a monospot test should be performed to rule out mononucleosis (Epstein-Barr virus). A throat culture and rapid antigen test are performed to help diagnose group A beta-hemolytic streptococcal infection. A Thayer-Martin plate test is performed to diagnose a gonococcal infection.

9-7 Answer C

A sexual history of oral-genital contact in a client presenting with pharyngitis is significant when infection with *Neisseria gonorrhoeae* is suspected. *N. gonorrhoeae* pharyngitis is a common sexually transmitted disease.

9-8 Answer B

When a practitioner places a vibrating tuning fork in the midline of a client's skull and asks if the tone sounds the same in both ears or is better in one, the examiner is performing the Weber test. The Weber test is valuable when a client states that hearing is better in one ear than the other. The Rinne test compares air conduction and bone conduction sound. The stem of a vibrating tuning fork is placed on the client's mastoid process and the client is asked to signal when the sound disappears. The fork is then quickly inverted so that the vibrating end is near the ear canal, at which time the client should still hear a sound. Normally, sound is heard twice as long by air conduction as by bone conduction. The caloric test, or oculovestibular test, assesses cranial nerves III, VI, and VIII. Ice water is instilled into the ear; if nerve function is normal, the eyes will deviate to that side. A hearing acuity test assesses the client's ability to hear the spoken word.

9-9 Answer C

Nasal stuffiness and epistaxis may occur during a normal pregnancy because of increased vascularization in the upper respiratory tract. The gums may also be soft and hyperemic and may bleed with normal toothbrushing. Additional laboratory tests are not necessary at this point. No treatment, other than teaching the client what to expect and do, is indicated.

9-10 Answer A

Bifid uvula, a condition in which the uvula is either partially or completely split, occurs in 18% of Native Americans and 10% of Asians and is rare in whites and blacks. There is no need for treatment.

9-11 Answer A

The most common cause of a white pupil (leukokoria or leukocoria) in a newborn is a congenital cataract. The incidence may be as high as 1 in every 500–1000 live births, and there is usually a family history. Some infants require no treatment; however, surgery may be performed on others during the first few weeks of life. Retinoblastoma, a common intraocular malignancy, is detected within the first few weeks of life and is the second most common cause of white pupil. Persistent hyperplastic primary vitreous is the third most common cause of white pupil and is a congenital developmental abnormality. Retinal detachment may occur as a result of trauma or disease and only rarely occurs in infancy.

9-12 Answer C

Treatment of amblyopia ("lazy eye") includes occluding the client's "good" (or better-seeing) eye and treating any underlying conditions such as cataracts or refractive errors. Treatment must be started by age 3 or 4 because amblyopia is irreversible after age 7. Amblyopia occurs in 50% of clients who have strabismus or misalignment of the eye muscles. Adults with strabismus frequently have double vision; however, young children learn to suppress or ignore double vision. As a result, young children have reduced central vision in the crossed eye from lack of use.

9-13 Answer C

Herpes simplex is associated with vesicular lesions on the lips and oral mucosa. The virus remains latent and may recur with sunlight exposure, stressful times, fever, trauma, and treatment with immunosuppressive drugs.

9-14 Answer C

Pruritus of the external ear canal is a common problem. In most cases, the pruritus is self-induced from enthusiastic cleaning or excoriation. The protective cerumen covering must be allowed to regenerate and may be helped to do so by application of a small amount of mineral oil, which helps to counteract dryness and reject moisture. The use of soap and water, as well as cotton-tipped swabs, should be avoided. The adage "you shouldn't put anything smaller than your elbow in your ear" holds true today. If an inflammatory component is present, a topical corticosteroid may be applied. Often, isopropyl alcohol may relieve ear canal pruritus.

9-15 Answer B

Test for near vision by using the Rosenbaum chart. Hold it about 12–14 in. from the client's eyes. A gross estimate of near vision may also be assessed by asking the client to read from a magazine or newspaper held about 12–14 in. away from the eyes. The Snellen eye chart tests vision at a distance of

20 ft. Testing the cardinal fields of gaze does not test for vision but rather for extraocular eye movements.

9-16   Answer C

When assessing the corneal light reflex, an abnormal finding indicates improper alignment of the eyes. It is noted when the reflections of the light are on different sites on the eyes. Some eye medications may cause unequal dilation, constriction, or inequality of pupil size that may be noted when assessing for direct and consensual pupil response. A neurological problem may be suspected if the pupils are unequal in size. Strabismus is noted during the cover-uncover test.

9-17   Answer A

When assessing the internal structure of the eye, absence of a red reflex may indicate the total opacity of the pupil because of a cataract or a hemorrhage into the vitreous humor. It may also be a result of improper positioning of the ophthalmoscope. Acute iritis is noted by constriction of the pupil accompanied by pain and circumcorneal redness (ciliary flush). If areas of hemorrhage, exudate, and white patches are present when the internal structure of the eye is assessed, they are usually a result of diabetes or long-standing hypertension.

9-18   Answer B

Corneas are harvested from the cadavers of uninfected persons younger than age 65 who die as the result of an acute trauma or illness. The client's question does not necessarily mean that she is thinking about dying, but it is natural for older adults to think about death, and their thoughts and feelings should be explored.

9-19   Answer A

Treatment for cleft lip and palate needs to be instituted immediately after birth by constructing a palatal obturator to help the infant feed. Cleft lip and palate rehabilitation is an extensive program involving multiple procedures. A cleft lip may be unilateral or bilateral and complete or incomplete. It may also occur with a cleft in the entire palate or just the anterior or posterior palate.

9-20   Answer C

The trachea deviates toward the unaffected side with an aortic aneurysm, unilateral thyroid lobe enlargement, and pneumothorax. It deviates toward the affected side with a large atelectasis or fibrosis.

9-21   Answer C

A child's head circumference is measured, using a measuring tape, at each well-child visit until age 2 years. At birth, head circumference measures about 32–38 cm and is 2 cm larger than the chest circumference. At age 2, both the head and chest measurements are equal. During childhood, the chest circumference exceeds the head circumference by 5–7 cm.

9-22   Answer C

Bell's palsy should be suspected if a client presents with a rapid-onset, complete paralysis of one-half of the face and the inability to raise the eyebrow, close the eye, whistle, or show the teeth. Bell's palsy is a lower motor neuron lesion resulting in cranial nerve VII paralysis. It is often a self-limiting condition, lasting a few days or weeks. Occasionally, facial paralysis may result from a tumor or physical trauma compromising the facial nerve. A cerebrovascular accident (CVA) would affect more than just the face. Trigeminal neuralgia, also called tic douloureux, is a painful disorder of the trigeminal nerve. It causes severe pain in the face and forehead on the affected side and is triggered by stimuli such as cold drafts, chewing, and drinking cold liquids.

9-23   Answer C

A child's central visual acuity is 20/30 by age 3. At birth, an infant can see about 12 in. away, an approximate 20/300 central visual acuity. It improves to 20/40 by age 2, 20/30 by age 3, and 20/20 by age 4.

9-24   Answer B

An explanation of 20/50 vision in a client's right eye would be: "You can see at 20 ft with your right eye what the normal person can see at 50 ft." Normal visual acuity is 20/20 on a Snellen eye chart. The larger the denominator, the poorer the vision. If vision is greater than 20/30, refer the client to an ophthalmologist or optometrist.

9-25   Answer C

The confrontation test is a gross measure of peripheral vision. It compares the client's peripheral vision with the practitioner's, assuming that the practitioner has normal peripheral vision. The cover test detects small degrees of deviated alignment by interrupting the fusion reflex that normally keeps both eyes parallel. The corneal light reflex test assesses the parallel alignment of the eye axes. The Snellen eye chart test assesses visual acuity.

9-26   Answer A

The normal ratio comparing the artery-to-vein ratio in the retinal vessels is 2:3 or 4:5, with the arterioles being a brighter red than the veins when viewed through the ophthalmoscope. The arterioles have a narrow light reflex from the center line of the vessel. Veins do not normally show a light reflex. Both arterioles and veins show a gradual and regularly diminishing diameter as you look at them from the disc to the periphery. When hypertension is present, the arterioles may be only about one-half the size of the corresponding vein, and they may appear opaque and lighter. With long-standing hypertension, nicking is present. This occurs when the underlying veins are concealed to some degree by the abnormally opaque arteriole wall at the vessel crossings.

9-27   Answer B

By age 3–4 months, an infant can fixate on, briefly follow, and then reach for a toy when the toy is placed in the infant's line of vision. At age 2–4 weeks, an infant can fixate on an object. By age 1 month, an infant can fixate on and follow a light or a bright toy. By age 6–10 months, an infant can fixate on and follow a toy in all directions.

9-28   Answer B

With ethmoid sinus problems, the pain is behind the eye and high on the nose. Maxillary sinus pain is over the cheek and into the upper teeth; frontal sinus pain is over the lower forehead; and sphenoid sinus pain is in the occiput, vertex, or middle of the head.

9-29   Answer D

In a pediatric client with acute epiglottitis, a number of symptoms can indicate that airway obstruction is imminent: stridor, restlessness, nasal flaring, as well as the use of accessory muscles of respiration. A reddened face does not indicate a lack of oxygenation. Although the child may scream and grab at the throat, these are not primary indicators of impending airway obstruction.

9-30   Answer C

Oral candidiasis (thrush) is distinctive because of the ability to rub off the white areas on the tongue with a tongue depressor. Leukoplakia cannot be removed by rubbing the mucosal surface; it appears as little white lesions on the tongue. Oral lichen planus is a chronic inflammatory autoimmune disease; it also has white lesions that do not rub off. Oral cancer must be ruled out in any lesion because early detection is the key to successful management and a good prognosis. Thrush may be seen in denture wearers, in debilitated clients, and in those who are immunocompromised or taking corticosteroids or broad-spectrum antibiotics.

9-31   Answer D

The easiest way to differentiate between otitis externa and otitis media is that with otitis externa, movement or pressure on the pinna is extremely painful. With otitis externa, there may also be tender swelling of the outer ear canal. Bilateral pain in the ears is more suggestive of otitis externa. Clients with acute mastoiditis present with severe pain in, and, especially behind, the ear.

9-32   Answer A

Presbyopia is the natural loss of accommodative capacity with age. In the mid-40s, persons note the inability to focus on objects at a normal reading distance. With hyperopia, objects at a distance are not seen clearly unless accommodation is used, and near objects may not be seen. This is corrected with plus or convex lenses. With myopia, the person is able to focus on very near objects without glasses. Far vision is difficult without the aid of corrective minus or concave lenses. With astigmatism, the refractive errors are different in the horizontal and vertical axes.

9-33   Answer A

The most frequent cause of laryngeal obstruction in an adult is a piece of meat that lodges in the airway. With a tumor, there would be a gradual growth, and treatment would probably be sought before there is a complete obstruction. Mucosal swelling from an allergic reaction may result in an obstruction, but this does not occur as frequently as a laryngeal obstruction from a piece of meat. Inhalation of a carcinogen would result only in an irritation of the mucosa, if anything.

9-34   Answer B

Nasal polyps are benign growths that occur frequently in clients with sinus problems, asthma, and allergic rhinitis. Polyps are neither neoplastic growths nor precancerous, but they do have the potential to affect the flow of air through the nasal passages. Clients who have asthma and have nasal polyps may have an associated allergy to aspirin, a syndrome that is referred to as Samter's triad.

9-35   Answer B

Dryness of the eyes and the appearance of "sunken" eyes are normal age-related changes. With hyperthyroidism, the eyes appear to bulge out (exophthalmos), but in hypothyroidism, the eyes do not appear any different. A moon face is apparent with Cushing's syndrome, and this might make the eyes appear to be sunken in, although on close examination, they are not. With a detached retina, the outward appearance is normal, but the client complains of seeing floaters or spots in the visual field and describes the sensation as like a curtain being drawn across the vision.

9-36   Answer D

Older adults are at a higher risk than middle-aged adults for developing an eye infection because of a decrease in tear production, which results in the inability of the tear ducts to wash out infectious organisms.

9-37   Answer B

A hordeolum (stye) is an abscess that may occur on the external or internal margin of the eyelid. It is typically caused by *Staphylococcus* bacteria.

9-38   Answer A

Xanthelasmas are soft, raised, yellow plaques on the eyelids at the inner eye canthus. They appear most frequently in women, beginning in the 50s. Xanthelasmas occur with both high and normal lipid levels and have no pathological significance. Pingueculae are yellowish, elevated nodules appearing on the sclera. They are caused by a thickening of the bulbar conjunctiva from prolonged exposure to the sun, wind, and dust. Arcus senilis appears as gray-white arcs or circles around the limbus as a result of deposits of lipid material that make the cornea look cloudy. Actinic keratoses are wartlike growths on the skin that occur in middle-aged or older adults and are caused by excessive exposure to the sun.

9-39   Answer C

Cranial nerve (CN) VIII, the vestibulocochlear (acoustic) nerve, is affected by sensorineural or perceptive hearing loss. Both the cochlear and vestibular branches have sensory pathways. CN II, the optic nerve, has sensory pathways. CN IV, the trochlear nerve, has both sensory and motor pathways. CN XI, the accessory nerve, has motor pathways.

9-40   Answer A

Although regular ocular pressure testing is indicated for all older adults on a routine basis, it is especially important for clients taking an extended regimen of high-dose inhaled glucocorticoids because prolonged continuous use increases the risk of ocular hypertension or open-angle glaucoma. NSAIDs and ACE inhibitors do not require ocular pressure monitoring. Older adults taking insulin need to have regular eye examinations because they are diabetic and have a risk of diabetic retinopathy, not because they are taking insulin.

9-41   Answer B

Presbyopia occurs in almost all persons beginning about the mid-40s. The lens loses elasticity and becomes hard and glasslike, decreasing its ability to change shape to accommodate for near vision. Arcus senilis, a gray-white arc or circle around the limbus from deposition of lipid material, does not affect vision. Cataracts and glaucoma may occur around age 50 or older.

9-42   Answer A

In older adults, the most common cause of decreased visual functioning is cataract formation (lens opacity), which should be expected by age 70. Glaucoma (increased ocular pressure) is the second most common cause of decreased visual functioning. It increases from age 46–60, then levels off. Macular degeneration (loss of central vision), which affects 30% of persons older than age 65, affects a person's ability to read fine print and do handiwork. Arcus senilis does not affect vision.

9-43   Answer B

Children ages 2½–3 years should have their vision screened using the Allen test, which uses picture cards. The Snellen E chart is used for preschoolers ages 3–6, whereas the Snellen letter chart is used for school-age and older clients. The Rosenbaum chart is used for a gross assessment of near vision by having the client hold reading material approximately 12–14 in. away.

9-44   Answer C

Esotropia is the inward turning of the eyes. Exotropia is the outward turning of the eyes. Strabismus, also called tropia, is the constant malalignment of the eye axes. It is likely to cause amblyopia. Pseudostrabismus has the appearance of strabismus because of the presence of epicanthic folds but is normal in young children.

9-45   Answer B

If a client has throbbing pain in the eye, an irregular pupil shape, marked photophobia, and redness (a deep, dull, red halo or ciliary flush) around the iris and/or cornea, suspect iritis. An immediate referral is warranted. The client may also have blurred vision. The client with conjunctivitis has redness more prominently at the periphery of the eye, along with tearing and itching. The client may also complain of a scratchy, burning, or gritty sensation but not pain, although photophobia may be present. The client with subconjunctival hemorrhage presents with a sudden onset of a painless, bright-red appearance on the bulbar conjunctiva that usually results from pressure exerted during coughing, sneezing, or Valsalva's maneuver. Other conditions that may result in a subconjunctival hemorrhage include uncontrolled hypertension and the use of anticoagulant medication. The client with acute glaucoma presents with circumcorneal redness, with the redness radiating around the iris, and a dilated pupil.

9-46   Answer B

Hypopyon is purulent matter in an inflamed anterior chamber. A hyphema is blood in the anterior chamber, the result of trauma or spontaneous hemorrhage. Anisocoria, common in 5% of the population, refers to unequal pupil size. In 95% of these persons, it indicates central nervous system disease. A pterygium is a painless, unilateral or bilateral, triangle-shaped encroachment onto the conjunctiva that appears on the nasal side and is caused by excessive ultraviolet light exposure.

9-47   Answer D

A common cause of conductive hearing loss in adults ages 20–40 is otosclerosis, a gradual hardening of the tympanic membrane that causes the footplate of the stapes to become fixed in the oval window. Presbycusis, a progressive, bilaterally symmetrical perceptive hearing loss arising from structural changes in the hearing organs, usually occurs after age 50. Trauma may result in a conductive hearing loss, but this is certainly not common.

9-48   Answer D

With bacterial conjunctivitis, there is purulent, thick discharge; with allergic conjunctivitis, a stringy mucoid discharge; and with viral conjunctivitis, there is usually a watery discharge. In a client with iritis, there is rarely a discharge.

9-49   Answer C

Acute otitis media is diagnosed when there is fluid in the middle ear accompanied by signs or symptoms of an ear infection, including fever and otalgia. During the acute stage, acute otitis media is very painful. Inappropriate or ineffective treatment can lead to otitis media with effusion, which is often painless. An acute infection implies a current, not chronic, problem.

9-50   Answer D

A client with acute glaucoma requires urgent treatment and usually presents with sudden onset of impaired vision, severe eye pain, vomiting, and headache. You may assess injected conjunctiva; steamy corneas; a fixed, partially dilated pupil; and a narrow chamber angle. A client with cataracts may present with decreased vision, and you would see an opacity, a cloudy lens, and a decreased view of the fundus. With macular degeneration, there is decreased central vision, and with presbyopia, there may be blurred vision but with a gradual onset. Only acute-angle glaucoma requires urgent treatment.

9-51   Answer C

Benzodiazepines like clonazepam (Klonopin) may be ordered for temporal mandibular joint disorders for a short course of therapy only (1–2 weeks). They may be helpful for acute pain secondary to masticatory muscle spasm or temporomandibular joint pain. Nonopioid analgesics may be ordered for inflammatory pain; anticonvulsants may be ordered for neuropathic pain; and skeletal muscle relaxants may be ordered for muscle relaxation.

9-52 Answer B

The antibiotic of choice for beta-lactamase coverage of otitis media is amoxicillin and potassium clavulanate (Augmentin). It is the first-line treatment for otitis media because it is effective against a wide range of bacteria, including beta lactamase. Amoxicillin (Amoxil) is not effective against beta lactamase. Azithromycin (Zithromax) for otitis media is usually reserved for more resistant strains of the common bacterial pathogens. Prednisone (Deltasone) is reserved for otitis media with effusion.

9-53 Answer A

Most perforated tympanic membranes seen with acute otitis media heal within several weeks. If it has not healed within 3–6 months, a surgical repair can be done, but not until age 7–9 years. Sam can swim on the surface with the use of an ear mold but must not dive, jump, or swim under water.

9-54 Answer A

If a child with otitis media with effusion has a change in the hearing threshold to less than or equal to 20 dB and has notable speech and language delays, more aggressive treatment is indicated. When the child's hearing examination reveals a change in the hearing threshold, it is extremely important that the provider evaluate the child's achievement of developmental milestones in speech and language. Any abnormal findings warrant referral.

9-55 Answer C

The immediate goal of myringotomy and tube placement in a child with recurrent episodes of otitis media is to allow removal of suppurative and mucoid material, thus releasing the pressure. This also prolongs the period of ventilation, allowing the middle ear mucosa to return to normal. Ventilation of the middle ear must be done to restore hearing and prevent aberrations in growth and development associated with hearing loss.

9-56 Answer A

A symptom cluster of severe throat pain with difficulty swallowing, copious oral secretions, respiratory difficulty and stridor, and fever but without pharyngeal erythema or cough is indicative of epiglottitis. Streptococcal pharyngitis presents with cervical adenitis, petechiae, a beefy-red uvula, and a tonsillar exudate. A mild case of tonsillitis may appear to be only a slight sore throat. A more severe case would involve inflamed, swollen tonsils; a very sore throat; and a high fever. Diphtheria starts with a sore throat, fever, headache, and nausea, then progresses to patches of grayish or dirty-yellowish membranes in the throat that eventually grow into one membrane.

9-57 Answer D

When teaching clients about mononucleosis (Epstein-Barr virus [EBV]), tell them to avoid contact sports, heavy lifting, and stress and that convalescence may take several weeks. Antibiotic therapy is not indicated for EBV. Bedrest is necessary only in severe cases.

9-58 Answer D

Currently, there is no effective treatment for atrophic macular degeneration. Laser photocoagulation may slow the exudative form of macular degeneration if performed early in the course of the disease. It seals leaking capillaries and stops the exudation. Clients cope with the disease by using large-print books and magazines, magnifying glasses, and high-intensity lighting.

9-59 Answer B

Using eardrops made of a solution of equal parts of alcohol and vinegar in each ear after swimming is effective in drying the ear canal and maintaining an acidic environment, therefore preventing a favorable medium for the growth of bacteria, the cause of swimmer's ear. It was previously mentioned that nothing smaller than your elbow should go in the ear. A hair dryer on the lowest setting several inches from the ear may be used to dry the canal.

9-60 Answer C

For a client who has had Ménière's disease for several years with some hearing loss but now has persistent vertigo, treatment by vestibular neurectomy might relieve the vertigo. In vestibular neurectomy, the portion of cranial nerve VIII controlling balance and sensations of vertigo is severed. Vertigo is usually relieved in 90% of the cases. A labyrinthectomy is the surgery of last resort for a client with Ménière's disease because the labyrinth is completely removed and cochlear function destroyed. This procedure is used only when hearing loss is nearly complete. Oral diuretics and a low-sodium diet may aid in maintaining a lower labyrinth pressure, which may help slightly. Wearing an earplug will not help and may aggravate the condition.

9-61 Answer C

There is no treatment for a subconjunctival hemorrhage other than to reassure the client that the blood will be reabsorbed within 2 weeks.

9-62 Answer C

The leading cause of blindness in persons ages 20–60 in the United States is diabetic retinopathy, a progressive microangiopathy with small-vessel damage and occlusion. Macular degeneration is the leading cause of blindness in persons older than age 60. Glaucoma may eventually lead to loss of vision, but the symptoms have a slow progression, usually leading the client to eventual surgery to correct the problem. Trauma rarely leads to blindness.

9-63 Answer C

When severe pain is elicited by tugging on a normal-appearing auricle, an acute infection of the external ear canal (otitis externa) is suspected. Otitis media, with or without effusion, cannot be diagnosed without examining the tympanic membrane. Otalgia is simply ear pain.

9-64 Answer A

Barotrauma of the auditory canal causing abnormal middle ear pressure may be relieved by the use of nasal steroids and oral decongestants. With barotrauma, there is no infection, just swelling of the airways, which causes the sensation of abnormal pressure; therefore, antibiotics are not indicated. This is certainly within the practitioner's scope of practice, and a referral is not indicated.

9-65 Answer B

Bruxism is grinding the teeth while sleeping and frequently occurs in young children. Bite blocks will prevent this until the child grows out of it.

9-66 Answer D

The most common cause of sensorineural hearing loss is presbycusis, a gradual decrease in cochlear function that occurs in most persons with advancing age. Otosclerosis (stapes fixation) and tympanic membrane sclerosis and scarring both result in a conductive hearing loss. Trauma would also result in a conductive hearing loss.

9-67 Answer A

In a young child, unilateral purulent rhinitis is most often caused by a foreign body. The key word is *unilateral*. Viral and bacterial infections and allergic reactions usually affect both nares.

9-68 Answer D

Because the cornea is an avascular organ, immune defenses have difficulty fighting off infections.

9-69 Answer A

Carbonic anhydrase inhibitors, such as acetazolamide (Diamox), act as diuretics to reduce the intraocular pressure in clients with glaucoma. A miotic causes contraction of the pupil and a mydriatic dilates the pupil. Because of the effect of pupil dilation on aqueous outflow in angle-closure glaucoma, medications such as atropine and other anticholinergics that have a mydriatic effect should be avoided. Miotics such as pilocarpine (Pilocar) may be given to cause contraction of the sphincter of the iris and to contract the ciliary muscle, which promotes accommodation for near vision and facilitates aqueous humor outflow by increasing drainage through the trabecular meshwork in open-angle glaucoma. But the question is asked about diuretics, which pilocarpine is not. It is a cholinergic agent.

9-70 Answer C

Flushing the ear with water is contraindicated when a client has a probable foreign body or insect in it. The water may cause the object to swell, making removal more difficult. Actions that may be taken include inspecting the ear canal with an otoscope, using a small suction device to try to remove the object, or instilling several drops of mineral oil in the ear.

9-71 Answer B

Approximately 10% of clients with a hearing loss are helped by medical or surgical treatment. If clients are sent for a hearing aid and not correctly identified as having a hearing loss, the underlying problem may not be resolved.

9-72 Answer D

The cervical lymphadenopathy associated with asymptomatic HIV infection may be described as cervical lymph nodes that are firm but not hard, nontender, and mobile. In a healthy person, cervical nodes are often palpable and are movable, discrete, soft, and nontender. In a client with an acute infection, the cervical nodes are bilateral, enlarged, warm, tender, and firm but freely movable. Cancerous nodes are hard, unilateral, nontender, and fixed. In a client with a chronic inflammation, such as tuberculosis, the nodes are clumped.

9-73 Answer A

Microtia refers to the size of the ears, specifically ears smaller than 4 cm vertically.

9-74 Answer B

With a chronic allergy, a client's mucosa appears swollen, boggy, pale, and gray. Redness indicates an acute process and the question asks about a chronic allergy.

9-75 Answer B

Cherry-red lips are a manifestation of carbon monoxide poisoning. They also occur with acidosis from aspirin poisoning or ketoacidosis. In light-skinned clients, circumoral pallor of the lips occurs with shock and anemia and cyanosis of the lips occurs with hypoxemia and chilling. Some lips are normally pale pink.

9-76 Answer C

In a client with mumps, the orifice of Stensen's duct appears red. The buccal mucosa in a normal client appears pink, smooth, and moist, although there may be some patchy hyperpigmentation in dark-skinned clients. Dappled brown patches are present with Addison's disease. Koplik's spots are a prodromal sign of measles.

9-77 Answer C

Tonsils that touch the uvula are graded 3+. A grade of 1+ indicates that the tonsils are visible; a 2+ indicates that the tonsils are halfway between tonsillar pillars and uvula; and 4+ indicates that the tonsils touch each other. Tonsils are enlarged to 2+, 3+, or 4+ with an acute infection.

9-78 Answer D

If a client is taking timolol maleate (Timoptic) drops for chronic open-angle glaucoma, you should be most concerned if the client is also taking atenolol (Tenormin), a beta blocker, for high blood pressure. Because timolol maleate drops are beta-adrenergic blockers, additional beta blockers can cause worsening of congestive heart failure or

reactive airway disease, as well as acute delirium. Aspirin therapy as prophylaxis for heart attack; ranitidine (Zantac) for gastroesophageal reflux disease; and alprazolam (Xanax), an anxiolytic for anxiety, do not interact adversely with eyedrops for glaucoma.

9-79 Answer A

The treatment for hyphema is strict bedrest, with the head elevated at least 20°. The client needs to see an ophthalmologist within 24 hours. In the meantime, the application of bilateral eye patches to minimize eye movement; the instillation of atropine 1%, two drops bid to reduce ciliary spasm; and the administration of appropriate aspirin-free pain medications are indicated.

9-80 Answer A

The symptoms of hay fever, also called allergic rhinitis, are similar to those of viral rhinitis but usually persist and are seasonal in nature. When assessing the nasal mucosa, you will observe that the turbinates are usually pale or violaceous because of venous engorgement with allergic rhinitis. With viral rhinitis, the mucosa is usually erythematous, and with nasal polyps, there are usually yellowish, boggy masses of hypertrophic mucosa. Nasal vestibulitis usually results from folliculitis of the hairs that line the nares.

9-81 Answer B

Management of influenza (flu) is generally symptomatic and includes rest, fluids, acetaminophen (Tylenol), and possibly a decongestant and an antitussive. The client should be advised to call in 4 days if symptoms have not resolved.

9-82 Answer D

For the client with flu, oseltamivir (Tamiflu) or zanamivir (Relenza) may be given. If the virus causing the flu is type A influenza, the client may benefit from either one of these drugs. They are most effective if started early in the course of the disease (within 48 hours), although reduction of symptoms and shortening the course of illness are still possible even if started 3–5 days after symptoms begin.

9-83 Answer B

Caution needs to be used when ordering a second-generation antihistamine for a client taking drugs such as cimetidine (Tagamet), erythromycin

(E-Mycin), clarithromycin (Biaxin), and ketoconazole (Nizoral) that can block cytochrome P450 metabolism or if the client has serious hepatic impairment.

9-84   Answer C

Painless, white, slightly raised patches in a client's mouth are probably caused by candidiasis (thrush). Aphthous ulcers (canker sores) are extremely painful. Herpes simplex (a viral infection), canker sores, and cancerous lesions are usually discrete and not spread over a large area.

9-85   Answer C

When ordering mycostatin (Nystatin) for an oral fungal infection, tell the client to swish the medication in the mouth to coat all the lesions and then to swallow it.

9-86   Answer D

Risk factors for oral cancers include age >50, smoking, use of alcohol, and chewing tobacco.

9-87   Answer C

Milk is the best storage and transport solution for avulsed teeth when one is planning on reimplanting them. If milk is not available, other solutions that might be used include saline (salt water), water, and saliva.

9-88   Answer B

Epstein's pearls are a normal finding in newborns and infants. They appear as small, yellow-white, glistening, pearly papules along the median raphe of the hard palate and on the gums. They look like teeth but are small retention cysts that disappear after a few weeks. Bednar's aphthae are traumatic areas or ulcers that appear on the posterior hard palate on either side of the midline. They result from abrasions while sucking. A buccal tumor is a tumor on the inside of the cheek. Exostosis (torus palatinus) is found in the midline of the posterior two-thirds of the hard palate and is benign. It is a smooth, symmetrical bony structure.

9-89   Answer C

Baby bottle caries, which occur in older infants and toddlers who take a bottle of milk, juice, or sweetened liquid to bed, destroy the upper deciduous teeth. The liquid pools around the upper front teeth, and the mouth bacteria act on the carbohydrates, especially sucrose, in the drink, forming metabolic acids that break down the tooth enamel and destroy its protein.

9-90   Answer C

A Weber test assesses hearing by bone conduction. With normal hearing, sound is heard equally well in both ears, meaning there is no lateralization. With conductive deafness, sound lateralizes to the defective ear because it is transmitted through bone rather than air. With perceptive deafness, sound lateralizes to the better ear.

9-91   Answer C

A smooth tongue may result from a vitamin deficiency. Normally, the dorsal surface of the tongue is rough because of papillae. The ventral surface near the floor of the mouth is smooth and shows large veins.

9-92   Answer D

Signs and symptoms of acute angle-closure glaucoma include seeing halos around lights, severe eye pain and redness, nausea and vomiting, headache, blurred vision, conjunctival injection, cloudy cornea, mid-dilated pupil, and an increased intraocular pressure. Acute angle-closure glaucoma is less common than primary open-angle glaucoma, accounting for about 10% of all glaucoma cases in the United States. Emergency treatment is indicated, so a prompt referral is necessary when these signs and symptoms occur.

9-93   Answer C

A client with retinal detachment complains of a sudden change in vision (either blurry vision, flashing lights, or floaters) but has no pain. On ophthalmoscopy, the retina appears pale, opaque, and folds in and undulates freely as the eye moves. Retinal detachment is an emergency and requires immediate surgery, usually scleral buckling, in which an encircling silicon band is used to keep the choroid in contact with the retina to promote attachment. Iritis is characterized by severe pain. Cataracts and most cases of glaucoma usually present as a gradual change in vision, not a sudden change.

9-94   Answer A

The most common offending allergens causing allergic rhinitis are, in descending order, pollens of grasses, trees, and weeds; fungi; animal allergens;

and dust mites. Rhinitis is the most troublesome allergic problem and affects 20% of the population.

9-95   Answer C

When trying to decide between a diagnosis of conjunctivitis and iritis, one of the distinguishing characteristics is a ciliary flush present in iritis. Photophobia is not usually present in conjunctivitis, but it is always present with iritis. Photophobia occurs with corneal inflammation, iritis, and angle-closure glaucoma. Clients with iritis and conjunctivitis both complain of eye discomfort, although in iritis the pain is moderately severe with intermittent stabbing. Both conditions generally produce a slowly progressive redness. Vision is normal with conjunctivitis and blurred with iritis.

9-96   Answer C

Clients with allergic conjunctivitis have a stringy, white discharge. Clients with bacterial conjunctivitis have a purulent discharge; those with viral conjunctivitis have serous or clear drainage and preauricular lymph node enlargement. A profuse mucoid or mucopurulent discharge is indicative of *chlamydial* conjunctivitis. Human papillomavirus (HPV) also is a risk factor for certain types of oral cancers.

9-97   Answer A

Hordeolum (stye) is the most common localized infection of one of the glands of the eyelids. Treatment includes warm compresses for 15 minutes four times a day and topical antibiotics. A chalazion is a chronic swelling of the eyelids not associated with conjunctivitis. Bacterial conjunctivitis does not involve one of the glands of the eyelids. Primary herpes simplex of the eye usually presents as conjunctivitis with a clear, watery discharge; vesicles on the lids; and preauricular lymphadenopathy.

9-98   Answer B

Keratoconjunctivitis sicca is dry eyes, a common disorder among older women. It is associated with dryness, redness, or a scratchy feeling in the eyes. On rare, severe occasions, there is marked discomfort and photophobia. Typically, it is caused by subtle abnormalities of the tear film and a reduced volume of tears. In most cases, tears can be replenished with the aqueous component of tears with over-the-counter artificial tears. Occasionally, mucomimetics are indicated when there is mucin deficiency. Viral conjunctivitis is caused by a virus and is associated with

pharyngitis, fever, malaise, and preauricular lymph node enlargement. Allergic eye disease is benign and usually occurs in late adolescence or early adulthood. It is usually seasonal, and allergy treatment may be effective. A corneal ulcer is most commonly the result of a bacterial, viral, or fungal infection.

9-99   Answer A

The classic sign of retinal detachment is a client stating that "a curtain came down over my eye." Typically, the person presents with blurred vision in one eye that becomes progressively worse, with no pain or redness. With acute angle-closure glaucoma, there is a rapid onset in older adults, with severe pain and profound visual loss. The eye is red, with a steamy cornea and a dilated pupil. With open-angle glaucoma, there is an insidious onset in older adults, a gradual loss of peripheral vision over a period of years, and perception of "halos" around lights. With a cataract, there is blurred vision that is progressive over months or years and no pain or redness.

9-100   Answer C

With external otitis, there is pain, an erythematous ear canal, and usually a history of recent swimming. Acute otitis media is also painful, is usually a result of cotton swab use or physical trauma, and usually follows an upper respiratory infection. Chronic otitis media is usually not painful, although during an exacerbation the ear may be painful. Ear pain may also be the result of temporomandibular joint dysfunction. It is usually made worse by chewing or grinding the teeth.

9-101   Answer C

Most recently, cognitive behavioral therapy has been recognized as an effective treatment for tinnitus. Therapy is focused on reducing the psychological distress associated with tinnitus and developing coping strategies for dealing with the problem. Antidepressants, such as nortriptyline 50 mg at bedtime, have proved to be effective especially if the tinnitus disrupts sleep. High doses of aspirin over a sustained period of time may actually cause tinnitus. Lidocaine given intravenously suppresses tinnitus in some individuals but is not suitable for long-term suppression. Corticosporin eardrops have proved to have no effect.

9-102   Answer A

The maxillary sinus is the largest of the paranasal sinuses and is the most commonly affected sinus.

There is usually pain and pressure over the cheek. Inability to transilluminate the cavity usually indicates a cavity filled with purulent material. Discolored nasal discharge, as well as a poor response to decongestants, may also indicate sinusitis. The ethmoid sinuses are usually nonpalpable and may not be transilluminated. The frontal sinuses are just below the eyebrows. Frontal sinusitis also includes pain and tenderness of the forehead.

9-103   Answer B

The palpebral fissures are the openings between the margins of the upper and lower eyelids. Someone who appears to be squinting is said to have narrow palpebral fissures. The nasolabial folds are the skin creases that extend from the angle of the nose to the corner of the mouth.

9-104   Answer B

Migraines classically are preceded by an aura and accompanied by nausea, vomiting sometimes, and photophobia. They are usually unilateral. Tension headaches are not associated with photophobia and are usually bilateral and associated with limited neck range of motion (ROM). Tension headaches are not preceded by an aura. Cluster headaches are unilateral, frequently occur at night, and bear some resemblance to migraines; however, cluster headaches are accompanied by tearing, nasal stuffiness, and sweating on the same side as the headache and they come in clusters. The client is not in the age range (older than 50) for temporal arteritis.

9-105   Answer B

The USPSTF found fair evidence that the thyroid-stimulating hormone test (TSH) can detect subclinical thyroid disease in people without symptoms of thyroid dysfunction, but it found poor evidence that treatment improves clinically important outcomes in adults with screen-detected thyroid disease. The USPSTF concluded that the evidence is insufficient to recommend for or against routine screening for thyroid disease in adults.

9-106   Answer C

Though there is not complete historical data, this client has no obvious risk factors for esophageal varices or esophageal cancer. She is a nondrinker and denies weight loss and changes in bowel function or color of stools, which could be a clue to a gastrointestinal bleed. The fact that her worse symptoms occur at night with regurgitation and heartburn is classic for GERD. Dysphagia is frequently a prominent symptom in GERD. She has no abdominal tenderness, and aside from the nighttime symptoms and dysphagia, she reports no symptoms with food or lack of food. Clients with peptic ulcer disease (PUD) frequently complain of clusters of pain separated by periods of no symptoms.

9-107   Answer D

The symptoms of GABS (group A beta-hemolytic streptococcus) are sudden onset of sore throat, exudative tonsillitis, tender anterior cervical lymph nodes, and history of fever. In this client, the sore throat has been present for 24 hours and did not come on suddenly and there is no exudate on the tonsils. Rhinitis, hoarseness, and dry cough are associated with a viral etiology. At this point, a rapid strep screen is appropriate and if the result is negative a strep culture should be done to rule out GABS. This client should not be treated with antibiotics until a positive GABS is reported.

9-108   Answer A

Trigeminal neuralgia is described as a sharp, piercing, shooting facial pain that is severe but usually lasts only a short time. The origin is the trigeminal nerve (CNV). TMJ is associated with pain on opening and closing the mouth and is also associated with crepitus of that joint. A goiter is generally painless. Preauricular adenitis (enlarged and inflamed preauricular nodes) would be sustained until the etiological cause is identified and treated.

9-109   Answer A

Though a change in sleeping habits (i.e., new bed pillows) is a possibility, in this case the character of the pain should lead the practitioner to inquire as to any traumatic event in the past involving her neck, such as a fall or motor vehicle accident or a history of repetitive activity involving the head or neck, such as a change in exercise routine or a new hobby. Spasm of the trapezius will cause difficulty in turning the head to one side or another. Difficulty swallowing, though significant in some clients, doesn't seem related to the presenting complaint.

9-110   Answer D

Cluster headaches come in clusters as this client describes, with exquisite pain awakening the client from sleep. Excessive lacrimation and sweating on the affected side is common. Though this client's pain is unilateral, he does not complain of photophobia and has never had an aura, facts that tend to lead away from a diagnosis of classic migraine. Because the pain is at night, tension headache is a less likely diagnosis. Sinus headache would usually be precipitated by allergies or cold symptoms with nasal congestion.

9-111   Answer B

An ESR may help confirm the diagnosis. An elevated ESR—anywhere from 50–100—may be seen in temporal arteritis; however, the ESR may also be normal. The temporal artery supplies the optic nerve, and if temporal arteritis is suspected due to the age of the client (50 and older) and the location and character of the pain, it is essential that a referral to a surgeon be made for immediate biopsy of the artery before damage to the optic nerve occurs.

9-112   Answer D

Because the herpes virus in this case seems to be along the ophthalmic branch of cranial nerve V, there is considerable risk that this client could develop permanent damage in that eye and an ophthalmological consult needs to be arranged promptly to ascertain damage and prevent any further damage.

9-113   Answer C

The ossicles seen on visualization of the tympanic membrane include the handle and short process of the malleus, and in some individuals you can see the incus through the drum. The pars flaccida is clearly visible. The stapes, cochlea, and round window are not visible.

9-114   Answer A

Sensorineural loss comes from exposure to loud noises, inner ear infections, tumors, congenital and familial disorders, and aging. The etiology of conductive loss includes ear infection, presence of a foreign body, perforated drum, and otosclerosis of the ossicles. The results of the Weber and Rinne test will assist in the diagnosis. Tinnitus is ringing in the ears, and vertigo is dizziness associated with inner ear dysfunction. The client does not complain of either of these symptoms.

9-115   Answer C

In hyperthyroidism the symptoms of rapid pulse, palpitations, and hypertension due to the excess production of T4 and T3 are common, whereas in hypothyroidism the opposite symptom complex is common. Velvety, warm, moist skin is a symptom of hyperthyroidism, whereas dry, coarse skin is a symptom of hypothyroidism. Hyperthyroidism is also characterized by exophthalmos, which is the term for the eyeball protruding forward. When it is bilateral, it may signify infiltrative ophthalmopathy of Graves' disease. There may be associated edema and conjectival injection as well.

9-116   Answer B

Bell's palsy affects the facial nerve resulting in weakness or paralysis of one side of the face. A stroke and shingles are unilateral in their presentation as well. A lesion affecting the sensory portion of the trigeminal nerve could be manifested by bilateral symptoms.

Bibliography

American Academy of Family Physicians, American Academy of Otolaryngology-Head and Neck Surgery, and American Academy of Pediatrics Subcommittee on Otitis Media With Effusion: Clinical practice guideline. *Pediatrics* 113(5):1412–1429, May 2005.

Aronson, AA: Pediatrics, otitis media. eMedicine, updated February 6, 2008. http://www.emedicine.com/EMERG/topic393.htm, accessed 9/2/08.

Bickley, LS: *Bates' Guide to Physical Examination and History Taking,* ed 9. Lippincott Williams & Wilkins, Philadelphia, 2007.

Brown, A, and Vega, C: Rapid strep test most cost-effective for pharyngitis workup in adults. Reuters Health Information, March 31, 2006. http://www.medscape.com/viewarticle/528883, accessed 3/31/06.

Conboy-Ellis, K, and Braker-Shaver, S: Intranasal steroids and allergic rhinitis. *The Nurse Practitioner* 32(4):44–49, 2007.

Daugherty, JA: The latest buzz on tinnitus. *The Nurse Practitioner* 32(10):42–47, 2007.

Diamond, S, and Feoktistov, A: Woman with short-lasting, strictly unilateral headaches. *Consultant* 10, 2007.

Dowdee, A, and Ossege, J: Assessment of childhood allergy for the primary care practitioner. *Journal of* the *American Academy of Nurse Practitioners* 19:53–62, 2007.

Dunphy, LM, et al: *Primary Care: The Art and Science of Advanced Practice Nursing,* ed 2. FA Davis, Philadelphia, 2007.

Guirguis-Blake, J, and Hales, CM: Putting prevention into practice, screening for thyroid disease. *American Family Physician* 71(7), 2005.

Jarvis, J: *Physical Examination and Health Assessment,* ed 3. WB Saunders, Philadelphia, 2000.

Kopes-Kerr, CP, and Alper, BS: Allergic conjunctivitis. *The Clinical Advisor* April, 2007.

Larkin, GL: Retinal detachment. eMedicine, updated April 7, 2008. http://www.emedicine.com/emerg/topic504.htm, accessed 9/2/08.

National Guidelines Clearinghouse: Acute pharyngitis. Institute for Clinical Systems Improvement, Bloomington, MN, May 2005. http://www. guideline.gov/, accessed 4/10/08.

Nootheti, S, and Bielory, L: Risk of cataracts and glaucoma with inhaled steroid use in children. *Comprehensive Ophthalmology Update* 7(11), 2006.

How well did you do?

85% and above, congratulations! This score shows application of test-taking principles and adequate content knowledge.

75%–85%, keep working! Review test-taking principles and try again.

65%–75%, hang in there! Spend some time reviewing concepts and test-taking principles and then try the test again.

Chapter 10: *Respiratory Problems*

JILL E. WINLAND-BROWN

Questions

10-1 *Marisa, who is pregnant, has just been given a diagnosis of tuberculosis. What do you do?*

A. Wait until Marisa delivers and then begin therapy immediately.

B. Begin therapy with isoniazid (Nydrazid), rifampin (Rimactane), and pyrazinamide now.

C. Begin therapy with isoniazid, rifampin, and ethambutol (Myambutol) now.

D. Begin therapy with isoniazid now, wait to see how Marisa tolerates it, and then add rifampin, pyrazinamide, or ethambutol.

10-2 *Which statement about chronic obstructive pulmonary disease (COPD) is true?*

A. The prevalence of COPD is directly related to increasing age.

B. The incidence of COPD is about equal in men and in women.

C. Cigar or pipe smoking does not increase the risk of developing COPD.

D. Environmental factors such as smoke do not affect the potential for COPD.

10-3 *Theophylline when given for COPD acts*

A. as a bronchodilator.

B. by decreasing and strengthening respirations.

C. to impede mucociliary clearance.

D. with a negative inotropic effect.

10-4 *Which bacterial agent is the most common pathogen in an acute exacerbation of chronic bronchitis?*

A. *Streptococcus pneumoniae*

B. *Haemophilus influenzae*

C. *Branhamella catarrhalis*

D. *Moraxella catarrhalis*

10-5 *Which statement is true regarding primary spontaneous pneumothorax?*

A. It usually occurs after individuals have recently started an exercise program.

B. It occurs more commonly in thin elderly men.

C. It usually occurs in healthy individuals without preexisting lung disease.

D. It frequently occurs in Marfan's syndrome.

10-6 *Which of the following is the most frequent contributor to the incidence of carcinoma of the lung?*

A. Chronic pneumonia

B. Exposure to materials such as asbestos, uranium, and radon

C. Chronic interstitial lung diseases

D. Cigarette smoking

10-7 *What would the tumor node metastasis (TNM) classification be for a lung tumor that had carcinoma in situ, metastasis to the lymph nodes in the peribronchial or the ipsilateral hilar region, and distant metastasis to the spine?*

A. T1SN1M1

B. T2N0M0

C. T3N1M1

D. T0N1M0

10-8 *Tina, age 49, is on multiple drug therapy for tuberculosis. She asks you how long she needs to take the drugs. You respond,*

A. "6 weeks to 2 months."

B. "4–6 months."

C. "6–9 months."

D. "1 year."

10-9 *When should well individuals be screened for tuberculosis?*

A. Every year

B. Every other year

C. At age 1 year, then again at entry to preschool or kindergarten, and then at some point during adolescence

D. Every 4 years

10-10 *Which drug category contains the drugs that are the first line of therapy for COPD?*

A. Corticosteroids

B. Inhaled beta-2 agonist bronchodilators

C. Inhaled anticholinergic bronchodilators

D. Xanthines

10-11 *What is a common inhaled allergen in allergic asthma (extrinsic asthma)?*

A. Smoke

B. Cold air

C. Strong smells

D. Pet dander

10-12 *When should a rescue course of prednisolone be initiated for an attack of asthma?*

A. When the client is in step 1 (intermittent stage)

B. When the client is in step 2 (mild persistent stage)

C. When the client is in step 4 (severe persistent stage)

D. Whenever the client needs it, at any time and at any step

10-13 *You are teaching Shawna, age 14 with asthma, to use a home peak expiratory flow meter daily to measure gross changes in peak expiratory flow. Which "zone" would rate her expiratory compliance as 50%–80% of her personal best?*

A. White zone

B. Green zone

C. Yellow zone

D. Red zone

10-14 *Which percentage of individuals for whom it is indicated typically receive the pneumococcus vaccine?*

A. 10%

B. 30%

C. 60%

D. 90%

10-15 *Of the nearly 46 million adults who smoke, 34% try to quit each year, but how many actually succeed?*

A. 2.5%

B. 10%

C. 20%

D. 50%

10-16 *What is the gold standard for the diagnosis of asthma?*

A. Validated quality-of-life questionnaires

B. Client's perception of 'clogged' airways

C. Spirometry

D. Bronchoscopy

10-17 *The well-established risk factor(s) for a nosocomial pneumonia caused by a multidrug-resistant organism is (are)*

A. antibiotic exposure and a hospital stay of more than 1 week.

B. age greater than 65 and having COPD.

C. having outpatient surgery.

D. having allergies to multiple antibiotics.

10-18 *Sally, age 49, has had asthma for several years but has never used a peak flow meter. Should you now recommend it?*

A. No, she has been managing fine without it.

B. Yes, she might recognize early signs of deterioration.

C. Present the options and let Sally decide.

D. No, at her age it is not recommended.

10-19 *You've been counseling your client about her asthma. You realize she doesn't understand your suggestions when she tells you that she'll do which of the following?*

A. Cover the mattress and pillows in airtight, dustproof covers.

B. Wash the bedding weekly and dry it on a hot setting for 20 minutes.

C. Avoid sleeping on natural fibers such as wool or down.

D. Open the windows and air out the room daily.

10-20 *Which of the following is considered a therapeutic indication for a bronchoscopy?*

A. To evaluate indeterminate lung lesions

B. To stage cancer preoperatively

C. To determine the extent of injury secondary to burns, inhalation, or other trauma

D. To remove a foreign body lodged in the trachea

10-21 *Jessica, age 9 months, is brought into the clinic by her mother. She has a low-grade fever, stridor with agitation, some retractions, and a cough, but no drooling. You diagnose viral croup. Your next step would be to*

A. hospitalize Jessica.

B. start antibiotic therapy.

C. order supportive treatment.

D. begin treatment with inhaled corticosteroids.

10-22 *Mr. Marks, age 54, has COPD. He has recently been experiencing difficulty in breathing. His arterial blood gas screening reveals pH 7.3, PaO_2 57 Hg, $PaCO_2$ 54 mm Hg, and oxygen saturation 84%. Mr. Marks has*

A. respiratory acidosis.

B. respiratory alkalosis.

C. metabolic acidosis.

D. metabolic alkalosis.

10-23 *When teaching a mother who has a child with cystic fibrosis, you emphasize that the most important therapeutic approach to promote the child's pulmonary function is to*

A. continuously administer low-flow oxygen.

B. administer bronchodilators on a regular basis.

C. perform chest physiotherapy with postural drainage, percussion, and vibration.

D. use maintenance antibiotic prophylactic therapy.

10-24 *A risk factor for pulmonary embolism in women includes which of the following?*

A. Extreme thinness

B. Alcohol intake

C. Cigarette smoking

D. Hypotension

10-25 *What is the normal ratio of the anteroposterior chest diameter to the transverse chest diameter?*

A. 1:1

B. 1:2

C. 2:3

D. 2:1

10-26 *To ease their breathing, clients with COPD often position themselves in*

A. an erect sitting position.

B. a tripod position.

C. a supine position.

D. a prone position.

10-27 *Increased tactile fremitus occurs with*

A. pleural effusion.

B. lobar pneumonia.

C. pneumothorax.

D. emphysema.

10-28 *Hyperresonance on percussion of the chest occurs with*

A. emphysema.

B. pneumonia.

C. pleural effusion.

D. lung tumor.

10-29 *The inspiratory rate equals the expiratory rate with which breath sound?*

A. Bronchial

B. Bronchovesicular

C. Vesicular

D. Tracheal

10-30 *With which voice sound technique do you normally hear a muffled "eeee" through the stethoscope on auscultating the chest when the client says "eeee"?*

A. Bronchophony

B. Egophony

C. Whispered pectoriloquy

D. Tonometry

10-31 *Mary, age 69, has COPD. Her oxygen saturation is less than 85%. She is to start on oxygen therapy to relieve her symptoms. How often must she be on oxygen therapy to actually improve her oxygen saturation?*

A. On an as-needed basis

B. Continuously

C. 6–12 hours per day

D. 18 hours per day

10-32 *Which is the accepted mass screening test for lung cancer?*

A. An annual physical examination

B. A chest x-ray

C. Sputum cytology

D. There is no accepted mass screening test for lung cancer.

10-33 *What is effective in the treatment of pneumonia, atelectasis, and cystic fibrosis?*

A. Deep breathing

B. Oxygen

C. Inhalers

D. Chest physiotherapy

10-34 *Which of the following medications commonly prescribed for tuberculosis cannot be taken by pregnant women?*

A. Isoniazid (INH)

B. Rifampin (RIF)

C. Pyrazinamide (PZA)

D. Ethambutol (EMB)

10-35 *Which of the following statements is true regarding weight and smoking cessation?*

A. Smokers weigh 10–20 lb less than nonsmokers.

B. When smokers quit, 90% of them gain weight.

C. Men gain more weight than women when they quit.

D. Smokers gain weight after smoking cessation because they replace cigarettes with food.

10-36 *When teaching smokers about using nicotine gum to aid in smoking cessation, tell them to*

A. chew the gum like regular gum.

B. discard the gum after 30 minutes.

C. drink a cup of coffee before chewing the gum because it assists in the nicotine absorption.

D. chew 6–9 pieces daily to help prevent nicotine withdrawal.

10-37 *Which of the following peripharyngeal upper respiratory tract infections occurs most often in children ages 2–5 years?*

A. Peritonsillar abscess

B. Epiglottitis

C. Laryngotracheobronchitis (croup)

D. Bacterial tracheitis

10-38 *Susie, age 10, has a cough that characteristically occurs all day long, but never during sleep. You suspect*

A. a psychogenic cough (or habit).

B. allergic rhinitis.

C. pertussis.

D. postnasal drip.

10-39 *Which of the following drugs causes a cough by inducing mucus production (bronchorrhea)?*

A. Tobacco and/or marijuana

B. Beta-adrenergic blockers

C. Aspirin and NSAIDs

D. Cholinesterase inhibitors

10-40 *The following figure shows a method of assessing for digital clubbing called*

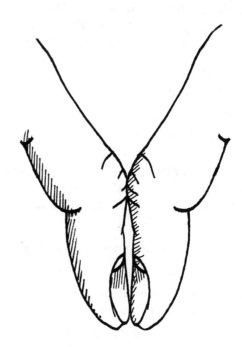

A. phalangeal depth ratio.

B. hyponychial angle.

C. the Schamroth sign.

D. the "diamond" test.

10-41 *What is the name of the horizontal groove in the rib cage at the level of the diaphragm, extending from the sternum to the midaxillary line that occurs normally in some children, as well as in children with rickets?*

A. The sternal groove

B. The rickettsial groove

C. The manubrial groove

D. Harrison's groove

10-42 *What would be the 1-minute Apgar score for a newborn in good condition who needs only* *suctioning of the nose and mouth and otherwise routine care?*

A. 7–10

B. 6–8

C. 3–6

D. 0–2

10-43   *In which age group does respiratory retraction occur more often?*

A. Newborn and infant

B. School-age child

C. Young adult

D. Older adult

10-44   *An infant who has periodic breathing with persistent or prolonged apnea (greater than 20 seconds) may have an increased risk of*

A. pneumonia.

B. left-sided congestive heart failure.

C. sudden infant death syndrome (SIDS).

D. anemia.

10-45   *Stridor can be heard on auscultation when a client has*

A. atelectasis.

B. asthma.

C. diaphragmatic hernia.

D. acute epiglottitis.

10-46   *The nursing diagnosis of "impaired gas exchange" may be demonstrated by*

A. clubbing of the fingers.

B. nasal flaring.

C. the use of accessory muscles.

D. a cough.

10-47   *Which irregular respiratory pattern has a series of three to four normal respirations followed by a period of apnea and is seen with head trauma, brain abscess, heat stroke, spinal meningitis, and encephalitis?*

A. Cheyne-Stokes respiration

B. Biot's breathing

C. Kussmaul's respiration

D. Hypoventilation

10-48   *What is the definition of the spirometric assessment of residual volume?*

A. The sum of the vital capacity and the residual volume

B. The amount of gas left in the lung after exhaling all that is physically possible

C. The volume that can be maximally exhaled after a passive exhalation

D. The measurement of the maximum flow rate achieved during the forced vital capacity maneuver

10-49   *Which of the following conditions is characterized by intermittent episodes of airway obstruction caused by bronchospasm, excessive bronchial secretion, or edema of bronchial mucosa?*

A. Asthma

B. Atelectasis

C. Acute bronchitis

D. Emphysema

10-50   *In which condition would you assess vesicular breath sounds, moderate vocal resonance, and localized crackles with sibilant wheezes?*

A. Bronchiectasis

B. Acute bronchitis

C. Emphysema

D. Asthma

10-51   *Which of the following statements is true regarding the recurrence of a spontaneous pneumothorax?*

A. A primary spontaneous pneumothorax is more likely to recur than a secondary one.

B. A secondary spontaneous pneumothorax is more likely to recur than a primary one.

C. Recurrence rates for both primary and secondary spontaneous pneumothorax are similar.

D. Spontaneous pneumothorax rarely recurs.

10-52   *Which of the following underlying lung diseases is the most common cause of a secondary spontaneous pneumothorax?*

A. COPD

B. Lung abscess

C. Cystic fibrosis

D. Tuberculosis

10-53 What is the term describing an auscultation sound at the mediastinum in the presence of a mediastinal "crunch" that coincides with cardiac systole and diastole?

A. Homans' sign

B. Hamman's sign

C. Manubrium's sign

D. Louis' sign

10-54 The causative agent of the community-acquired pneumonia seen most often in the client with an alcohol problem is

A. *Pneumococcus.*

B. *Mycoplasma.*

C. *Legionella.*

D. *Haemophilus influenzae.*

10-55 Increased severity of underlying illness, presence of an indwelling urethral catheter, and use of broad-spectrum antibiotics are risk factors predisposing clients to the development of

A. tuberculosis.

B. decreased mobility.

C. pressure ulcers.

D. nosocomial pneumonia.

10-56 What do you include in your teaching about Spiriva (tiotropium) when you initially prescribe it for your client with COPD?

A. Use it every time you use your beta-2 agonist.

B. Stop taking all your other COPD medications.

C. Use this once per day.

D. Stop taking Spiriva if you develop the adverse effect of dry mouth.

10-57 Mark, age 72, has been living in a shelter for 4 months. Today he appears at the clinic complaining of productive cough, weight loss, weakness, anorexia, night sweats, and generalized malaise. These have been bothering him for 8 weeks. What would be one of the first tests you order?

A. Mantoux test

B. Chest x-ray

C. Complete blood work

D. Sputum culture

10-58 Harvey is taking theophylline for his COPD. Which of the following increases the clearance rate and might indicate the need for a higher dosage of theophylline to be ordered?

A. Cigarette smoking

B. Hepatic insufficiency

C. Allopurinol (Zyloprim)

D. Cimetidine (Tagamet)

10-59 Which of the following statements about sarcoidosis is true?

A. It commonly occurs in persons in their 50s.

B. It is more common in whites than in blacks.

C. Many organs may be involved, but the most involved organ is the lung.

D. It occurs more frequently in men than in women.

10-60 Marci, age 15, has been given a diagnosis of step 1 (mild intermittent) asthma. What long-term control therapy is indicated?

A. None

B. A single agent with anti-inflammatory activity

C. An inhaled corticosteroid with the addition of long-acting bronchodilator if needed

D. Multiple long-term control medications with oral corticosteroids if needed

10-61 What is the normal respiratory rate of an 18-month-old child while awake?

A. 58–75 breaths per minute

B. 30–40 breaths per minute

C. 23–42 breaths per minute

D. 19–36 breaths per minute

10-62 A definitive test for cystic fibrosis is

A. the sweat test.

B. a sputum culture.

C. a fecal fat test.

D. a Chymex test for pancreatic insufficiency.

10-63 What is the most common cause of sudden and unexpected death in infants, accounting for 80% of post-neonatal infant mortality with a peak incidence at 6 months?

A. Choking

B. Shaken baby syndrome

C. Infantile pneumonia

D. Sudden infant death syndrome (SIDS)

10-64 *The two most predominant organisms constituting the normal flora of the oropharynx are*

A. *Streptococci* and *Staphylococci.*

B. *Streptococci* and *Moraxella catarrhalis.*

C. *Staphylococci* and *Candida albicans.*

D. various protozoa and *Staphylococci.*

10-65 *What early acid-base disturbance occurs in a teenager admitted for an aspirin overdose?*

A. Respiratory acidosis

B. Respiratory alkalosis

C. Metabolic acidosis

D. Metabolic alkalosis

10-66 *Which of the following statements regarding the respiratory status of the pregnant woman is false?*

A. The thoracic cage may appear wider.

B. The costal angle may feel wider.

C. Respirations may be deeper.

D. Oxygenation is decreased.

10-67 *Which shape of the thorax is normal in an adult?*

A. Elliptical

B. Funnel

C. Pectus carinatum

D. Barrel

10-68 *Which of the following workers is at risk for developing pneumoconiosis?*

A. Farmers

B. Coal miners

C. Construction workers

D. Potters

10-69 *Cough and congestion result when breathing*

A. carbon monoxide.

B. sulfur dioxide.

C. tear gas.

D. carbon dioxide.

10-70 *A cough caused by a postnasal drip related to sinusitis is more prevalent at what time of day?*

A. Continuously throughout the day

B. In the early morning

C. In the afternoon and evening

D. At night

10-71 *In which condition would the trachea be deviated toward the normal side?*

A. Pleural effusion and thickening

B. Pneumonia

C. Bronchiectasis

D. Pulmonary fibrosis

10-72 *Which sympathomimetic agents are the drugs of choice for asthma?*

A. Alpha agonists

B. Beta-1 agonists

C. Beta-2 agonists

D. Alpha antagonists

10-73 *Jamie has her asthma well controlled by using only a beta-adrenergic metered-dose inhaler. Lately, however, she has had difficulty breathing during the night and her sleep has been interrupted about three times a week. What do you do?*

A. Prescribe a short course of steroid therapy.

B. Prescribe an inhaled steroid.

C. Prescribe a longer-acting bronchodilator.

D. Prescribe oral theophylline.

10-74 *Community-acquired bacterial pneumonia is most commonly caused by*

A. *Streptococcus pneumoniae.*

B. *Mycoplasma pneumoniae.*

C. *Haemophilus influenzae.*

D. *Staphylococcus aureus.*

10-75 *The antibiotic of choice for the treatment of* Streptococcus pneumoniae *infection is*

A. dicloxacillin.

B. erythromycin.

C. penicillin.

D. ampicillin clavulanate.

10-76 *Martin, age 76, has just been given a diagnosis of pneumonia. Which of the following is an indication that he should be hospitalized?*

A. Inability to take oral medications and multilobar involvement on chest x-ray

B. Alert and oriented status, slightly high but stable vital signs, and no one to take care of him at home

C. Sputum with gram-positive organisms

D. A complete blood count (CBC) showing leukocytosis

10-77 *Which of the following statements is true regarding pulmonary tuberculosis?*

A. Manifestations are usually confined to the respiratory system.

B. Dyspnea is usually present in the early stages.

C. Crackles and bronchial breath sounds are usually present in all phases of the disease.

D. Night sweats are often noted as a manifestation of fever.

10-78 *Which group is at the highest risk for tuberculosis?*

A. Racial and ethnic minorities

B. Foreign-born individuals

C. Substance abusers

D. Nursing home residents

10-79 *Which of the following individuals most likely will have a false-negative reaction to the Mantoux test?*

A. Marvin, age 59

B. Jane, who is on a short course of corticosteroid therapy for an acute exacerbation of asthma

C. Jerry, who has lymphoid leukemia

D. Mary, who recently was exposed to someone coughing

10-80 *The diagnosis of tuberculosis does not need to be reported when*

A. the client's Mantoux test shows an induration of 15 mm.

B. a case of tuberculosis is only suspected.

C. an asymptomatic client has a positive chest x-ray for pulmonary tuberculosis.

D. the Mantoux test shows a raised injected or red area without induration.

10-81 *The most common cause of a persistent cough in children of all ages is*

A. an allergy.

B. recurrent viral bronchitis.

C. asthma.

D. an upper respiratory infection.

10-82 *Which of the following differential diagnoses should be considered with a chronic cough in children ages 1–5 years after the more common causes have been ruled out?*

A. Allergic rhinitis

B. Chronic sinusitis

C. Enlarged adenoids

D. Cystic fibrosis

10-83 *Unexplained nocturnal cough in an older adult should suggest*

A. allergies.

B. asthma.

C. congestive heart failure.

D. viral syndrome.

10-84 *Evidenced-based practice has shown that clients with COPD will benefit the most from which of the following single modalities?*

A. Nutritional supplementation

B. Routine use of inspiratory muscle training

C. Pulmonary rehabilitation

D. Psychosocial interventions

10-85 *Which of the following statements is true when trying to differentiate pulmonary from cardiac causes of dyspnea on exertion?*

A. When the cause is pulmonary, the rate of recovery to normal respiration is slow, and dyspnea abates eventually after cessation of exercise.

B. Clients with dyspnea from cardiac causes remain dyspneic much longer after cessation of exercise.

C. In dyspnea arising from cardiac causes, the heart rate will return to preexercise levels within a few minutes after cessation of exercising.

D. Clients with pulmonary dyspnea have minimal dyspnea at rest.

10-86 *Laura, age 36, has an acute onset of dyspnea. Associated symptoms include chest pain, faintness, tachypnea, peripheral cyanosis, low blood pressure, crackles, and some wheezes. Her history reveals that she is taking birth control pills and that she smokes. What do you suspect?*

A. Asthma

B. Bronchitis

C. Pulmonary emboli

D. Pneumothorax

10-87 *What percentage of persons who smoke one pack of cigarettes per day or more have a cough?*

A. 10%–25%

B. 40%–60%

C. 75%

D. 100%

10-88 *The most common reason for a chronic cough in children is*

A. asthma.

B. a postinfection.

C. a postnasal drip.

D. an irritant.

10-89 *A pulmonary function test, such as spirometry, is helpful in the diagnosis of*

A. chronic bronchitis.

B. lung cancer.

C. pneumonia.

D. tuberculosis.

10-90 *Which drug contributes to a decreased response to tuberculin skin testing (TST)?*

A. Antibiotics

B. Inhaled allergy medications

C. Corticosteroids

D. Birth control pills

10-91 *Which is the most notable clinical manifestation of glottis (tongue) cancer?*

A. Earache

B. Halitosis

C. Hoarseness

D. Frequent swallowing

10-92 *After a total laryngectomy for laryngeal cancer, the client will have a*

A. permanent tracheostomy.

B. temporary tracheostomy until the internal surgical incision heals.

C. temporary tracheostomy until an implant can be done.

D. patent normal airway.

10-93 *Michael, age 52, has a dry cough, dyspnea, chills, fever, general malaise, headache, confusion, anorexia, diarrhea, myalgias, and arthralgias. Which diagnosis do you suspect?*

A. Bronchopneumonia

B. Legionnaires' disease

C. Primary atypical pneumonia

D. *Pneumocystis jiroveci* pneumonia

10-94 *In trying to differentiate between chronic bronchitis and emphysema, you know that chronic bronchitis*

A. usually occurs after age 50 and has insidious progressive dyspnea.

B. usually presents with a cough that is mild and with scant, clear sputum, if any.

C. presents with adventitious sounds, wheezing and rhonchi, and a normal percussion note.

D. results in an increased total lung capacity with a markedly increased residual volume.

10-95 *James, age 12, just moved here from Texas. He presents with a headache, cough, fever, rash on the legs and arms, myalgias, and dysuria. His white blood cell count is 12.9 with 8% bands and 7%–10% eosinophils. Electrolyte levels are normal. Blood cultures are negative. Sputum is not available. A Mantoux skin test so far is negative. What do you suspect?*

A. Pulmonary tuberculosis

B. Lymphoma

C. Asthma

D. Coccidioidomycosis

10-96 *In inner-city children, an important cause of asthma-related illness and hospitalizations is*

A. heredity and genetics.

B. vitamin deficiencies.

C. cockroaches.

D. playing on asphalt playgrounds.

10-97   *Jill, age 49, has daily symptoms of asthma. She uses her inhaled short-acting beta-2 agonist daily. Her exacerbations affect her activities, and they occur at least twice weekly and may last for days. She is affected more than once weekly during the night with an exacerbation. Which category of asthma severity is Jill in?*

A. Mild intermittent

B. Mild persistent

C. Moderate persistent

D. Severe persistent

10-98   *What should be considered in all clients with adult-onset asthma or in clients with asthma that worsens in adulthood?*

A. Occupational asthma

B. A suppressed immune system

C. Another immunologic disease

D. Concurrent COPD

10-99   *How does pregnancy affect asthma?*

A. During pregnancy, asthma usually improves.

B. During pregnancy, asthma usually worsens.

C. Symptoms in about one-third of pregnant women with asthma improve, about one-third are unchanged, and about one-third worsen.

D. Symptoms in about one-half of pregnant women improve; those of the other half worsen.

10-100   *Other than smoking cessation, which of the following slows the progression of COPD in smokers?*

A. Making sure the environment is free of all pollutants

B. Eliminating all pets from the environment

C. Engaging in moderate to high levels of physical activity

D. Remaining indoors with air conditioning as much as possible

10-101   *During the history portion of a respiratory assessment, it's particularly important to ask if the client takes which of the following drugs?*

A. Beta-2 agonists

B. Calcium channel blockers

C. Angiotensin-converting enzyme (ACE) inhibitors

D. Birth control pills

10-102   *Coughing up blood or sputum that is streaked or tinged with blood is known as*

A. hemoptysis.

B. regurgitation.

C. bloody sputum.

D. rhinorrhea.

10-103   *When you teach clients about using steroid inhalers for asthma or COPD, what information is essential?*

A. Keep the inhaler in the refrigerator.

B. Do not use another inhaler for 10 minutes after the steroid inhaler.

C. Rinse your mouth after using.

D. Be careful not to shake the container prior to using.

10-104   *The most common mode of transmission of the common cold in adults is*

A. hand-to-hand transmission.

B. persons coughing into the air.

C. environmental pollutants.

D. unclean food utensils.

10-105   *Persons requiring home oxygen will have an oxygen saturation below*

A. 90%.

B. 85%.

C. 80%.

D. 75%.

10-106   *The definitive test for sleep apnea is*

A. a Holter monitor.

B. a trial period of a continuous positive air pressure (CPAP) appliance.

C. an overnight polysomnogram.

D. an ear, nose, and throat (ENT) specialist confirming an abnormal uvula.

Answers

10-1   Answer C

Treatment of tuberculosis in pregnant women is essential and should not be delayed; therefore,

Marisa's treatment should begin now. The preferred initial treatment is isoniazid (Nydrazid), rifampin (Rimactane), and ethambutol (Myambutol). The teratogenicity of pyrazinamide is undetermined, so it is not wise to use this drug unless resistance to the other drugs is demonstrated or is likely.

10-2   Answer A

The prevalence of chronic obstructive pulmonary disease (COPD) is directly related to increasing age. Men are affected much more often than women because the percentage of men who smoke is greater than that of women. The risk of developing COPD is related to the number of cigarettes smoked and the duration of smoking. Cigar or pipe smoking also increases the risk of developing COPD, but to a lesser extent than does cigarette smoking. Environmental factors, including secondhand smoke, also affect the potential for COPD. The usual client with COPD is one who is older than age 50 and has smoked one pack of cigarettes per day for more than 20 years.

10-3   Answer A

Theophylline, a methylxanthine derivative, acts as a bronchodilator, decreases dyspnea, improves mucociliary clearance, improves gas exchange, enhances respiratory muscle performance, increases neuroinspiratory drive, and has a positive inotropic effect. The decision to institute theophylline therapy must be individualized and should not be universally made in all clients with COPD. It should be added to the treatment plan in clients who have not achieved an optimal clinical response to beta agonists and ipratropium (Atrovent) metered-dose inhalers.

10-4   Answer A

While viral bronchitis requiring only supportive care is the most common etiology of acute exacerbations of chronic bronchitis, bacterial involvement must be considered when there is increased sputum production lasting over a week or new chest x-ray findings. *Streptococcus pneumoniae* is the most common agent, followed by *Haemophilus influenzae* and *Moraxella catarrhalis*, similar to the causative agents of sinusitis and community-acquired pneumonia. *Branhamella catarrhalis* and *Moraxella catarrhalis* are the same organism.

10-5   Answer C

A primary spontaneous pneumothorax usually occurs in healthy individuals without preexisting lung disease. It occurs more commonly in young, tall, asthenic men and is an accumulation of air in the normally airless pleural space between the lung and chest wall. Persons with Marfan's syndrome are more prone to aortic aneurysms, not to pneumothorax.

10-6   Answer D

The following contribute to the incidence of carcinoma of the lung: cigarette smoking; exposure to materials such as asbestos, uranium, and radon; and chronic interstitial lung diseases such as pulmonary fibrosis arising from scleroderma. It is estimated that approximately 2 million persons will develop carcinoma of the lung in each of the next several years; 85% of all lung carcinomas are secondary to cigarette use.

10-7   Answer A

A T1SN1M1 indicates that the lung carcinoma is in situ, has metastasis to the lymph nodes in the peribronchial or the ipsilateral hilar region, and has distant metastasis to the spine. Although the TNM system is generalized for all solid tumors, it is often adapted for specific types of cancers. T is for the relative tumor size, N indicates the presence and extent of lymph node involvement, and M denotes distant metastases. For specific lung cancer staging, the T may range from 0, with no evidence of primary tumor, to 4, which indicates that the tumor has invaded the mediastinum or involves the heart, great vessels, trachea, esophagus, vertebral body, or carina and there is presence of malignant pleural effusion. The N may range from 0, indicating no regional lymph node metastasis, to 3, indicating metastasis to the contralateral, mediastinal, scalene, or supraclavicular nodes. The M is either X, indicating that the presence of distant metastasis cannot be assessed, or 1, meaning that distant metastasis is present.

10-8   Answer C

With the use of multiple drug therapy for tuberculosis, the duration of the therapy has shortened from 1 year to a standard of 6–9 months. If the client has a drug-resistant organism or is immunodeficient, the precise duration of therapy is uncertain but may extend from 1–2 years in some cases.

10-9   Answer C

Current recommendations for well individuals suggest screening for tuberculosis (TB) using an intradermal or multipuncture skin test at age 1 year, then again at entry to preschool or kindergarten, and then at some point during adolescence. TB testing should be considered for all new immigrants, as well as for young people planning to study or travel extensively in areas where TB is endemic.

10-10   Answer B

All the drugs listed may be appropriate for COPD, but inhaled short-acting beta-2 agonist bronchodilators are the first line of therapy in the Global Initiative for Chronic Obstructive Lung Disease (GOLD) in stage 1.

10-11   Answer D

Allergic asthma (extrinsic asthma) is a chronic inflammatory disorder of the airways. The symptoms of allergic and nonallergic asthma are the same, but the triggers are not. Allergic asthma is triggered by inhaled exposure to allergens. The most common of these are dust mites, pet dander, pollens, mold, grass, and ragweed. Nonallergic asthma triggers generally don't cause inflammation but can aggravate airways, especially if they're already inflamed. Nonallergic triggers include smoke, exercise, cold air, strong smells like chemicals and perfume, air pollutants, and intense emotions.

10-12   Answer D

A rescue course of prednisolone should be initiated for an attack of asthma whenever the client needs it, at any time and at any step. Attempts should be made to use systemic corticosteroids in an acute or rescue fashion: a short burst followed by tapering to the lowest dose possible and preferably discontinued, with inhaled steroids prescribed for chronic or maintenance therapy.

10-13   Answer C

Shawna should perform a peak expiratory flow meter reading daily during a 2-week period when she feels well. The highest number recorded during this period is her "personal best." A green zone (80%–100% of her personal best) is when no asthma symptoms are present and she should continue with her normal medication regimen. A yellow zone (50%–80% of her personal best) occurs when asthma symptoms may be starting and signals caution. A red zone (below 50% of her personal best) indicates that an asthma attack is occurring and that Shawna should take her inhaled beta-2

agonist and repeat the peak flow assessment. There is no white zone.

10-14   Answer B

Despite widespread endorsement by numerous medical and nursing organizations, the pneumococcal polysaccharide vaccine is administered to only 30% of individuals for whom it is indicated. Experts from the Advisory Committee on Immunization Practices estimate that as many as 90% of deaths attributed to *Streptococcus pneumoniae* could be prevented if use of the currently available vaccine were more common. Pneumococci account for more deaths than any other vaccine-preventable disease. The pneumococcal vaccine should be considered for the following persons: persons aged 65 and older; children older than age 2 with chronic heart and lung disorders; children older than age 2 with spleen dysfunction; persons with leukemia, kidney failure, organ transplantation, or immunosuppressive disorders; and Alaskan natives and certain Native American populations. If an elective splenectomy or immunosuppressive therapy is planned, the vaccine should be given 2 weeks prior to the procedure.

10-15   Answer A

Of the nearly 46 million adults who smoke, 34% try to quit each year, but only 2.5% succeed. Although the overall success rate of smoking cessation is disappointing, smoking cessation programs have been extremely helpful. Motivation is the key to a successful effort, along with making every clinical encounter an opportunity to discuss the topic. At the very least, every client should be asked about his or her smoking history. Clinicians should advise smokers to quit, assist them in setting a quitting date, provide self-help materials, and evaluate them for nicotine replacement therapy (patches, nasal spray, or gum) or pharmacological therapies.

10-16   Answer C

Spirometry remains the gold standard for the diagnosis of asthma, as well as for periodic monitoring of the condition. Routine use of validated quality-of-life questionnaires may detect impairment and severity of the disease.

10-17   Answer A

Treatment of nosocomial pneumonia is complicated by the frequent involvement of multidrug-resistant organisms. Prior exposure to antibiotics and a hospital stay of more than 1 week are well-established risk factors for infection with these organisms.

10-18   Answer B

Daily peak flow monitoring has long been recommended for clients with asthma. The new guidelines from the National Asthma Education and Prevention Program of the National Heart, Lung, and Blood Institute increase the flexibility of this recommendation and suggest that the use of peak flow measurements be individualized. The guidelines recommend that all clients with persistent asthma assess peak flow each morning. Subsequent assessments are necessary during the day when the morning measurement is less than 80% of the client's personal best peak expiratory flow (PEF) measurement. The goal of daily PEF monitoring is to recognize early signs of deterioration in airway function so that corrective steps can be initiated.

10-19   Answer D

To control the common asthma trigger of dust mites, the following measures are recommended: Cover the mattress and pillows in airtight, dust-proof covers; wash the bedding weekly and dry it on a hot setting for 20 minutes; avoid sleeping on natural fibers such as wool or down; remove all carpeting from bedrooms; and reduce indoor humidity to less than 50%. Opening the windows daily would allow allergens to enter.

10-20   Answer D

There are both diagnostic and therapeutic indications for a bronchoscopy. The therapeutic uses include removal of mucous plugs, secretions, and foreign bodies; assistance with difficult endotracheal intubations; and treatment of endobronchial neoplasms. Diagnostic uses include evaluation of indeterminate lung lesions (abnormal chest film); preoperative staging of cancer; determination of the extent of injury secondary to burns, inhalation, or other trauma; assessment of airway patency, including problems associated with endotracheal tubes, wheeze, and stridor; investigation of unexplained symptoms (cough, hemoptysis, stridor, and so on) or unexplained findings (recurrent laryngeal nerve paralysis, recent diaphragmatic paralysis); evaluation of suspicious or malignant sputum cytology; bronchoalveolar lavage for interstitial lung disease; and specimen collection for selective cultures or suspected infection.

10-21   Answer C

The treatment of viral croup is supportive. Mist therapy, oral hydration, and minimal handling are recommended. The presence of stridor at rest requires hospitalization. Antibiotic therapy is not indicated because this condition is viral. The use of corticosteroids remains controversial in this instance. A short course may be tried if the client is unresponsive to epinephrine, but the corticosteroid is given orally or parentally. Nebulized steroids may also be effective, but they are not available in the United States.

10-22   Answer A

Respiratory acidosis results when the serum $PaCO_2$ exceeds 45 mm Hg and the serum pH is less than 7.35. It occurs when there is a reduction in the rate of alveolar ventilation in relation to the rate of carbon dioxide production. The end result is an accumulation of dissolved carbon dioxide or carbonic acid. Mr. Marks' COPD leads to alveolar hypoventilation with an acute retention of carbon dioxide, resulting in acute respiratory acidosis. With respiratory alkalosis, hyperventilation is usually evident, the $PaCO_2$ is less than 35 mm Hg, and the pH is greater than 7.45. In metabolic acidosis, the HCO_3 is less than 22 mEq/L and the pH is less than 7.35. In metabolic alkalosis, the HCO_3 is more than 26 mEq/L and the pH is greater than 7.45.

10-23   Answer C

Daily performance of chest physiotherapy with postural drainage, percussion, and vibration to remove the abnormally viscous mucus is essential for the client with cystic fibrosis. With cystic fibrosis, the problem lies at the level of the epithelial cells of the small airways, not the bronchi; therefore, bronchodilators do not help. Antibiotics should be administered during an infectious process, not prophylactically. Oxygen therapy may be required for hypoxemia, but not continuously.

10-24   Answer C

A large prospective study in women showed that obesity, cigarette smoking, and hypertension increased their risk for pulmonary embolism. Alcohol intake does not predispose a woman to pulmonary embolism.

10-25   Answer B

The normal anteroposterior diameter of the chest as compared with the transverse diameter is approximately 1:2. An anteroposterior measurement that equals the transverse measurement is defined as a barrel chest, which usually indicates some obstructive lung disease.

10-26 Answer B

Clients with COPD often sit in a tripod position: leaning forward with their arms braced against their knees, a chair, or a bed. This provides clients with leverage so that their rectus abdominal, intercostal, and accessory neck muscles can all assist with expiration.

10-27 Answer B

Increased tactile fremitus occurs with compression or consolidation of lung tissue, such as occurs in conditions like lobar pneumonia. Decreased tactile fremitus occurs when anything obstructs the transmission of vibrations, such as occurs in conditions like pleural effusion, pneumothorax, and emphysema or with an obstructed bronchus.

10-28 Answer A

Hyperresonance on percussion of the chest is found when too much air is present, such as occurs with emphysema or a pneumothorax. A dull sound on percussion indicates an abnormal density in the lungs, such as occurs with pneumonia, pleural effusion, a lung tumor, or atelectasis.

10-29 Answer B

With bronchovesicular breath sounds, the inspiratory rate equals the expiratory rate. With bronchial or tracheal breath sounds, the inspiratory rate is shorter than the expiratory rate, and with vesicular breath sounds, the inspiratory rate is greater than the expiratory rate.

10-30 Answer B

Hearing a muffled (and sometimes nondistinct) "eeee" through the stethoscope when auscultating the chest when the client says "eeee" is known as egophony. When consolidation is present, the "eeee" sound changes to an "aaaaa" sound. With bronchophony, when the client repeats "99-99-99," normally you can hear a soft, muffled, indistinct sound but cannot distinguish what is being said. With whispered pectoriloquy, when the client whispers "1-2-3," a normal response is faint, muffled, and almost inaudible. Tonometry measures intraocular pressure.

10-31 Answer D

To decrease mortality in clients with COPD whose oxygen saturations are less than 85%, oxygen must be used at least 18 hours per day to be of more than symptomatic benefit. The oxygen can be either a specific concentration delivered by mask or a flow rate administered through a nasal cannula. It is needed to maintain adequate oxygenation levels during both activity and rest.

10-32 Answer D

Currently, there is no accepted mass screening test for lung cancer. Because of cost, mass screening for lung cancer in healthy individuals with no risk factors is not recommended. Individuals who are at high risk (those who are cigarette smokers, have been exposed to radon or asbestos, and have a strong family history) should be periodically screened through the use of an annual physical examination, chest x-ray, and possibly sputum cytology. Suspicious chest x-rays should be followed by further diagnostic tests.

10-33 Answer D

Chest physiotherapy is effective in the treatment of pneumonia; atelectasis; and diseases resulting in weak or ineffective coughing, such as cystic fibrosis. This technique uses percussion and postural drainage along with coughing and deep breathing exercises. It is performed by positioning the client so that the involved lobes of the lung are placed in a dependent drainage position and then using a cupped hand or vibrator to percuss the chest wall. Nasotracheal suctioning is quite uncomfortable but still useful in the appropriate clinical setting in the absence of significant coagulopathy.

10-34 Answer C

Pyrazinamide (PZA) should not be taken by pregnant women. Active tuberculosis should be treated with isoniazid and ethambutol and continued for at least 18 months to prevent relapse. Two-drug regimens are not recommended if isoniazid resistance is suspected. If a third drug or a more potent drug is necessary due to extensive or severe disease, rifampin could be added. Because of the risk of ototoxicity, streptomycin should not be prescribed. Isoniazid is the safest drug during pregnancy.

10-35   Answer D

Smokers weigh 5–10 lb less than nonsmokers of comparable age and height. When smokers quit, 80% of them gain weight; the average weight gain is 5 lb, but about 10% of that 80% who gain weight gain more than 25 lb. On average, women gain more weight than men: 8 lb as compared with 5 lb. Heavy smokers (those who smoke two packs per day or more) gain more weight than light smokers. This weight gain is caused by replacing the habit of smoking cigarettes with eating to satisfy the need for oral gratification.

10-36   Answer B

When teaching smokers about using nicotine gum to aid in smoking cessation, tell them to discard the gum after 30 minutes. The gum should not be chewed like regular gum. A piece is chewed only long enough to release the nicotine, which produces a peppery taste, and then "parked" between the gums and buccal mucosa to allow for nicotine absorption. Drinking liquids while the gum is in the mouth should be avoided. Acidic beverages such as coffee should be avoided for 1–2 hours before the use of the gum. The smoker should be instructed to chew 9–12 pieces daily to help prevent nicotine withdrawal.

10-37   Answer B

The peripharyngeal upper respiratory tract infection that occurs most often in children ages 2–5 years is epiglottitis. Peritonsillar abscess occurs more frequently during the teenage years; laryngotracheobronchitis (croup) in children ages 3 months to 3 years; and bacterial tracheitis in children ages 3–10 years.

10-38   Answer A

If a cough characteristically occurs all day long but never during sleep, suspect that it is a psychogenic cough (or habit). Allergic rhinitis results in a cough that is seasonal; pertussis in a cough that is followed by a "whoop"; and a postnasal drip results in a throat-clearing cough.

10-39   Answer D

Cholinesterase inhibitors cause a cough by inducing mucus production (bronchorrhea). Tobacco and marijuana cause a cough by being direct irritants. Beta-adrenergic blockers, aspirin, and NSAIDs

cause a cough by potentiating reactive airway disease.

10-40   Answer C

The Schamroth sign is useful as a quick method of assessing for digital clubbing. The dorsal surfaces of the terminal phalanges of similar fingers are placed together. With clubbing, the normal diamond-shaped window at the bases of the nailbeds disappears and a prominent distal angle forms between the end of the nails. Normally, this angle is minimal or nonexistent. The phalangeal depth ratio measures the ratio of the distal phalangeal depth to the interphalangeal depth. It is normally less than 1 but increases to more than 1 with finger clubbing. *Hyponychial* refers to the nailbed, and there is no such thing as a diamond test.

10-41   Answer D

Harrison's groove is the name of the horizontal groove in the rib cage at the level of the diaphragm, extending from the sternum to the midaxillary line. It occurs normally in some children and also occurs in children with rickets. The other grooves are just listed as distractors.

10-42   Answer A

A 1-minute Apgar score of 7–10 indicates that the newborn is in good condition, needing only suctioning of the nose and mouth and otherwise routine care. A 1-minute Apgar score of 3–6 indicates a moderately depressed newborn requiring more resuscitation and close monitoring. A 1-minute Apgar score of 0–2 indicates a severely depressed newborn requiring full resuscitation, ventilator support, and intensive care. The interpretation of Apgar scores is 7–10, good to excellent; 4–6, fair; and less than 4, poor.

10-43   Answer A

Retractions occur more often in the newborn and infant than at other ages because the intercostal tissues are weak and underdeveloped. Supraclavicular or suprasternal retractions suggest upper airway obstruction, while retraction of intercostals or subcostal muscles suggests lower airway obstruction.

10-44   Answer C

An infant who has periodic breathing with persistent or prolonged apnea (greater than 20 seconds) may have an increased risk of sudden infant death syndrome. Rapid respiratory rates accompany pneumonia, anemia, fever, pain, and heart disease. Tachypnea (a very rapid respiratory rate of 50–100 breaths per minute) during sleep may be an early sign of left-sided congestive heart failure.

10-45 Answer D

Stridor, a high-pitched inspiratory crowing sound, can be heard on auscultation when a client has acute epiglottitis or croup. Persistent fine crackles can be heard with atelectasis, expiratory wheezes with asthma, and persistent peristaltic sounds with diminished breath sounds on the same side with a diaphragmatic hernia.

10-46 Answer A

The nursing diagnosis of "impaired gas exchange" may be demonstrated by clubbing of the fingers. Nasal flaring and cough are present if the client has a nursing diagnosis of "ineffective airway clearance" or "ineffective breathing pattern." The use of accessory muscles to assist breathing may indicate a nursing diagnosis of "ineffective breathing pattern."

10-47 Answer B

Biot's breathing is the term for an irregular respiratory pattern of a series of three to four normal respirations followed by a period of apnea. It is seen with head trauma, brain abscess, heat stroke, spinal meningitis, and encephalitis. Cheyne-Stokes respiration is similar, except that the pattern is regular. The most common cause of Cheyne-Stokes respiration is severe congestive heart failure, followed by renal failure, meningitis, drug overdose, and increased intracranial pressure. This regular pattern occurs normally in infants and older adults during sleep. Kussmaul's respiration is hyperventilation with an increase in both the rate and depth of the breaths. Hypoventilation is a reduced rate and depth of breathing that causes an increase in carbon dioxide in the bloodstream.

10-48 Answer B

The definition of the spirometric assessment of residual volume is the amount of gas left in the lung after exhaling all that is physically possible. This measurement is expressed as a ratio of total lung capacity to vital capacity. The total lung capacity is the sum of the vital capacity and the residual volume. The expiratory reserve volume is the volume that can be maximally exhaled after a passive exhalation. The peak flow is the measurement of the maximum flow rate achieved during the forced vital capacity maneuver.

10-49 Answer A

Asthma is characterized by intermittent episodes of airway obstruction caused by bronchospasm, excessive bronchial secretion, or edema of bronchial mucosa. Atelectasis is a collapse of alveolar lung tissue, and findings reflect the presence of a small, airless lung. It is caused by complete obstruction of a draining bronchus by a tumor, thick secretions, or an aspirated foreign body. Acute bronchitis is an inflammation of the bronchial tree characterized by partial bronchial obstruction and secretions or constrictions. It results in abnormally deflated portions of the lung. Emphysema is a permanent hyperinflation of lung beyond the terminal bronchioles with destruction of the alveolar walls.

10-50 Answer B

In acute bronchitis, the breath sounds are vesicular, vocal resonance is moderate, and the adventitious sounds are localized crackles with sibilant wheezes. In bronchiectasis, the breath sounds are usually vesicular, but vocal resonance is usually muffled and crackles are the adventitious sounds. In emphysema, the breath sounds are of decreased intensity and often with prolonged expiration, vocal resonance is muffled or decreased, and the adventitious sounds are occasional wheezes and often fine crackles in late inspiration. In asthma, the breath sounds are distant, vocal resonance is decreased, and wheezes are the adventitious sounds.

10-51 Answer C

Recurrence rates for both primary and secondary spontaneous pneumothorax are similar. Recurrence rates range from 10%–50%, and about 60% of those clients will have a third recurrence. After three episodes, the recurrence rate exceeds 85%. Repeated spontaneous pneumothorax should be treated by pleurodesis or surgical intervention, including parietal pleurectomy.

10-52 Answer A

Secondary spontaneous pneumothoraces are most often due to underlying emphysematous COPD or HIV-associated *Pneumocystis jiroveci* (formerly known as *Pneumocystis carinii*) pneumonia (PCP). Other predisposing conditions include lung abscess, cystic fibrosis, and tuberculosis.

10-53   Answer B

An auscultation sound at the mediastinum in the presence of a mediastinal "crunch" that coincides with cardiac systole and diastole is known as Hamman's sign, named after the American physician Louis Hamman. It is present with spontaneous mediastinal emphysema or pneumomediastinum. Homans' sign is pain in the calf when the foot is passively dorsiflexed; it is a possible sign of deep vein thrombosis (DVT) in the calf. There is no manubrium or Louis sign.

10-54   Answer A

The community-acquired pneumonia seen most often in the client with or without an alcohol problem is pneumococcal, which is caused by the gram-positive bacteria *Pneumococcus* (also called *Streptococcus pneumoniae*). Alcoholics are at risk for the usual pathogens, but they also have a higher incidence of pneumonia caused by gram-negative organisms (including *Klebsiella pneumoniae*, *Legionella*, and *Haemophilus influenzae*) and anaerobic pneumonia secondary to aspiration than do people who are not alcohol abusers.

10-55   Answer D

Risk factors predisposing clients to the development of nosocomial (hospital-acquired) pneumonia include increased severity of the underlying illness, presence of an indwelling urethral catheter, use of broad-spectrum antibiotics (which increase the risk of superinfection), previous hospitalization, presence of intravascular catheters, intubation (especially prolonged intubation), and recent thoracic or upper abdominal surgery.

10-56   Answer C

Spiriva (tiotropium) is a once-daily, long-acting anticholinergic. It results in improved lung function studies and reduction in the use of rescue medication and in COPD exacerbations. The most frequently reported adverse side effect is that of dry mouth, which is easily remedied with increased hydration.

10-57   Answer A

Although all of these tests might be indicated, the first test that should be ordered for a client presenting with productive cough, weight loss, weakness, anorexia, night sweats, and generalized malaise for 8 weeks' duration would be a Mantoux skin test for tuberculosis (TB). The client is at high risk for developing TB because of his residence in a shelter and his low socioeconomic status.

10-58   Answer A

Cigarette smoking increases the clearance rate of theophylline and may result in the need for a larger dose. Hepatic insufficiency, allopurinol (Zyloprim), and cimetidine (Tagamet) all decrease the clearance rate of theophylline and may result in the need for a smaller dose.

10-59   Answer C

Sarcoidosis is a multisystem disorder of unknown cause that has a prevalence of about 20 cases in 10,000. It usually occurs in clients ages 20–40, but it can occur at any age. Sarcoidosis occurs more frequently in women than in men, and in the United States, it is more common in blacks than in whites (about 10:1). Although many organs may be involved, the most involved organ is the lung (90%).

10-60   Answer A

No long-term control therapy is indicated for all clients with step 1 (mild intermittent) asthma, be they adolescents, children, or adults. Clients with step 1 asthma need only quick relief with a beta-2 agonist as needed. There is no indication for long-term control until they approach step 2 (mild persistent) asthma.

10-61   Answer B

The normal respiratory rate of an 18-month-old child (age 1–2 years) while awake is 30–40 breaths per minute. Between ages 6 and 12 months, the awake child breathes between 58 and 75 times per minute. An awake child age 2–4 years breathes between 23 and 42 times per minute; and a child age 4–6 years breathes between 19 and 36 times per minute.

10-62   Answer A

The definitive tests for cystic fibrosis (CF) are the sweat test and DNA analysis. The diagnosis is confirmed by a positive sweat test or by confirming the presence of two of the recognized CF mutations in DNA, one each on the maternally and paternally derived chromosome 7. Sweat testing can be performed at any age. However, newborns in the first few weeks of life may not produce a large enough volume of sweat to analyze, but in those who do, the results will be accurate. Immunoreactive trypsinogen (IRT) levels are elevated in most infants with CF for the first several weeks of life; however, this test has relatively poor specificity because as many as 90% of the positives on the initial screen are false positives. Early diagnosis of CF improves the poor prognosis for untreated CF. If untreated, most clients die by age 1–2 years. With current care, median survival is age 29.

A sputum or throat culture positive for mucoid *Pseudomonas aeruginosa* is suggestive of CF. An abnormal Chymex test for pancreatic insufficiency is a supportive laboratory test to diagnose CF. A fecal fat test, while reliable, is not specific to CF; any condition affected by malabsorption or maldigestion will be associated with increased fecal fat.

10-63 Answer D

Sudden infant death syndrome (SIDS) is the most common cause of sudden and unexpected death in infants; 40%–50% of postneonatal infant mortality is caused by SIDS. The peak incidence of SIDS is at ages 2–4 months; 95% of all SIDS deaths occur by age 6 months.

10-64 Answer A

Streptococci (especially *Streptococcus viridans*) and *Staphylococci* (especially *Staphylococcus aureus*) are the two most predominant types of organisms constituting the normal flora of the oropharynx. They are followed by *Streptococcus pyogenes*, *Streptococcus pneumoniae*, *Moraxella catarrhalis*, *Neisseria* species, and lactobacilli.

10-65 Answer B

Respiratory alkalosis is the early acid-base disturbance that occurs in an aspirin overdose (salicylate intoxication). It results from direct stimulation of the respiratory center in the medulla, which causes an increase in pH and a decrease in $PaCO_2$. This leads to metabolic acidosis as the body compensates by renal excretion of bicarbonate to normalize the pH.

10-66 Answer D

In the pregnant woman, the thoracic cage may appear wider and the costal angle may feel wider than in the nonpregnant state. Respirations may be

deeper, although this can be quantified only with pulmonary function tests. Oxygenation is not decreased.

10-67 Answer A

The normal adult has a thorax that has an elliptical shape with an anteroposterior:transverse diameter ratio of 1:2 or 5:7. Funnel breast (pectus excavatum) is a markedly sunken sternum and adjacent cartilages; it is congenital and usually not symptomatic. Pigeon breast (pectus carinatum) is a forward protrusion of the sternum with ribs sloping back at either side and vertical depressions along the costochondral junctions; it is less common than pectus excavatum and requires no treatment. A barrel-shaped chest is present when the anteroposterior and transverse diameters of the chest are equal and the ribs are horizontal instead of in the normal downward slope; it is associated with normal aging and with chronic emphysema and asthma caused by hyperinflation of the lungs.

10-68 Answer B

Coal miners are at risk for developing pneumoconiosis. Pneumoconiosis is caused by the inhalation of dust particles and is an occupational hazard in mining and stone cutting. Farmers may be at risk for grain and/or pesticide inhalation. Construction workers handling asbestos may develop asbestosis. Potters, stonecutters, and miners are at risk for silicosis from inhaling silica (quartz) dust. A related respiratory disease, histoplasmosis is a systemic fungal respiratory diseased caused by fungus in the soil with a high organic content and undisturbed bird droppings, such as those around old chicken coops, caves, and so on.

10-69 Answer B

Cough and congestion result when breathing sulfur dioxide. Carbon monoxide produces dizziness, headache, and fatigue. Tear gas irritates the conjunctiva and produces a flow of tears. Carbon dioxide produces sleepiness.

10-70 Answer D

Some conditions have a characteristic timing of a cough. A cough caused by a postnasal drip related to sinusitis is more prevalent at night. A cough associated with an acute illness, such as a respiratory infection, is continuous throughout the day. A cough in the early morning is usually caused by chronic bronchial inflammation from habitual smoking. A cough in the afternoon and/or evening may reflect exposure to irritants at work.

10-71   Answer A

With pleural effusion and thickening, the trachea would be deviated toward the normal side because of fluid displacing the pleural space. The trachea is usually not displaced with pneumonia. With bronchiectasis, the trachea is midline or deviated toward the affected side, and with pulmonary fibrosis, the trachea is deviated to the most affected side.

10-72   Answer C

The sympathomimetic agents that are the first-line drugs of choice for hyperreactive airway disease—asthma—are the beta-2 agonists. There are different adrenergic receptors in different tissues. Beta-2 adrenergic agents (agonists) are more specific in their action to promote bronchodilation and are less likely to be associated with side effects. In addition to promoting bronchodilation, these agents also increase secretion of electrolytes by the airways and enhance mucociliary activity. Protein kinase A levels increase within the smooth muscle cells, resulting in inhibition of myosin phosphorylation and smooth muscle cell relaxation. Alpha agonists cause vasoconstriction and beta-1 adrenergic agents (agonists) increase cardiac contractility and heart rate, effects that are undesirable in clients with asthma. Alpha antagonist is not a drug class.

10-73   Answer B

If a client develops moderate asthma, defined as more than two episodes per week, an inhaled steroid should be prescribed and used in conjunction with the beta-2 adrenergic metered-dose inhaler. With no improvement, a longer-acting bronchodilator, such as salmeterol xinafoate (Serevent), may be added. If the asthma worsens, then a short course of oral steroids may be tried. Theophylline is no longer used except in extremely resistant cases.

10-74   Answer A

Streptococcus pneumoniae causes 30%–75% of all community-acquired bacterial pneumonia, followed by *Mycoplasma pneumoniae* (5%–35%); *Haemophilus influenzae* (6%–12%), and *Staphylococcus aureus* (3%–10%).

10-75   Answer C

The antibiotic of choice for the treatment of *Streptococcus pneumoniae* pneumonia is penicillin. Alternative choices are erythromycin and clindamycin. Dicloxacillin is the antibiotic of choice for infections caused by *Staphylococcus aureus*; erythromycin is the antibiotic of choice for infections caused by *Mycoplasma pneumoniae*; and ampicillin clavulanate is the antibiotic of choice for *Moraxella catarrhalis* infections. Once therapy has been started, the client's respiratory and cardiovascular status should be monitored, along with his or her general overall status, including level of energy, appetite, and temperature. Most clients on the appropriate antibiotic therapy improve within 48–72 hours. Fever that continues more than 24 hours after initiating therapy usually does not indicate failure of the antibiotic; rather, the usual response to therapy is a gradual reduction in the maximum daily temperature.

10-76   Answer A

For a client diagnosed with pneumonia, the following are indications for hospitalization: inability to take oral medications; multilobar involvement on chest x-ray; acute mental status changes; a severe vital sign abnormality (pulse rate greater than 140 per minute, systolic blood pressure less than 90 mm Hg, or a respiratory rate greater than 30 per minute); a secondary suppurative infection such as empyema, meningitis, or endocarditis; or a severe acute electrolyte, hematological, or metabolic abnormality.

10-77   Answer D

In the client with pulmonary tuberculosis, night sweats are often noted as a manifestation of fever. With pulmonary tuberculosis, systemic manifestations are usually present; symptoms are not confined to the respiratory system. Fever occurs in 50%–80% of cases, and symptoms such as malaise and weight loss are frequent. Dyspnea, an ominous feature, usually occurs with widespread advanced disease. Crackles and bronchial breath sounds may be present, but more often there are no abnormal findings, even in well-developed pulmonary disease.

10-78   Answer A

Groups at high risk for tuberculosis include racial and ethnic minorities (70% of all reported cases in the United States); foreign-born individuals

(24% of all cases in the United States); substance abusers (5–20 times normal); individuals with HIV infection (40–100 times normal); and residents of prisons, nursing homes, and shelters (2–10 times normal).

10-79   Answer C

Individuals predisposed to have a false-negative reaction to the Mantoux test include newborns and those older than age 60; those in an immunosuppressive state, such as persons taking corticosteroids and anticancer agents or those with HIV infection or chronic renal failure; persons with a neoplasm, especially lymphoid leukemia and lymphomas; and persons with an acute infection, such as measles, mumps, chickenpox, typhoid fever, brucellosis, typhus, and pertussis. Tuberculosis had been close to eradication until HIV appeared. Coughing alone is not predictive of TB.

10-80   Answer D

Tuberculosis is a reportable disease. Every potential case must be reported to the local health department. This includes when the client's Mantoux test shows an induration of 15 mm; when a case of tuberculosis is merely suspected; and when an asymptomatic client has a positive chest x-ray for pulmonary tuberculosis. Screening tests in higher-risk areas with suspected infection that do not have a positive reaction do not need to be reported. These include the appearance of a red area with an induration of less than 10 mm on the first test (less than 5 mm on employees with a yearly screen).

10-81   Answer B

The most common cause of a persistent cough in children of all ages is recurrent viral bronchitis. Recurrent viral bronchitis is most prevalent in preschool and young school-age children, and there may be a genetically determined host susceptibility to frequently recurring bronchitis. The key words are persistent cough. Young clients with recurrent cough often have asthma, but it is not usually persistent. Providers should be suspicious of underlying asthma contributing to a recurrent cough when there is a family history of allergies, atopy, or asthma. Similarly, allergies and an upper respiratory infection do not present with a persistent cough; rather, they present with an intermittent one.

10-82   Answer D

A chronic cough in children ages 1–5 years should suggest bronchiectasis or cystic fibrosis after the more common causes—allergic rhinitis, chronic sinusitis, and enlarged adenoids—have been ruled out. Although rare, chronic cough in children younger than age 1 should suggest congenital malformations or neonatal infections, including viral and *chlamydial* pneumonias. Other relatively rare causes of chronic cough in young infants include recurrent aspiration of milk, saliva, or gastric contents.

10-83   Answer C

Unexplained nocturnal cough in an older adult should suggest congestive heart failure. Older adults, whose physical activity may be restricted by arthritis or other associated diseases, may not present with the usual symptom of dyspnea on exertion. The main complaint instead may be a chronic unexplained cough that may occur only at night while the client is recumbent or a cough that may worsen at night.

10-84   Answer C

The joint American College of Chest Physicians (ACCP) and American Association of Cardiovascular and Pulmonary Rehabilitation (AACVPR) evidence-based clinical practice guidelines for pulmonary rehabilitation offer new evidence that pulmonary rehabilitation is beneficial for clients with COPD and those with other chronic lung conditions. Pulmonary rehab improves the symptom of dyspnea, improves the health-related quality of life, reduces the number of hospital days and other measures of health-care utilization, and is cost effective. Evidence is insufficient to support the routine use of nutritional supplementation in pulmonary rehabilitation of clients with COPD. Current practice and expert opinion support including psychosocial interventions as a component of comprehensive pulmonary rehabilitation programs for clients with COPD, but clients benefit the most from pulmonary rehabilitation.

10-85   Answer B

When trying to differentiate pulmonary from cardiac causes of dyspnea on exertion, it is important to remember that clients with dyspnea from cardiac causes remain dyspneic much longer after cessation of exercise. The heart rate also takes longer to return to preexercise levels. When the cause is pulmonary, the rate of recovery to normal respiration is fast and the dyspnea is gone a few minutes after the cessation of exercise. Clients with pulmonary dyspnea usually do not have dyspnea at rest. Clients with severe cardiac dyspnea demonstrate a volume of respiration that is greater than normal at every level of exercise, and they experience the dyspnea sooner after beginning the exertion.

10-86   Answer C

If a client presents with an acute onset of dyspnea with associated symptoms of chest pain, faintness, tachypnea, peripheral cyanosis, low blood pressure, crackles, and some wheezes, and has a history of taking birth control pills and smoking, suspect pulmonary emboli. Other signs and symptoms associated with pulmonary emboli include loss of consciousness and a pleural friction rub. Precipitating and aggravating factors include the use of oral contraceptives and prolonged recumbency. Acute dyspnea would also occur with asthma, but the physical findings would include bilateral wheezing; sibilant, whistling sounds; and prolonged expiration. With bronchitis, dyspnea is not necessarily the presenting symptom. A cough precedes the dyspnea, and there would be rhonchi present on auscultation. With a pneumothorax, there is an acute onset of dyspnea, and the physical findings would include decreased or absent breath sounds with a tracheal shift.

10-87   Answer B

Of persons who smoke one pack of cigarettes per day or more, 40%–60% have a cough. It is defined as chronic bronchitis if the cough has been productive for at least 3 months during each of 2 consecutive years.

10-88   Answer B

The most common reason for a chronic cough in children is a postinfection. The other reasons, in order of frequency, are asthma, a postnasal drip, and irritants. Uncommon causes include other respiratory infections, pertussis, a foreign body, cystic fibrosis, congenital abnormalities, and psychogenic reasons.

10-89   Answer A

A pulmonary function test, such as spirometry, is helpful in the diagnosis of restrictive lung disease and obstructive lung disease, including chronic

bronchitis and asthma. Clients with postinfectious or cough-variant asthma may show mild obstruction, but they often have normal spirometry. A chest x-ray confirms the diagnosis of pneumonia. While spirometry may show a decrease in lung capacity with advanced lung cancer, it is not diagnostic.

10-90   Answer C

Drugs such as corticosteroids and other immunosuppressive agents contribute to a decreased response to TST. Other factors that may contribute to a decreased response to TST include viral infections (measles, mumps, chickenpox, HIV), bacterial infections (typhoid fever, pertussis), nutritional factors (severe protein depletion), diseases affecting lymphoid organs, and stress (surgery, burns).

10-91   Answer C

Clinical manifestations of cancer of the larynx include earache, halitosis, hoarseness, change in the voice, painful swallowing, dyspnea, and a palpable lump in the neck. The most notable manifestation of glottic (tongue) cancer is hoarseness or a change in the voice because the tumor prevents complete closure of the glottis during speech.

10-92   Answer A

After a total laryngectomy for laryngeal cancer, the client will have a permanent tracheostomy because no connection exists between the trachea and the esophagus.

10-93   Answer B

If a client has a dry cough, dyspnea, chills, fever, general malaise, headache, confusion, anorexia, diarrhea, myalgias, and arthralgias, suspect Legionnaires' disease. Legionnaires' disease has a gradual onset. Bronchopneumonia has a gradual onset with a cough, scattered crackles, minimal dyspnea and respiratory distress, and a low-grade fever. Primary atypical pneumonia has a gradual onset with a dry, hacking, nonproductive cough; fever; headache; myalgias; and arthralgias. *Pneumocystis jiroveci* pneumonia occurs in clients with AIDS. It has an abrupt onset with a dry cough, tachypnea, shortness of breath, significant respiratory distress, and fever.

10-94   Answer C

In trying to differentiate between chronic bronchitis and emphysema, remember that chronic bronchitis presents with adventitious sounds, wheezing and rhonchi, and a normal percussion note. Chronic bronchitis usually occurs after age 35, with recurrent respiratory infections. There is usually a persistent, productive cough of copious mucopurulent sputum, and pulmonary function studies show normal or decreased total lung capacity with a moderately increased residual volume. In a client with emphysema, the onset is usually after age 50. There is an insidious progressive dyspnea and the cough is usually absent or mild with scant, clear sputum, if any. There are also distant or diminished breath sounds and a hyperresonant percussion note. The pulmonary function studies show an increased total lung capacity with a markedly increased residual volume.

10-95   Answer D

Coccidioidomycosis is the leading mycotic (fungal) infection in the southwestern United States, with an annual morbidity estimated at 35,000 cases. Although the majority of those infected recover spontaneously without antibiotic intervention, for immunocompromised persons, the disseminated disease can lead to high morbidity and a greater than 50% mortality rate. Providers should suspect coccidioidomycosis in clients presenting with pulmonary complaints, particularly those who may have recently visited an endemic area. An influenza-like syndrome appears 7–28 days after inhalation of *Coccidioides immitis* in less than half of clients infected. Symptoms, in descending order of frequency, include fever, cough, chest pain, chills, sputum production, sore throat, and hemoptysis. Cutaneous manifestations occur in 10% of clients, particularly younger ones, and present as generalized maculopapular erythematous eruptions. Coccidioidomycosis is readily treatable if recognized at an early stage. For the majority of infected individuals, the prognosis is excellent even without therapy. Systemic antifungal therapy should be considered in infants, older adults, debilitated persons, those with prolonged primary disease, and populations at high risk of dissemination. Intravenous amphotericin B is the mainstay of therapy.

10-96   Answer C

In an inner-city study of 476 children, researchers determined that the combination of cockroach allergy and exposure to the insects is an important cause of asthma-related illness and hospitalizations among that group of children. Levels of cockroach, dust mite, and cat allergens in the children's homes were measured and allergy skin tests were performed on the children. Of these children, 37% were allergic to cockroaches, 35% to dust mites, and 23% to cats. The study then assessed the severity of the children's asthma over 12 months and found that children who were both allergic to cockroaches and exposed to high cockroach allergen levels were hospitalized for their asthma 3.3 times more often than children who were allergic but not exposed to high levels of cockroach allergen, or children who were exposed to high levels of cockroach allergen but who were not allergic.

10-97   Answer C

Jill has daily symptoms of asthma. She uses her inhaled short-acting beta-2 agonist daily. Her exacerbations affect her activities, and they occur at least twice weekly and may last for days. She is affected more than once weekly during the night with an exacerbation. Jill is in the step 3 (moderate persistent) category of asthma severity. This is because she has daily symptoms along with exacerbations affecting her activity and nocturnal symptoms that occur more than once per week. In step 1 (mild intermittent) asthma, symptoms are no more frequent than twice weekly and nocturnal symptoms are no more frequent than twice per month. In step 2 (mild persistent) asthma, symptoms are more frequent than twice weekly but less than once a day, exacerbations may affect activity, and nocturnal symptoms are more frequent than twice per month. In step 4 (severe persistent) asthma, the client has continuous symptoms with limited physical activity, frequent exacerbations, and frequent nocturnal symptoms.

10-98   Answer A

Occupational asthma should be considered in all clients with adult-onset asthma or in clients with asthma that worsens in adulthood. As many as one in five cases of asthma may be a result of exposure to chemicals in the workplace. Approximately 250 chemicals have been found to cause occupational asthma symptoms, which usually appear soon after a worker is first exposed to the asthma-inducing chemical but sometimes may appear months to years later.

10-99   Answer C

Symptoms in about one-third of pregnant women with asthma will improve during pregnancy; about one-third will be unchanged; and about one-third will worsen. Pregnancy is associated with changes in lung volume. There is an increase in tidal volume and a 20%–50% increase in minute ventilation. The clinical course of asthma during pregnancy may be predicted by the course during the first trimester, and most clients have the same pattern of response with repeated pregnancies. The treatment of asthma during pregnancy follows the same principles as with other clients. Medications not specifically required should not be given in the first trimester, and all medications should be given at their minimal effective dose and frequency.

10-100   Answer C

Research has shown that engaging in moderate to high levels of physical activity slows the decline in smokers' lung function and may help prevent as many as 21% of COPD cases.

10-101   Answer C

A cough occurs in about 10% of clients who take ACE inhibitors such as captopril (Captoten) and enalapril (Vasotec). A complete history of prescribed and over-the-counter (OTC) drugs, including any herbal preparations, should be taken. Knowing all drugs taken is important, but because of the potential for ACE inhibitors to cause a cough, it is particularly important to ask about this category of drugs when doing a respiratory assessment.

10-102   Answer A

Hemoptysis is defined as expectoration of blood. The client often reports coughing up blood or sputum that is streaked or tinged with blood. In addition, hemoptysis may be manifested as fresh (bright red) or old blood or, in the case of bleeding from an infected lung cavity, it may present as slow oozing or frank bleeding. In cases of profuse hemoptysis, blood clots may be expectorated.

10-103   Answer C

After using a steroid inhaler, always rinse your mouth to prevent oral candidiasis ("thrush"). Brushing the teeth will get rid of any bad taste. The inhaler or diskus should be shaken first. If the client is also taking a beta-2 agonist, tell him or her to take that first, as that will open the airway, allowing more of the steroid medication to be administered.

10-104   Answer A

Hand-to-hand transmission (after handling fomites serving as reservoirs of infection) is the most common mode of transmission of the common cold in adults, underscoring the importance of frequent hand washing in the prevention of new cases. Colds are also caused by viruses spread through direct inhalation of airborne droplet sprays aerosolized by the infected person while speaking, coughing, or sneezing.

10-105   Answer B

Requirements for home oxygen include (1) a PaO_2 of 55 mm Hg or less or an oxygen saturation (Sa) below 85% and (2) a PaO_2 of 55–59 mm Hg if erythrocytosis (hematocrit of 56% or more) or cor pulmonale (P wave more than 3 mm in leads II and III) is present. Because hypoxia leads to pulmonary hypertension and increases the work of the right ventricle, low-flow oxygen may help prevent or deter development of cor pulmonale. The goal of therapy is a PaO_2 of 60 mm Hg or SaO_2 of 90%, which usually can be accomplished with 1–2 L of oxygen per minute for 15 hours per day.

10-106   Answer C

The definitive test for sleep apnea is an overnight polysomnogram. This all-night recording of the client's sleep, performed in a sleep center, is the "gold standard" for identifying the presence, type, and severity of sleep apnea.

Bibliography

Barclay, L, and Vega, C: New guidelines highlight benefits of pulmonary rehabilitation. Medscape Medical News. http://www.medscape.com/viewarticle/558167, accessed 6/20/07.

Cui, DJ: The new asthma guidelines—What primary care clinicians need to know. *Clinician Reviews* 17(5):26–32, May 2007.

Dillon, PM: *Nursing Health Assessment—A Critical Thinking, Case Studies Approach*, ed 2. FA Davis, Philadelphia, 2007.

Dunphy, LM, et al: *Primary Care: The Art and Science of Advanced Practice Nursing*, ed 2. FA Davis, Philadelphia, 2007.

Freeman, D, Lee, A, and Price, D: Efficacy and safety of tiotropium in COPD patients in primary care: The SPiRiva Usual CarE (SPRUCE) Study. *Respiratory Research*, 2007.

Garcia-Aymerich, J, et al: Regular physical activity modifies smoking-related lung function decline and reduces risk of chronic obstructive pulmonary disease: A population cohort study. *American Journal of Respiratory and Critical Care Medicine* 175:458–463, 2007.

Rance, K: The asthma-allergy connection. Complex companions. *Advance for Nurse Practitioners* 15(4):31–33, April 2007.

Youngkin, EQ, et al: *Pharmacotherapeutics: A Primary Care Guide*, ed 2. Upper Saddle River, NJ, Pearson-Prentice Hall, NJ, 2005.

How well did you do?

85% and above, congratulations! This score shows application of test-taking principles and adequate content knowledge.

75%–85%, keep working! Review test-taking principles and try again.

65%–75%, hang in there! Spend some time reviewing concepts and test-taking principles and try the test again.

Pyle, K, et al: Keeping cardiac arrest patients alive with therapeutic hypothermia. *American Nurse Today* 2(7):32–36, July 2007.

U.S. Department of Health and Human Services: *Healthy People 2010: Understanding and Improving Health*. U.S. Department of Health and Human Services, Washington, DC, 2000.

Yaakob,W, and Schabel, S: Photo quiz—Upper extremity swelling in a smoker. *Consultant* 47(4):381–388, April 2007.

Youngkin, EQ, et al: *Pharmacotherapeutics: A Primary Care Guide*, ed 2. Pearson-Prentice Hall, Upper Saddle River, NJ, 2005.

How well did you do?

85% and above, congratulations! This score shows application of test-taking principles and adequate content knowledge.

75%–85%, keep working! Review test-taking principles and try again.

65%–75%, hang in there! Spend some time reviewing concepts and test-taking principles and try the test again.

Chapter 12: *Abdominal Problems*

Questions

12-1 *Marcie just returned from Central America with traveler's diarrhea. Which antibiotic do you order?*

A. Ampicillin (Polycillin)

B. Tetracycline (Achromycin)

C. Ciprofloxacin (Cipro)

D. Azithromycin (Zithromax)

12-2 *Which protozoal infection is the most common intestinal infection in the United States that also occurs worldwide?*

A. Salmonellosis

B. Giardiasis

C. Botulism

D. Shigellosis

12-3 *Which laboratory value would you expect to be increased in the presence of significant diarrhea?*

A. Serum potassium

B. Serum sodium

C. Serum chloride

D. Bicarbonate

12-4 *Martina, age 34, has AIDS and currently suffers from diarrhea. You suspect that she has which protozoal infection of the bowel?*

A. Giardiasis

B. Amebiasis

C. Cryptosporidiosis

D. *Escherichia coli*

12-5 *Cydney has been given a diagnosis of ascariasis. Which symptoms would you expect to see?*

A. Low-grade fever, productive cough with blood-tinged sputum, wheezing, and dyspnea

B. Nocturnal perianal and perineal pruritus

C. Diarrhea, cramps, and malaise

D. Ascites and facial and extremity edema

12-6 *Sam has ulcerative colitis and is on a low-residue diet. Which foods do you recommend that Sam should avoid?*

A. Potato skins, potato chips, and brown rice

B. Vegetable juices and cooked and canned vegetables

C. Ground beef, veal, pork, and lamb

D. White rice and pasta

12-7 *Martin has had an ileostomy for ulcerative colitis. Which self-care measures do you teach him to relieve food blockage?*

A. Lie in a supine position.

B. Massage the peristomal area.

C. Take a hot shower or tub bath.

D. Drink cold fluids.

12-8 *Olive has an acute exacerbation of Crohn's disease. Which laboratory test value(s) would you expect to be decreased?*

A. Sedimentation rate

B. Liver enzyme levels

C. Vitamins A, B complex, and C levels

D. Bilirubin level

12-9 *Clients with sprue usually have*

A. a large-in-stature appearance.

B. accelerated maturity.

C. polycythemia.

D. steatorrhea.

12-10 *Sandra has celiac disease. You place her on which diet?*

A. A low-fat diet

B. A low-residue diet

C. A gluten-free diet

D. A high-protein diet

12-11 *Timothy, age 68, complains of an abrupt change in his defecation pattern. You evaluate him for*

A. constipation.

B. colorectal cancer.

C. irritable bowel syndrome.

D. acute appendicitis.

12-12 *After treating a patient for Helicobacter pylori infection, what test do you order to see if it has been cured?*

A. An enzyme-linked immunosorbent assay titer

B. A urea breath test

C. A rapid urease test (*Campylobacter*-like organism)

D. A repeat endoscopy

12-13 *Marian, age 52, is obese. She complains of a rapid onset of severe right upper quadrant abdominal cramping pain, nausea, and vomiting. Your differential diagnosis might be*

A. appendicitis.

B. irritable bowel syndrome.

C. cholecystitis.

D. Crohn's disease.

12-14 *Which oral medication might be used to treat a client with chronic cholelithiasis who is a poor candidate for surgery?*

A. Ursodiol (Actigall)

B. Ibuprofen (Advil)

C. Prednisone (Deltasone)

D. Methyltertbutyl ether

12-15 *The most common cause of elevated liver function tests is*

A. hepatitis.

B. biliary tract obstruction.

C. chronic alcohol abuse.

D. a drug-induced injury.

12-16 *You are doing routine teaching with a patient who has a family history of colorectal cancer. You know she misunderstands the teaching when she tells you she will*

A. decrease her fat intake.

B. increase her fiber intake.

C. continue her daily use of aspirin.

D. increase her fluid intake.

12-17 *Lucy, age 49, has pain in both the left and right lower quadrants. What might you suspect?*

A. A gastric ulcer

B. Gastritis

C. Pelvic inflammatory disease

D. Pancreatitis

12-18 *Which of the following antibiotics causes more episodes of nausea and/or vomiting than the others?*

A. Azithromycin (Zithromax)

B. Erythromycin (E-Mycin)

C. Penicillin (Pen-Vee K)

D. Tetracycline (Achromycin)

12-19 *All of the following medications are used for the control of nausea and vomiting. Which medication works by affecting the chemoreceptor trigger zone, thereby stimulating upper gastrointestinal motility and increasing lower esophageal sphincter pressure?*

A. Anticholinergics such as scopolamine (Donnatal)

B. Antidopaminergic agents such as prochlorperazine (Compazine)

C. Antidopaminergic and cholinergic agents such as metoclopramide (Reglan)

D. Tetrahydrocannabinols such as dronabinol (Marinol)

12-20 *To differentiate among the different diagnoses of inflammatory bowel diseases, you look at the client's histological, culture, and radiological features. Mary has transmural inflammation, granulomas, focal involvement of the colon with some skipped areas, and sparing of the rectal mucosa. What do you suspect?*

A. Crohn's disease

B. Ulcerative colitis

C. Infectious colitis

D. Ischemic colitis

12-21 *Which of the following treatments for ulcerative colitis is contraindicated?*

A. A high-calorie, nonspicy, caffeine-free diet that is low in high-residue foods and milk products

B. Corticosteroids in the acute phase

C. Antidiarrheal agents

D. Colectomy with permanent ileostomy in severe cases

12-22 *In a 2-month-old infant with vomiting and diarrhea, the most effective way of determining a fluid deficit is to check for*

A. decreased peripheral perfusion.

B. hyperventilation.

C. irritability.

D. hyperthermia.

12-23 *You suspect that Harry has a peptic ulcer and tell him that it has been found to be strongly associated with*

A. anxiety and panic attacks.

B. long-term use of NSAIDs.

C. infection by *Helicobacter pylori*.

D. a family history of peptic ulcers.

12-24 *The American Cancer Society recommends a sigmoidoscopy for colon cancer screening in persons at average risk every*

A. year, beginning at age 50 for 2 years, then every 3–5 years thereafter.

B. 3 years, beginning at age 40.

C. other year for clients with a family history of colon cancer.

D. 2 years, beginning at age 45.

12-25 *A false-positive result with the fecal occult blood test can result from*

A. ingestion of large amounts of vitamin C.

B. a high dietary intake of rare-cooked beef.

C. a colonic neoplasm that is not bleeding.

D. stool that has been stored before testing.

12-26 *Which area(s) of Jill's gastrointestinal tract may be affected by her Crohn's disease?*

A. All areas from the mouth to the anus

B. The colon

C. The sigmoid colon

D. The small intestine

12-27 *Harvey just came back from Mexico. Which pathogen do you suspect is responsible for his diarrhea?*

A. Enterococci

B. *Escherichia coli*

C. *Klebsiella*

D. Staphylococci

12-28 *The most common causes of upper gastrointestinal hemorrhage are*

A. esophagitis and carcinomas.

B. erosive gastritis and peptic ulcer disease.

C. peptic ulcer disease and esophageal varices.

D. carcinomas and arteriovenous malformations.

12-29 *Sigrid, age 82, has irritable bowel, chronic constipation, and diverticulitis. Which pharmacological agent do you recommend?*

A. Bulking agents

B. Stool softeners

C. Laxatives

D. Lubricants

12-30 *The metabolism of which drug is not affected in Marsha, age 74?*

A. Alcohol

B. Anticonvulsants

C. Psychotropics

D. Oral anticoagulants

12-31 *Sidney has ulcerative colitis and asks you about a Koch pouch. You respond,*

A. "It's a method of bowel training for clients with chronic diarrhea."

B. "It's a name for a continent ileostomy."

C. "It's a packet of daily pills to take to relieve diarrhea."

D. "It's like a sanitary pad and it's used to contain any rectal leakage."

12-32 *Stacy, a nursing student, is to begin her series of hepatitis B vaccinations. You test her for a serological marker and the results show hepatitis B surface antibodies (HbsAb). You tell Stacy that she*

A. needs to begin the hepatitis B series as soon as possible.

B. needs to be tested again because one reading is not indicative of immunity.

C. is permanently immune to hepatitis B.

D. has an acute hepatitis B infection.

12-33 *Maura had a less than 7% value on her Schilling test. What medication do you anticipate that Maura might need?*

A. Folic acid

B. Vitamin B_{12}

C. Thyroid medication

D. Hormone replacement therapy

12-34   *Tina has a chronic hepatitis C infection. She asks you how to prevent its transmission. You respond,*

A. "Do not donate blood until 1 year after diagnosis."

B. "A vaccine is available to prevent transmission."

C. "There is no possibility of transmission through razors or toothbrushes."

D. "Abstain from sex during your period."

12-35   *You suspect that Nikki has a gastroduodenal ulcer caused by Helicobacter pylori and plan to treat her empirically. What medications should you order?*

A. Bismuth subsalicylate (Pepto-Bismol), tetracycline (Tetracap) or amoxicillin (Amoxil), and metronidazole (Flagyl)

B. Bismuth subsalicylate (Pepto-Bismol) and omeprazole (Prilosec)

C. Amoxicillin (Amoxil) and omeprazole (Prilosec)

D. Clarithromycin (Biaxin) and metronidazole (Flagyl)

12-36   *Nausea is difficult to discern in a young child. What question might you ask to determine if the child has nausea?*

A. "Are you sick to your tummy?"

B. "Are you hungry?"

C. "Are you eating the way you normally eat?"

D. "Are you nauseous?"

12-37   *A mother is bringing in her 4-year-old child, whom she states has acute abdominal pain and a rash. Which of the following do you initially rule out?*

A. Rocky Mountain spotted fever

B. Measles

C. Appendicitis

D. A food allergy

12-38   *Bobby, age 6, has constant periumbilical pain shifting to the right lower quadrant, vomiting, a small volume of diarrhea, absence of headache, a mild elevation of the white blood cell count with an early left shift, and white blood cells in the urine. You suspect*

A. appendicitis.

B. gastroenteritis.

C. acute pancreatitis.

D. Rocky Mountain spotted fever.

12-39   *The most common viral infection causing diarrhea in the United States is*

A. enteric adenovirus.

B. a Norwalk-like virus.

C. rotavirus.

D. *Giardia lamblia.*

12-40   *For an uncomplicated Salmonella infection, the antibiotic of choice is*

A. ampicillin (Polycillin).

B. amoxicillin (Amoxil).

C. trimethoprim-sulfamethoxazole (Bactrim).

D. No antibiotic is indicated.

12-41   *The proper order of assessing the abdomen is*

A. palpation, percussion, auscultation, inspection.

B. inspection, palpation, auscultation, percussion.

C. inspection, auscultation, percussion, palpation.

D. percussion, auscultation, inspection, palpation.

12-42   *You assess for Cullen's sign in Dan, age 62, after surgery. Cullen's sign may indicate*

A. intra-abdominal bleeding.

B. a ventral hernia.

C. appendicitis.

D. jaundice.

12-43   *Striae most commonly occur with*

A. pregnancy.

B. excessive weight gain.

C. diabetes.

D. ascites.

12-44   *When percussing the abdomen, hyperresonance is present*

A. when there is gaseous distention.

B. over a distended bladder.

C. over adipose tissue.

D. over fluid or a mass.

12-45   *You elicit costovertebral angle tenderness in Gordon, age 29. Which condition do you suspect?*

A. Cirrhosis

B. Inflammation of the kidney

C. Inflammation of the spleen

D. Peritonitis

12-46 *Which organ structure produces and secretes bile to emulsify fats?*

A. Salivary glands

B. Pancreas

C. Liver

D. Gallbladder

12-47 *Rebound tenderness may indicate*

A. peritoneal inflammation.

B. a ventral hernia.

C. portal hypertension.

D. Crohn's disease.

12-48 *How do you respond when Andrea, who is taking her newborn home from the hospital, asks you when her baby's umbilical cord stump will fall off?*

A. "Within 7 days"

B. "In 10–14 days"

C. "In 14–21 days"

D. "In 21–30 days"

12-49 *By what age do abdominal respirations cease in a child?*

A. 2 years

B. 5 years

C. 7 years

D. 13 years

12-50 *Hyperactive bowel sounds (borborygmi) are present in which of the following conditions?*

A. Cirrhosis

B. Laxative use

C. Late mechanical bowel obstruction

D. Pancreatic cancer

12-51 *Which of the following signs or symptoms indicates biliary obstruction with liver disease?*

A. Pruritus

B. Increased abdominal girth

C. Right upper quadrant pain

D. Easy bruising

12-52 *Sally had an ileostomy performed for inflammatory bowel disease. What type of fecal output can Sally expect?*

A. Hard, formed stool

B. Semisoft stool

C. Semisoft to very soft stool

D. A continuous, soft-to-watery effluent

12-53 *Shelby has recently been diagnosed with pancreatitis. Which of the following objective findings, also known as Grey Turner's sign, can result from the pancreatic inflammatory process that you might find on a rare occasion?*

A. Left-sided pleural effusion

B. Bluish discoloration over the flanks

C. Bluish discoloration over the umbilicus

D. Jaundice

12-54 *Which is the most common presenting symptom of gastric cancer?*

A. Weight loss

B. Dysphagia

C. Hematemesis

D. Gastrointestinal bleeding

12-55 *Once gastric cancer has been diagnosed, which test should be ordered to accurately determine the correct staging?*

A. Computed tomography

B. Magnetic resonance imaging

C. Endoscopic ultrasound

D. Ranson's test

12-56 *Margie, age 52, has an extremely stressful job and was just given a diagnosis of gastric ulcer. She tells you that she is sure it is going to be malignant. How do you respond?*

A. "Don't worry, gastric ulcers are not gastric cancer."

B. "About 95% of gastric ulcers are benign."

C. "You have about a 50:50 chance of having gastric cancer from your ulcer."

D. "Even if it is cancer, surgery is 100% successful."

12-57 *Jonas, age 34, had a Billroth II (hemigastrectomy and gastrojejunostomy with vagotomy) performed 1 week ago and just started eating a bland diet. What do you suspect when he complains of epigastric fullness, distention, discomfort, abdominal cramping, nausea, and flatus after eating?*

A. Obstruction

B. Dumping syndrome

C. Metabolic acidosis

D. Infectious colitis

12-58 *When Sammy asks you what he can do to help his wife, who has dumping syndrome, what do you suggest he tell her to do?*

A. Eat foods higher in carbohydrates.

B. Eat three large meals plus three snacks per day.

C. Eat foods with a moderate fat and protein content.

D. Drink fluids with each meal.

12-59 *Marvin, a known alcoholic, has alcoholic cirrhosis, is frequently admitted for coagulopathies, and occasionally receives blood transfusions. His wife asks you why he has bleeding problems. How do you respond?*

A. "Occasionally he accumulates blood in the gut."

B. "There is an interruption of the normal clotting mechanisms."

C. "Long-term alcohol abuse has made his vessels very friable."

D. "His bone marrow has been affected."

12-60 *Your client's 2-month-old daughter is admitted with gastroenteritis with dehydration after 2 days of vomiting and diarrhea. When she asks you what is causing the diarrhea, how do you respond?*

A. "She must be lactose intolerant from the formula, and this alters the fluid balance."

B. "Her body's telling you that it's time to initiate some solids into her system."

C. "The virus is causing irritation of the gastrointestinal lining, which causes an increase in gastrointestinal motility."

D. "The infectious agent invaded the gastrointestinal mucosa and affected the balance of water and electrolytes."

12-61 *An infant who is ruminating should be diagnosed and treated for*

A. cystic fibrosis.

B. esophagitis.

C. Meckel's diverticulum.

D. intussusception.

12-62 *A palpable spleen 2 cm or less below the left costal margin in a 2-year-old child is*

A. indicative of splenomegaly.

B. a sign of internal hemorrhaging.

C. normal.

D. a sign of infection.

12-63 *Mona is breastfeeding her 5-day-old daughter, who has just been found to have physiological jaundice with a bilirubin level of more than 20 mg/dL. You should tell Mona that she*

A. should stop breastfeeding altogether.

B. can continue breastfeeding.

C. should discontinue breastfeeding for 24 hours.

D. should alternate breast milk with formula for every other feeding.

12-64 *You are trying to differentiate between functional (acquired) constipation and Hirschsprung's disease in a neonate. Distinguishing features of Hirschsprung's disease includes which of the following?*

A. Small ribbonlike stools

B. Obvious abdominal pain

C. Female gender

D. Small weight gain

12-65 *Ellie, age 42, has a seizure disorder and has been taking phenytoin (Dilantin) for years. Which supplement should she also be taking if no other problems exist?*

A. Vitamin B_{12}

B. Iron

C. Folic acid

D. Calcium

12-66 *In counseling Maria, age 24, who is healthy, you advise her to limit her intake of sugar to prevent*

A. dental caries.

B. obesity.

C. diabetes.

D. hyperactivity.

12-67 *The most common cause of mechanical bowel obstruction in all ages is*

A. volvulus.

B. intussusception.

C. cancer.

D. a hernia.

12-68 *Nora, age 78, has terminal cancer and is wasting away. What should you order to stimulate her appetite?*

A. Megestrol (Megace)

B. Sertraline (Zoloft)

C. Vitamin C

D. Alprazolam (Xanax)

12-69 *Which physical examination maneuver for diagnosing appendicitis is done by deep palpation over the left lower quadrant (LLQ) with a sudden, unexpected release of pressure?*

A. Rovsing's sign

B. Psoas sign

C. Obturator sign

D. McBurney's sign

12-70 *Zena just had a hemorrhoidectomy. You know she hasn't understood your teaching when she tells you that she'll*

A. take a sitz bath after each bowel movement for 1–2 weeks after surgery.

B. drink at least 2000 mL of fluids per day.

C. decrease her dietary fiber for 1 month.

D. take stool softeners as prescribed.

12-71 *You auscultate Julie's abdomen and hear a peritoneal friction rub. Which condition do you rule out?*

A. Peritonitis

B. A liver or spleen abscess

C. A liver or spleen metastatic tumor

D. Irritable bowel syndrome

12-72 *Lipids are broken down in which area of the gastrointestinal tract?*

A. Esophagus

B. Stomach

C. Small intestine

D. Large intestine

12-73 *When George tells you that his feces are foul smelling, you suspect which of the following?*

A. Blood in the stool

B. Ingestion of a low-fat diet

C. Prostate cancer

D. Appendicitis

12-74 *Simon states that he is worried because he has a bowel movement only every third day. You respond,*

A. "You should have two to three stools per day."

B. "You should defecate once a day."

C. "You should have at least three stools per week."

D. "There is no such thing as a 'normal' pattern of defecation."

12-75 *Anson tells you that he thinks his antacids are causing his diarrhea. You respond,*

A. "Antacids contain fructose that may not be totally absorbed and results in fluid being drawn into the bowel."

B. "Antacids contain sorbitol or mannitol, sugars that aren't absorbed and can cause fluid to be drawn into the bowel."

C. "Antacids contain caffeine, which decreases bowel transit time."

D. "Antacids may contain magnesium, which decreases bowel transit time and may contain poorly absorbed salts that draw fluid into the bowel."

12-76 *How do diphenoxylate (Lomotil) and loperamide (Imodium) help relieve diarrhea?*

A. They reduce bowel spasticity and acid secretion in the stomach.

B. They decrease the motility of the ileum and colon, slowing the transit time and promoting more water absorption.

C. They increase motility to assist in removing all of the stool.

D. By decreasing the sensations of the gastric nerves, they send a message to the brain to slow down peristalsis.

12-77 *Sara is taking polyethylene glycol (GoLYTELY) in preparation for a barium enema. What do you teach her about the medication?*

A. Drink the solution at room temperature.

B. Take the medication with food so that it will be absorbed better.

C. Take the medication in the early evening so as not to interfere with sleep.

D. Drink all of the solution in one sitting.

12-78 *Which laxative is safe for long-term use?*

A. Mineral oil

B. Bisacodyl (Dulcolax)

C. Methylcellulose (Citrucel)

D. Magnesium hydroxide (milk of magnesia)

12-79 *Steve, age 79, has gastroesophageal reflux disease (GERD). When teaching him how to reduce his lower esophageal sphincter pressure, which substances do you recommend that he avoid?*

A. Apples

B. Peppermint

C. Cucumbers

D. Popsicles

12-80 *Rebound tenderness at McBurney's point would alert you to*

A. appendicitis.

B. peritonitis.

C. a spleen injury.

D. irritable bowel syndrome.

12-81 *Marisa, age 42, has celiac disease. She is prone to osteopenic bone disease as a result of impaired calcium absorption because of*

A. increased calcium absorption by the small intestine.

B. increased absorption of the fat-soluble vitamin D.

C. the binding of calcium and magnesium in the intestinal lumen by unabsorbed dietary fatty acids.

D. decreased magnesium absorption.

12-82 *The most important diagnostic test for celiac disease is*

A. confirming malabsorption by laboratory tests.

B. a barium enema.

C. a peroral biopsy of the duodenum.

D. a gluten-free diet trial with an accompanying improvement in mucosal histological response.

12-83 *Dottie brings in her infant who has gastrointestinal reflux. What do you tell her about positioning her infant?*

A. Always position infants on their back to prevent sudden infant death syndrome.

B. Rotate your infant between lying on the back and on the stomach.

C. The infant should be placed on the left side.

D. Place the infant in whatever position the infant remains quiet.

12-84 *Which of the following findings is not associated with diverticulitis?*

A. Left lower quadrant abdominal pain

B. A history of irritable bowel syndrome

C. A tender mass in the left lower quadrant

D. An elevated temperature

12-85 *A common complication of viral gastroenteritis in children is*

A. dehydration.

B. gastrointestinal bleeding.

C. peritonitis.

D. bacterial sepsis.

12-86 *Tenesmus refers to*

A. projectile vomiting.

B. severe lower abdominal pain.

C. constipation.

D. a persistent desire to empty the bowel or bladder.

12-87 *You are counseling Lillian, who is lactose intolerant, about foods to avoid. You know she misunderstands the teaching when she tells you she can have*

A. yogurt.

B. foods containing whey.

C. prehydrolyzed milk.

D. oranges.

12-88 *Which type of hepatitis is transmitted by the fecal-oral route, sewage, contaminated water, shellfish, and possibly blood?*

A. Hepatitis A (HAV)

B. Hepatitis B (HBV)

C. Hepatitis C (HCV)

D. Hepatitis D (HDV)

12-89 *While you are obtaining Henry's history, he tells you that he had a portacaval shunt done in the past. What does this imply?*

A. A history of liver cancer

B. A history of alcohol abuse

C. A congenital biliary problem

D. Heavy tobacco use

12-90 *Samantha is 100 lb overweight and wants to have a gastroplasty performed. In discussing this with her, you explain that by having this procedure she may*

A. develop diarrhea.

B. lose too much weight.

C. develop hemorrhoids.

D. vomit after she eats.

12-91 *What is the most common cause of melena?*

A. Colon cancer

B. Upper GI bleeding

C. Drug abuse

D. Smoking

12-92 *Ruby has a colostomy and complains that her stools are too loose. What food(s) do you suggest to help thicken the stools?*

A. Cheese

B. Leafy green vegetables

C. Raw fruits and vegetables

D. Dried beans

12-93 *Which type of hernia usually occurs at a previous surgical incision site?*

A. Umbilical

B. Congenital

C. Hiatal

D. Ventral

12-94 *Rose has gastroesophageal reflux disease. You know she misunderstands your teaching when she tells you that she will*

A. avoid coffee, alcohol, chocolate, peppermint, and spicy foods.

B. eat smaller meals.

C. have a snack before retiring so that the esophagus and stomach are not empty at bedtime.

D. stop smoking.

12-95 *Rose, your client with gastroesophageal reflux disease, has many other concurrent conditions. She wants to know if there are any medications she should not take. You tell her to avoid*

A. antibiotics.

B. NSAIDs.

C. oral contraceptives.

D. antifungals.

12-96 *Treatment for achalasia may include*

A. balloon dilation of the lower esophageal sphincter.

B. beta blockers.

C. a fundoplication.

D. an esophagogastrectomy.

12-97 *Matt, age 26, recently returned from a camping trip and has gastroenteritis. He says that he has been eating only canned food. Which of the following pathogens do you suspect?*

A. *Campylobacter jejuni*

B. *Clostridium botulinum*

C. *Clostridium perfringens*

D. *Staphylococcus*

12-98 *Duodenal and gastric ulcers have many of the same manifestations. Which is more common with gastric ulcers rather than duodenal ulcers?*

A. Epigastric or abdominal pain

B. Vomiting

C. Possibility of perforation

D. Obstruction of the gastrointestinal tract

12-99 *Martha has a Cushing's ulcer. What might have precipitated this?*

A. Her house burned down when she was not at home.

B. She was in a bad auto accident in which she sustained a head injury.

C. She spent the weekend deep-sea diving.

D. She was on an overseas airline flight that lasted more than 24 hours.

12-100 *Which procedure enlarges the opening between the stomach and duodenum to improve gastric emptying?*

A. Billroth I

B. Total gastrectomy

C. Pyloroplasty

D. Vagotomy

12-101 *Sylvia, age 59, has acute hepatitis. You're told it's from a drug overdose. Which drug do you suspect?*

A. Flagyl

B. Acetaminophen

C. Sumatriptan

D. Hydrocortisone

12-102 *The majority of the population of the United States has antibodies against which type of hepatitis?*

A. Hepatitis A

B. Hepatitis B

C. Hepatitis C

D. Hepatitis D

E. Hepatitis E

12-103 *Sandy, age 52, presents with jaundice, dark urine, and light-colored stools, stating that she is slightly improved over last week's symptoms. Which stage of viral hepatitis do you suspect?*

A. Incubation

B. Prodromal

C. Icteric

D. Convalescent

12-104 *Which of the following statements about cirrhosis is true?*

A. Biliary cirrhosis is the most common type of cirrhosis in the United States.

B. Alcoholic cirrhosis occurs only in malnourished alcoholics.

C. Cirrhosis is reversible if diagnosed and treated at an early stage.

D. Women tend to develop cirrhosis more quickly with less alcohol intake than men.

12-105 *Marty, age 52, notices a bulge in his midline every time he rises from bed in the morning. You tell him it's a ventral hernia, also known as*

A. inguinal hernia.

B. epigastric hernia.

C. umbilical hernia.

D. incisional hernia.

12-106 *You suspect appendicitis in Andrew, who is 18. With his right hip and knee flexed, you slowly rotate his right leg internally to stretch a muscle. He states that it is painful over his right lower quadrant. Which sign did you elicit?*

A. Rovsing's sign

B. Psoas sign

C. Obturator sign

D. McBurney's sign

12-107 *Susan, age 59, has no specific complaints when she comes in for her annual examination. She does, however, have type 2 diabetes, slight hypertension, dyslipidemia, and central obesity. You diagnose her as having*

A. a cardiovascular emergency.

B. a glycemic event.

C. metabolic syndrome.

D. multiple organ dysfunction

12-108 *Which modality/ies is/are the most effective in patients with metabolic syndrome?*

A. Specific vitamin and mineral supplements

B. Diet and exercise

C. Specific pharmacological therapy

D. Eliminating alcohol and smoking from their lifestyle

12-109 *Which of the following is a hospital-based nosocomial infection that has seen a serious rise in the past decade?*

A. Pneumonia

B. Hepatitis B

C. *Staphylococcus* infection

D. *C. difficile*

12-110 *A second-generation cephalosporin, cefmeta-zole is to be given to your patient undergoing colorectal surgery. You know that the dosing recommendation to prevent an incisional surgical site infection (SSI) is*

A. three doses prior to surgery.

B. one dose prior to surgery.

C. a weekly course of therapy.

D. therapy beginning after surgery.

12-111 *Sally, age 21, is to undergo a tonsillectomy. She has heard that when this surgery is performed in adults, it is extremely difficult. She's heard about taste changes after a tonsillectomy. What do you tell her?*

A. "As the tongue is responsible for sweet, sour, salty, and bitter taste abilities, they will all be affected somewhat."

B. "You will have some alterations, but we'll have to wait and see how you are affected personally."

C. "You may notice a slight difference initially, but there are no lasting changes in taste."

D. "About half of the patients have some permanent alterations in the sense of taste."

12-112 *A concern with older patients having abdominal surgery is*

A. older patients have an increased peristalsis, and bowel sounds must be checked very frequently.

B. older adults have a diminished response to painful stimuli that may mask abdominal health problems.

C. because older adults are prone to diarrhea after surgery, you must be vigilant about skin breakdown.

D. because of liver enlargement, postoperative medications are processed faster.

Answers

12-1   Answer C

Traveler's diarrhea caused by *Escherichia coli* is treated with a 3- to 5-day course of ciprofloxacin (Cipro), norfloxacin (Noroxin), or trimethoprim-sulfamethoxazole (Bactrim). Ampicillin (Polycillin) may be used to treat salmonellosis caused by *Salmonella* bacteria and shigellosis caused by *Shigella* bacteria. Ampicillin and tetracycline (Achromycin) are used to treat cholera, which is caused by *Vibrio cholerae*. Azithromycin (Zithromax) is a good choice for treating community-acquired pneumonia.

12-2   Answer B

Giardiasis, a protozoal infection of the upper small intestine, is caused by *Giardia lamblia*. It is the most common intestinal protozoal infection in the United States that also occurs worldwide. *Clostridium botulinum*, which causes botulism, is an enterotoxin, whereas *Salmonella*, causing salmonellosis, and *Shigella*, causing shigellosis, are both bacteria.

12-3   Answer C

Serum chloride level is increased with significant diarrhea when the diarrhea causes sodium loss that is greater than chloride loss. However, when there is severe diarrhea and vomiting, serum chloride levels may be decreased. Serum potassium and chloride levels are decreased as a result of loss through stool, and bicarbonate level is decreased in a metabolic acidotic state.

12-4   Answer C

Cryptosporidiosis, a common protozoal infection of the bowel, is common in immunocompromised clients. It causes villous atrophy and mild inflammatory changes and may secrete an enterotoxin. Giardiasis and amebiasis are also protozoal infections affecting the intestine, but because the question mentioned that Martina has AIDS, the answer must be cryptosporidiosis. *Escherichia coli* (*E. coli*) is a gram-negative bacterium.

12-5   Answer A

Ascariasis is the most common of the intestinal helminths (parasitic worms). It causes pulmonary manifestations such as low-grade fever, productive cough with blood-tinged sputum, wheezing, and dyspnea because the larvae are transmitted to the lungs from the vascular system. The larvae burrow through alveolar walls, migrating up the bronchial tree to the pharynx, and then down the esophagus back to the intestines. Nocturnal perianal and perineal pruritus occur with enterobiasis (pinworm infection). Diarrhea, cramps, and malaise are common with trichinosis. Ascites and facial and extremity edema are common with trichuriasis.

12-6   Answer A

Potato skins, potato chips, fried potatoes, brown rice, and whole-grain pasta products should be avoided if a client with ulcerative colitis is on a low-residue diet that was ordered to reduce intestinal motility and allow the bowel to rest.

12-7 Answer B

Self-care measures to teach a client with an ileostomy how to relieve food blockage include massaging the peristomal area, which may stimulate peristalsis and fecal elimination; assuming a knee-chest position to reduce intra-abdominal pressure; taking a warm shower or tub bath to relax the abdominal muscles; and drinking warm fluids or grape juice to produce a mild cathartic effect.

12-8 Answer C

Folic acid and serum levels of most vitamins, including A, B complex, C, and the fat-soluble vitamins, are decreased in Crohn's disease as a result of malabsorption. The sedimentation rate and liver enzymes and bilirubin levels are all increased.

12-9 Answer D

Celiac disease, also known as celiac sprue, may begin during early childhood or adulthood. Clients with sprue usually have steatorrhea, abdominal bloating and cramps, and diarrhea. Clients with celiac disease are often small in stature and have delayed maturity. The malabsorption that results may cause deficiencies such as anemia.

12-10 Answer C

Clients with celiac disease have an allergy to gliadin, a component of gluten; therefore, they are placed on a gluten-free diet in which wheat and other grains containing analogues to wheat gluten, such as oats, barley, and rye, must be avoided.

12-11 Answer B

A middle-aged or older client with an abrupt change in defecation pattern must be evaluated for colorectal cancer.

12-12 Answer B

A urea breath test is the easiest, least expensive, and most reliable test for *Helicobacter pylori*, which causes peptic ulcers. Its average sensitivity is 96% and specificity is 98%. An enzyme-linked immunosorbent assay titer, a rapid urease test (*Campylobacter*-like organism [CLO]) test, and an endoscopy may also be used. The CLO test and endoscopy require biopsy specimens and are therefore more invasive.

12-13 Answer C

A rapid onset of severe right upper quadrant (RUQ) abdominal cramping pain with nausea and vomiting is a classic presentation of acute cholecystitis; 90%–95% of clients with acute cholecystitis also have gallstones. Other symptoms include low-grade fever, epigastric tenderness, guarding, and pain on inspiration during palpation of the RUQ (Murphy's sign). Pain associated with appendicitis would typically be near the navel progressing to the right lower quadrant. In irritable bowel syndrome and Crohn' disease, the pain and cramping is more diffuse in the abdomen and is not usually accompanied by nausea and vomiting. The pain with IBS originates over some area of the colon, with the lower left quadrant (LLQ) being most often affected.

12-14 Answer A

Ursodiol (Actigall) is an oral bile acid that dissolves gallstones. For dissolution, 8–10 mg/kg per day is given in two to three divided doses; for prevention, 300 mg bid is given. The safety of its use after 24 months has not been established. NSAIDs such as ibuprofen (Advil) may be very irritating to the gastrointestinal mucosa. Steroids such as prednisone (Deltasone) may mask an infection, as well as be irritating to the gastric mucosa. Methyltertbutyl ether (MTBE) is a lipid solvent that is infused directly into the gallbladder via a T-tube.

12-15 Answer C

Hepatocellular damage from chronic alcohol abuse is the most frequent cause of elevated liver function tests (LFTs) in adults. Other causes include biliary tract obstruction, hepatitis, drug-induced injuries, vascular changes caused by anoxia, and congestive heart failure; however, chronic alcohol abuse remains the number one cause of abnormal LFTs.

12-16 Answer D

Increasing fluid intake has not been shown to decrease the risk of colorectal cancer. Current recommendations to aid in preventing colorectal cancer include decreased fat and increased fiber consumption and the daily use of aspirin. The daily use of aspirin has been shown to decrease the incidence of colorectal cancer, as well as dramatically decrease the incidence of metastasis.

12-17   Answer C

The pain associated with pelvic inflammatory disease can be palpated in both the right and left lower quadrants. Pain in the left upper quadrant may signify a gastric ulcer, gastritis, pancreatitis, splenic abscess, or pleurisy.

12-18   Answer B

Erythromycin (E-Mycin) is the antibiotic that causes the most cases of gastrointestinal upset such as nausea or vomiting. Other medications that commonly cause nausea and vomiting are opiates, estrogen, ipecac, digitalis, chemotherapy, and theophylline.

12-19   Answer C

Metoclopramide (Reglan) is used for diabetic gastroparesis and postoperative nausea and vomiting. It works by affecting the chemoreceptor trigger zone, thereby stimulating upper gastrointestinal motility and increasing lower esophageal sphincter pressure. Anticholinergics work at the site of the labyrinth receptors and the chemoreceptor trigger zones—that is, the vomiting center. Antidopaminergic agents work at the chemoreceptor trigger zone. The site and mechanism of tetrahydrocannabinols are unknown.

12-20   Answer A

Crohn's disease would show transmural inflammation, granulomas, focal involvement of the colon with some skipped areas, and sparing of the rectal mucosa. Ulcerative colitis would show acute inflammatory infiltrates, depleted goblet cells, negative cultures, and involvement of the rectum. Infectious colitis, because of the toxic products released, may induce periportal inflammation, mild hepatomegaly, and low-grade liver enzyme abnormalities, but usually without trophozoites in the liver. Ischemic colitis seen on colonoscopy reveals segmental inflammatory changes most often in the rectosigmoid and the splenic flexure, where there is more collateral circulation.

12-21   Answer C

Antidiarrheal agents are contraindicated in the presence of ulcerative colitis because they may precipitate colonic dilation. Sulfasalazine (Azulfidine) is often prescribed for its antibiotic and inflammatory effects; however, it interferes with folate metabolism, and therefore folate supplements may be required. A high-calorie, nonspicy, caffeine-free diet that is low in high-residue foods and milk products; corticosteroids in the acute phase; and a colectomy with permanent ileostomy in severe cases are all treatments for ulcerative colitis.

12-22   Answer A

In a 2-month-old infant with vomiting and diarrhea, the most effective way of determining a fluid deficit is to check for decreased peripheral perfusion, dry oral mucous membranes, and sunken fontanels. The body compensates for loss of fluid by shifting the interstitial fluid into the intravascular space, thereby maintaining perfusion of vital organs. If the fluid loss continues, circulating volume is diminished, and vasoconstriction occurs in the peripheral vessels, resulting in decreased perfusion.

12-23   Answer C

Although stress-related conditions such as anxiety and panic attacks and long-term use of NSAIDs may contribute to and aggravate peptic ulcer disease, about 90% of the cases of peptic ulcers have been found to be caused by infection with the bacteria *Helicobacter pylori*.

12-24   Answer A

The American Cancer Society (ACS) recommends a sigmoidoscopy for colon cancer screening in persons at average risk every year, beginning at age 50 for 2 years, then every 3–5 years thereafter. The ACS also recommends an annual digital rectal examination beginning at age 40 and checking the stool for occult blood every year beginning at age 50.

12-25   Answer B

A false-positive result with the fecal occult blood test can result from a high dietary intake of rare-cooked beef or fruits and vegetables that contain peroxidases. Oral iron preparations have also been shown to produce a false-positive result in some, but not all, studies. False-negative results can occur in clients who ingest large amounts of vitamin C or have a colon neoplasm that is not bleeding. A false-negative result can also occur if the stool has been stored before testing.

12-26   Answer A

Although the colon is the major site of gastrointestinal involvement in Crohn's disease (inflammatory bowel disease), the disease can affect all areas from the mouth to the anus.

12-27   Answer B

Escherichia coli is the pathogen most often responsible for traveler's diarrhea (infectious diarrhea). Other causes may include viruses, other bacteria, protozoa, or parasites.

12-28   Answer C

The most common causes of upper gastrointestinal hemorrhage, in descending order, are peptic ulcer disease, esophageal varices, esophagitis, erosive gastritis, carcinomas, and arteriovenous malformations.

12-29   Answer A

Bulking agents such as psyllium preparations or methylcellulose preparations are used for irritable bowel, chronic constipation, and diverticulitis. Stool softeners such as docusate sodium are frequently used for the prevention of constipation but most likely are not effective for chronic use. Saline laxatives such as magnesium hydroxide are indicated for intermittent use in chronic constipation and as a bowel preparation; stimulant irritant laxatives such as bisacodyl, senna, and cascara are used in acute constipation and should not be used for chronic constipation. Lubricants such as mineral oil are used in intermittent chronic constipation.

12-30   Answer A

Although drug metabolism by the liver is usually impaired in older adults, the metabolism of alcohol is unchanged.

12-31   Answer B

Performed for clients with ulcerative colitis, a Koch pouch (continent ileostomy) is the surgical removal of the rectum and colon and construction of an internal ileal reservoir, nipple valve, and stoma, allowing for intermittent drainage of ileal contents.

12-32   Answer C

The marker for permanent immunity, hepatitis B surface antibodies in the serum will be present 4–10 months after exposure and immunity to hepatitis B. Hepatitis B surface antigen is the earliest indicator of the presence of an acute infection and is present 4–12 weeks after exposure. This marker is also indicative of a chronic infection.

12-33   Answer B

A Schilling test is a timed urine test that evaluates the ability to absorb vitamin B_{12} from the gastrointestinal tract. It is used to diagnose pernicious anemia and malabsorption syndromes. The normal values range from 10%–40%. A value less than 7% indicates pernicious anemia and some gastric lesions.

12-34   Answer D

Because the hepatitis C virus is transmitted in blood, including menstrual blood, clients should abstain from sex during menstruation. Clients should not donate blood, and there is a possibility of transmission through razors, toothbrushes, and tattoo instruments. No vaccine is available.

12-35   Answer A

All of the drugs listed are used in the eradication of *Helicobacter pylori*. Traditional 14-day "triple therapy" with bismuth subsalicylate (Pepto-Bismol), tetracycline (Tetracap) or amoxicillin (Amoxil), and metronidazole (Flagyl) has consistently produced eradication rates of approximately 90% and is the least expensive therapy.

12-36   Answer B

To elicit information concerning nausea in a young child, ask the child about hunger because a young child cannot usually differentiate between hunger and mild nausea. Young children sometimes equate being "sick to their tummy" with vomiting and thus might answer no when questioned about nausea.

12-37   Answer C

There are many systemic causes of acute abdominal pain that also result in a rash. In the infectious category, these include Rocky Mountain spotted fever, measles, mumps, anaphylaxis, acute rheumatic fever, and infectious mononucleosis. A food allergy may also present itself as abdominal pain along with dermatitis. Appendicitis does not present with a rash.

12-38   Answer A

Constant periumbilical pain shifting to the right lower quadrant; vomiting following the pain; a small volume of diarrhea; no systemic symptoms such as a headache, malaise, or myalgia; a mild elevation of the white blood cell count with an early left shift; and white blood cells (WBCs) or red blood cells (RBCs) in the urine are indications of appendicitis. The WBC count becomes high only with gangrene or perforation of the appendix. The urine may have WBCs or RBCs if the bladder is irritated and ketonuria if there is prolonged vomiting.

12-39   Answer C

Rotavirus causes 15%–35% of all the cases of diarrhea in the United States. It is followed by enteric adenovirus and Norwalk-like viruses. *Giardia lamblia* is a parasite that causes a high incidence of diarrhea in day-care centers.

12-40   Answer D

Antibiotic therapy is not indicated for an uncomplicated salmonellosis because it is generally a self-limiting illness.

12-41   Answer C

The proper order of assessing the abdomen is inspection, auscultation, percussion, and palpation. It is important to inspect the abdomen first before percussion or palpation to avoid causing any discomfort that might alter the client's position. Auscultation is important before percussion and palpation because both of these techniques can increase peristalsis, which would give a false interpretation of bowel sounds on auscultation.

12-42   Answer A

Cullen's sign is a bluish periumbilical color that may indicate intra-abdominal bleeding.

12-43   Answer A

Striae are silvery-white, linear, jagged marks (stretch marks) about 1–6 cm in length that result when elastic fibers in the reticular layer of the skin are broken as a result of rapid or prolonged stretching. This stretching most commonly occurs with pregnancy but may also occur with excessive weight gain, or ascites.

12-44   Answer A

Hyperresonance is present when there is gaseous distention. Dullness occurs over a distended bladder or adipose tissue and when there is fluid or a mass present.

12-45   Answer B

Costovertebral angle tenderness occurs when one hand is "thumped" with the ulnar edge of the other fist over the 12th rib at the costovertebral angle on the back and tenderness or sharp pain occurs. It indicates inflammation of the kidney.

12-46   Answer C

The liver produces and secretes bile to emulsify fats. The salivary glands moisturize food and release enzymes that initiate the digestion process. The pancreas secretes cells that regulate blood sugar levels, store carbohydrates, and inhibit insulin and glucagon secretion. The gallbladder stores and concentrates bile.

12-47   Answer A

Rebound tenderness is present when there is pain on release of pressure to the abdomen and is a reliable indicator of peritoneal inflammation.

12-48   Answer B

An infant's umbilical cord stump dries within 7 days, then hardens and falls off in 10–14 days. It then takes 3–4 weeks for skin to cover the area.

12-49   Answer C

Abdominal respirations cease by age 7 years. The absence of abdominal respirations in children younger than age 7 indicates peritoneal inflammation.

12-50   Answer B

Hyperactive bowel sounds (borborygmi) are present with laxative use, early mechanical bowel obstruction, gastroenteritis, and brisk diarrhea.

12-51   Answer A

Pruritus indicates that biliary obstruction is present with the liver disease. Increased abdominal girth indicates ascites is present from portal hypertension or hypoalbuminemia. Right upper quadrant pain may indicate hepatitis, cholecystitis, hepatocellular carcinoma, or abscess. Easy bruising may indicate splenomegaly secondary to portal hypertension with platelet sequestration, or coagulopathy secondary to decreased synthesis of clotting factors.

12-52   Answer D

Fecal output from an ileostomy is a malodorous, continuous, soft-to-watery effluent material that contains intestinal enzymes, which are very irritating to the skin around the stoma. Stomas farther along the large colon will have more formed stools, and a sigmoid colostomy will result in stools that are almost normal in consistency.

12-53   Answer B

Grey Turner's sign is a bluish discoloration over the flanks. Cullen's sign is a bluish discoloration around the umbilicus. Other findings that can result from the pancreatic inflammatory process include left-sided pleural effusion, jaundice caused by impingement on the common bile duct, and an epigastric mass secondary to pseudocyst development.

12-54   Answer A

Weight loss is usually the presenting symptom of gastric cancer, followed by dysphagia. Hematemesis occurs in 10%–15% of all clients with gastric cancer. Gastrointestinal bleeding is uncommon with gastric cancer, although common with colorectal cancer.

12-55   Answer C

Once gastric cancer has been diagnosed, accurate staging can be determined by an endoscopic ultrasound. Ranson's criteria is a classification system to assess the severity of pancreatitis.

12-56   Answer B

About 95% of gastric ulcers are benign, even though some of these seem to look malignant on x-ray.

12-57   Answer B

Dumping syndrome may occur 1–3 weeks after gastric surgery when the client starts to consume larger meals. Food enters the intestine faster and in larger quantities than before the surgery, causing the client to experience epigastric fullness, distention, discomfort, abdominal cramping, nausea, and increased flatus.

12-58   Answer C

To help clients with dumping syndrome, suggest that they eat foods with a moderate fat and protein content. These foods tend to leave the stomach more slowly and do not draw fluid into the intestine. Also suggest that they reduce the amount of carbohydrates consumed, eat six small meals per day, and take fluids between meals and not at mealtime.

12-59   Answer B

Because of Marvin's alcoholism and his resulting dietary insufficiencies, there is an inadequate amount of vitamin K in the liver for the thrombin to convert fibrinogen to fibrin; thus, the sequence of coagulation is disrupted.

12-60   Answer D

In 80% of the cases, gastroenteritis is viral in nature. This viral infection causes diarrhea by stimulating the secretion of electrolytes into the intestine. This is rapidly followed by water along the osmotic gradient, resulting in watery stools.

12-61   Answer B

In the process of rumination, food is regurgitated, mouthed, or chewed, and then reswallowed. It may be psychogenic or self-stimulated. In some cases when there is an attempt to stimulate the gag reflex in infants, esophagitis has been shown to be present and the rumination is in response to the pain in the throat.

12-62   Answer C

A palpable spleen 2 cm or less below the left costal margin is a normal finding in a child younger than age 3 and may be a normal finding in an older child. Other symptoms would have to be present to warrant further evaluation.

12-63   Answer C

No treatment is necessary for physiological jaundice unless the bilirubin level exceeds 20 mg/dL. With slightly lower levels, it may take longer for the jaundice to disappear if the mother is breastfeeding and she may want to supplement with formula after each feeding. With a high level of bilirubin, if the mother discontinues breastfeeding for 24 hours, the level will probably decrease. The mother should pump her breasts during this time so she can keep producing breast milk and start nursing again once the MD is satisfied with the bilirubin level.

12-64   Answer A

Hirschsprung's disease is common in male infants, results in small ribbonlike stools, usually has no accompanying abdominal pain unless there is obstruction, and may be accompanied by failure to thrive. The infant with functional (acquired) constipation is usually male and has very large stools and abdominal pain, but failure to thrive is uncommon.

12-65   Answer C

Clients taking phenytoin (Dilantin) should also be taking 0.4–1 mg/day of folic acid because Dilantin promotes a folate deficiency. Phenytoin may also contribute to demineralization of the bone, so the serum calcium levels should also be checked. If demineralization is detected, then vitamin D should be added.

12-66   Answer A

Reducing sugar intake is one of the preventive measures to take against dental caries. Other measures include regular brushing and flossing. Sugar has not been correlated with hyperactivity, and simple sugars do not cause diabetes. Dietary fat, rather than sugar, is the culprit in obesity.

12-67   Answer D

Hernias account for more cases of mechanical bowel obstruction in all ages than do volvulus, intussusception, or cancer.

12-68   Answer A

Although depression might be a contributing factor to Nora's wasting away, megestrol (Megace) can produce weight gain by stimulating appetite and food intake and by decreasing the nausea and vomiting that usually accompany terminal cancer.

12-69   Answer A

All these are physical examination maneuvers for diagnosing appendicitis. If pain is elicited during the examination, appendicitis is suspected. Rovsing's sign is deep palpation over the LLQ with sudden, unexpected release of pressure. Psoas sign is pain when the patient is instructed to try to lift the right leg against gentle pressure applied by the examiner or pain when the patient is placed in the left lateral decubitus position and the right leg is extended at the hip. The obturator sign occurs when the patient with the right hip and knee flexed experiences pain when the examiner slowly rotates the right leg internally, which stretches the obturator muscle. McBurney's sign is pain elicited when pressure is applied to McBurney's point, which is located halfway between the umbilicus and the anterior spine of the ilium.

12-70   Answer C

For the client who has just had a hemorrhoidectomy, teaching would include advising the client to maintain an adequate intake of dietary fiber to maintain stool bulk; to take a sitz bath after each bowel movement for 1–2 weeks after surgery to promote relaxation and aid with discomfort; to drink at least 2000 mL of fluids per day; to take stool softeners as prescribed (for short-term relief only); and to exercise regularly to maintain stool bulk, softness, and regularity.

12-71   Answer D

A peritoneal friction rub, which sounds like a rough, grating sound, occurs over organs with a large surface area in contact with the peritoneum when there is peritoneal inflammation (peritonitis). When a peritoneal friction rub is heard over the lower right rib cage, it may be caused by an abscess or tumor of the liver. When heard over the lower left rib cage in the left anterior axillary line, it may indicate infection of the spleen or an abscess or tumor of the spleen. Irritable bowel syndrome does not produce a friction rub.

12-72   Answer C

Lipids are broken down in the small intestine by the pancreatic lipases. Carbohydrates, proteins, and nucleic acids are also broken down in the small intestines by various enzymes.

12-73   Answer A

A distinct foul odor to the stool may indicate blood in the stool, ingestion of a high-fat diet, or colon cancer.

12-74   Answer D

There is no such thing as a "normal" pattern of defecation. Patterns of defecation vary widely and may in part be affected by dietary habits, fluid intake, bacteria in the stool, psychological stress, or voluntary postponement of defecation.

12-75   Answer D

Antacids may contain magnesium, which decreases bowel transit time and may contain poorly absorbed salts that result in an osmotic draw of fluid into the bowel. Fructose, sorbitol, and caffeine are not usually contained in antacids. Fructose is present in apple juice, pear juice, grapes, honey, dates, nuts, figs, and fruit-flavored soft drinks. Sorbitol or mannitol is present in apple juice, pear juice, sugarless gums, and mints. Caffeine is present in coffee, tea, cola drinks, and over-the-counter analgesics.

12-76   Answer B

Diphenoxylate (Lomotil) and loperamide (Imodium), like all opiates and opium derivatives, help to relieve diarrhea by decreasing the motility of the ileum and colon, slowing the transit time, and promoting more water absorption. Anticholinergics such as atropine (Donnatal) and other belladonna alkaloids (Donnagel) reduce bowel spasticity and acid secretion in the stomach.

12-77   Answer C

Polyethylene glycol (GoLYTELY) should be taken in the early evening so as not to interfere with sleep because the first bowel movement begins within 1 hour and continues until the sigmoid colon is clear. The solution should be chilled to enhance palatability, taken on an empty stomach, and administered in 8-oz servings every 10 minutes until 1 gallon is consumed.

12-78   Answer C

Bulk-forming agents such as methylcellulose (Citrucel) are the only laxatives that are safe for long-term use. They contain natural vegetable fiber that is not absorbed. This creates bulk and draws water into the intestine, thus softening the stool. Mineral oil reduces the absorption of the fat-soluble vitamins A, D, E, and K and may cause damage to the liver and spleen because of systemic absorption. Irritant or stimulant laxatives, such as bisacodyl (Dulcolax), work by stimulating the motility and secretion of the intestinal mucosa. Osmotic and saline laxatives and cathartics, such as magnesium hydroxide (milk of magnesia), when used over the long term, may suppress normal bowel reflexes.

12-79   Answer B

Food substances that reduce the lower esophageal sphincter pressure or irritate the gastric mucosa include alcohol, caffeinated beverages, chocolate, citrus fruits, decaffeinated coffee, fatty foods, onions, peppermint and spearmint, tomatoes, and tomato-based products. Nonfood substances that irritate GERD include anticholinergic drugs, beta-adrenergic blocking agents, calcium channel blockers, Diazepam, estrogens, nicotine, and theophylline.

12-80   Answer A

Rebound tenderness at McBurney's point, located midway between the umbilicus and the anterior iliac crest in the right lower quadrant, would alert you to appendicitis.

12-81   Answer C

Osteopenic bone disease may occur in celiac disease because there is decreased calcium absorption by the small intestine, decreased absorption of the fat-soluble vitamin D, and binding of calcium and magnesium in the intestinal lumen by unabsorbed dietary fatty acids. Clients should be identified as having celiac disease before menopause so that therapy to increase bone mass can be instituted before clients develop osteopenia.

12-82   Answer D

The diagnosis of celiac disease is classically established by a trial period of a gluten-free diet with an accompanying improvement in the mucosal histological response. Laboratory tests may confirm malabsorption, but they are not diagnostic of celiac disease. A barium enema may show dilation of the small intestine, but in mild celiac disease, the enema results may be normal. A peroral biopsy showing the gross absence of duodenal folds on endoscopy is a clue to the presence of celiac disease, but it is not diagnostic because this symptom may also occur in tropical sprue, intestinal lymphoma, Zollinger-Ellison syndrome, and other diseases.

12-83   Answer C

Infants with gastrointestinal reflux should be placed on their left side to prevent aspiration. They should be fed a formula thickened with rice cereal while being held in an upright position and kept in an elevated prone position for 1 hour after feeding so that gravity helps prevent reflux.

12-84   Answer B

A history of irritable bowel syndrome has no association with diverticulitis. A client with diverticulitis would have left lower quadrant abdominal pain, a tender mass in the left lower quadrant, and an elevated temperature.

12-85   Answer A

Dehydration is the most common complication of viral gastroenteritis in children. Gastrointestinal bleeding is uncommon. Peritonitis and bacterial sepsis are other causes of diarrhea.

12-86   Answer D

Tenesmus is the spasmodic contraction of the anal or bladder sphincters, producing pain and the persistent desire to empty the bowel or bladder via involuntary, ineffectual straining efforts. Rectal tenesmus is often experienced in ulcerative colitis.

12-87 Answer B

Advise clients who are lactose intolerant to avoid foods containing whey. Whey is a lactose-rich ingredient found in some foods; therefore, labels need to be read on all foods for clients who are lactose intolerant. To control symptoms, dietary lactose should be reduced or restricted by using lactose-reduced and lactose-free dairy products or by eating lactose-rich food in small amounts or in combination with low-lactose or lactose-free foods. Fermented dairy products such as aged or hard cheeses and cultured yogurt are easier to digest and contain less lactose than other dairy products. Most stores carry milk that has been pretreated with lactase, making it more than 70% lactose free. Lillian can eat oranges.

12-88 Answer A

Hepatitis A (HAV) is transmitted by the fecal-oral route, sewage, contaminated water and shellfish, and possibly by blood. Hepatitis B (HBV) is transmitted by the percutaneous route (permucosal) through infected blood and body fluids and sexual contact. Hepatitis C (HCV) is transmitted by the percutaneous route, in the community, and a large percentage of those infected have no known risk factors. Hepatitis D (HDV) is transmitted by the percutaneous route, but most have coinfection with HBV. Hepatitis E (HEV) is transmitted by the fecal-oral route.

12-89 Answer B

A portacaval shunt is the surgery often performed for bleeding esophageal varices. They are associated with alcoholic cirrhosis and portal hypertension, commonly the result of a history of alcohol abuse. Bleeding esophageal varices occur when the small esophageal veins become distended and rupture from increased pressure in the portal system.

12-90 Answer A

Diarrhea is a common problem after a gastroplasty because of the induced malabsorption. Clients usually do not end up losing too much weight because sometimes the only foods they can tolerate are high-caloric foods (simple sugars) such as ice cream.

12-91 Answer B

Melena is defined as black, tarry stools that test positive for occult blood. The most common cause of melena is upper GI bleeding, but bleeding in the small bowel or the right colon can also produce melena. It is the action of gastric acid and intestinal secretions that reduces bright red blood to black, tarry stools. To produce melena, about 100–200 mL of blood must be present. Because of GI transit time, it is possible for melena to continue for several days, after the acute bleeding has stopped.

12-92 Answer A

Cheese, bread, pasta, rice, pretzels, and yogurt all help to thicken stools. Leafy green vegetables, raw fruits and vegetables, and dried beans may all loosen stools.

12-93 Answer D

An incisional or ventral hernia may develop at a previous surgical incision site. An umbilical hernia may be congenital or acquired as the tissue around the umbilical ring weakens. Conditions resulting in umbilical hernias include pregnancy, including multiple pregnancies with prolonged labor; obesity; ascites; and large intra-abdominal tumors.

12-94 Answer C

She should not have a snack before retiring. Clients with gastroesophageal reflux disease should be instructed to avoid coffee, alcohol, chocolate, peppermint, and spicy foods; eat smaller meals; stop smoking; remain upright for 2 hours after meals; elevate the head of the bed on 6–8 in. blocks; and refrain from eating for 3 hours before retiring.

12-95 Answer B

The client with gastroesophageal reflux disease should avoid taking NSAIDs because they tend to aggravate the already-irritated gastric mucosa.

12-96 Answer A

Achalasia is an absence of peristalsis of the esophagus and a high gastroesophageal sphincter pressure. After initial noninvasive treatments, clients may require a balloon dilation of the lower esophageal sphincter. Calcium channel blockers, not beta blockers, may be used to decrease symptoms of dysphagia. A fundoplication is done for a hiatal hernia. An esophagogastrectomy is performed for esophageal cancer.

12-97   Answer B

Clostridium botulinum is an anaerobic gram-positive bacillus that produces toxins. The primary source is canned foods. *Campylobacter jejuni* is found primarily in eggs and poultry but may be found in domestic animals. *Clostridium perfringens* is found in soil, feces, air, and water. Outbreaks are caused most often by contaminated meat. *Staphylococcus* is a common cause of food poisoning. It is caused by the ingestion of an enterotoxin found in improperly handled or stored foods.

12-98   Answer B

Vomiting is more common with gastric ulcers than duodenal ulcers. Stools are more often altered with duodenal ulcers. The possibility of perforation and obstruction of the gastrointestinal tract is present in both types of ulcers. Approximately half of the clients report relief of pain with food or antacids (especially with duodenal ulcers). Many clients deny the relationship of meals to the pain. Two-thirds of clients with duodenal ulcers and one-third with gastric ulcers have nocturnal pain that awakens them.

12-99   Answer B

Cushing's ulcers are stress ulcers that occur after a head injury or intracranial disease. A Cushing's ulcer may also occur after a severe burn.

12-100   Answer C

A pyloroplasty surgically enlarges the opening between the stomach and duodenum to improve gastric emptying. A Billroth I is a gastroduodenostomy. A total gastrectomy is removal of the entire stomach and is rarely performed. It results in an anastomosis connecting the esophagus to the duodenum or jejunum. A vagotomy severs a portion or all of the vagus nerves to the stomach.

12-101   Answer B

The following drugs may cause acute hepatitis: acetaminophen, allopurinol, aspirin in high doses, captopril, carbamazepine, isoniazid, ketoconazole, methyldopa, NSAIDs, procainamide, and sulfonamides.

12-102   Answer A

The majority of the population in the United States has antibodies against hepatitis A (HAV). Besides immunity, there is also a vaccine available.

12-103   Answer C

During the incubation period of viral hepatitis, there are no subjective or objective complaints. During the prodromal stage, there is anorexia, nausea, vomiting, malaise, upper respiratory infection (nasal discharge, pharyngitis), myalgia, arthralgia, easy fatigability, fever (HAV), and abdominal pain. In the icteric stage of viral hepatitis, there is jaundice, dark urine, and light-colored stools. There are continued prodromal complaints with gradual improvement. During the convalescent stage, there is an increased sense of well-being; the appetite returns; and the jaundice, abdominal pain, and fatigability abate.

12-104   Answer D

Women tend to develop cirrhosis more quickly with less alcohol intake than men, which suggests that a smaller, leaner body mass and enhanced absorption are both factors in the development of alcoholic cirrhosis. Alcoholic cirrhosis, also known as Laënnec's, portal, fatty, or micronodular cirrhosis, is the most common type of cirrhosis in the United States. Alcoholic cirrhosis is often associated with nutritional and vitamin deficiencies but occurs in well-nourished individuals, as well as alcoholics. Cirrhosis is the irreversible end stage of liver injury and may be caused by a variety of insults.

12-105   Answer B

A ventral hernia, also known as an epigastric hernia, occurs along the midline between the xiphoid process and the umbilicus. The fibers along the linea alba are brought together in a patchwork-type closure; the defect exists within this decussation. As these fibers weaken, the contents can herniate through the abdomen. Epigastric hernias are three times more likely to occur in men than women. Umbilical hernias that develop in adulthood occur through a weakening in the abdominal wall around the umbilical ring. Incisional hernias can occur anywhere along a surgical incision into the abdomen. An inguinal hernia may be indirect or direct. Indirect inguinal hernias result when tissue herniates through the internal inguinal ring, which extends the length of the spermatic cord. A direct inguinal hernia occurs when the transversus abdominis and internal oblique muscles are attached, forming a high arch on the inferior border that results in a faulty shutter mechanism.

12-106   Answer C

The obturator sign is elicited when, with the patient's right hip and knee flexed, the examiner slowly rotates the right leg internally, which stretches the obturator muscle. Pain over the RLQ is considered a positive sign. Rovsing's sign is pain elicited with deep palpation over the LLQ with sudden, unexpected release of pressure. This causes tenderness over the RLQ and is considered a positive finding. Psoas sign is pain when the patient is instructed to try to lift the right leg against gentle pressure applied by the examiner or by placing the patient in the left lateral decubitus position and extending the patient's right leg at the hip. An increase in pain is considered positive and is an indication of the inflamed appendix irritating the psoas muscle. McBurney's sign is pain elicited when pressure is applied to McBurney's point, which is located halfway between the umbilicus and the anterior spine of the ilium.

12-107   Answer C

Susan has a constellation of symptoms known as metabolic syndrome. The World Health Organization (WHO), National Cholesterol Education Program Adult Treatment Panel (NCEP-ATP III), and the International Diabetes Federation (IDF) have slightly different criteria for this diagnosis. They all, however, include hypertension, dyslipidemia, and central obesity.

12-108   Answer B

Several studies show that intensive lifestyle changes in the form of diet and exercise can go miles in reducing death and events in high-risk patients. Studies on managing diabetes show that these modifications are more effective than drug therapy. Exercise, for example, is a strong deterrent for developing diabetes and heart disease. Some easy fixes in the diet are staying away from high-fructose corn syrup and trans fats, which are two of the biggest metabolic syndrome antagonists. Patients need to understand the association of what goes in the mouth and what goes on with their blood chemistry. Teaching must help patients understand and manage all the factors that put them in the metabolic danger zone.

12-109   Answer D

The rate of C. *difficile* colitis has increased 109% in the past decade. The case fatality rate among C. *difficile* colitis patients climbed as well. Awareness of this must be heightened if we are to help control the public health ramifications of this important and morbid nosocomial infection.

12-110   Answer A

Three-dose cefmetazole administration is significantly more effective for prevention of incisional surgical site infection (SSI) than single-dose administration for patients undergoing colorectal surgery. Use of prophylactic antibiotics in elective colorectal surgery is essential. The incidence of incisional SSI among patients undergoing colorectal surgery may be as high as 30%–50% without prophylactic antibiotics.

12-111   Answer C

Although some patients report a significant subjective drop in taste function following surgery, none of the patients have ongoing taste dysfunction. Sweet, sour, salty, and bitter taste abilities may be temporarily affected, but there is no lasting change in taste seen after a tonsillectomy.

12-112   Answer B

Older adults have a diminished response to painful stimuli that may mask abdominal health problems. Older adults may have difficulty assuming some positions necessary for the physical examination, so positions may need to be modified to meet their needs. As people age, many of their body systems slow down and become less efficient. In the GI tract, there is a reduction of saliva, stomach acid, gastric motility, and peristalsis that causes problems with swallowing, absorption, and digestion. These changes, along with a general reduction of muscle mass and tone, also contribute to constipation. The liver becomes smaller and liver function declines, making it harder to process medications.

Bibliography

Barclay, L, and Lie, D: Three-dose cefmetazole may be better than a single dose for colorectal surgery. http://www.medscape.com/viewarticle/560045, accessed 7/20/07.

Dillon, PM: *Nursing Health Assessment—A Critical Thinking, Case Studies Approach*, ed 2. FA Davis, Philadelphia, 2007.

Dunphy, LM, et al: *The Art and Science of Advanced Practice Nursing,* ed 2. FA Davis, Philadelphia, 2007.

Landsmann, MA: Weighing in on metabolic syndrome. *Healthy Aging* 2(5):54–59, January/February 2007.

No lasting change in taste seen after tonsillectomy. http://www.medscape.com/viewarticle/560045, accessed 7/20/07.

Rise in serious cases of C. *difficile* colitis seen over 11-year period. http://www.medscape.com/viewarticle/559865, accessed 7/20/07.

How well did you do?

85% and above, congratulations! This score shows application of test-taking principles and adequate content knowledge.

75%–85%, keep working! Review test-taking principles and try again.

65%–75%, hang in there! Spend some time reviewing concepts and test-taking principles and try the test again.

Chapter 13: *Renal Problems*

Questions

13-1 *Clinical manifestations including microscopic or gross hematuria, a palpable abdominal mass, fever, and flank pain may indicate a*

A. pancreatic tumor.

B. liver tumor.

C. colon mass.

D. renal tumor.

13-2 *Cardiovascular failure is a major cause of which type of acute renal failure?*

A. Prerenal

B. Intrarenal

C. Postrenal

D. Perirenal

13-3 *If a client with acute renal failure (ARF) excretes 400 mL of urine on Tuesday, how much fluid intake (both oral and intravenous) should the client have on Wednesday?*

A. 400 mL

B. 600 mL

C. 900 mL

D. 1200 mL

13-4 *Dietary management for the client in acute renal failure includes*

A. decreasing carbohydrate intake.

B. increasing dietary sodium intake.

C. limiting protein intake.

D. increasing potassium.

13-5 *Goodpasture's syndrome is*

A. characterized by glomerulonephritis and pulmonary hemorrhage resulting from immune complex damage to the glomerular and alveolar basement membranes.

B. characterized by massive proteinuria, hypoalbuminemia, hyperlipidemia, and edema.

C. an inflammatory autoimmune disorder affecting the connective tissue of the body with

inflammatory lesions involving the supportive tissues of the glomerulus.

D. typically the end stage of other glomerular disorders, such as rapidly progressive glomerulonephritis, lupus nephritis, or diabetic nephropathy.

13-6 *What is the most common cause of chronic renal failure (CRF)?*

A. Glomerulonephritis

B. Hypertension

C. Diabetic nephropathy

D. A combination of urological diseases

13-7 *The most frequent complication during hemodialysis is*

A. bleeding.

B. infection.

C. dialysis dementia.

D. hypotension.

13-8 *You should be concerned about the use of diuretics, chronic renal failure, a high-protein diet, gout, leukemia, or lymphoma when a serum uric acid level is*

A. 4.0 mg/dL.

B. 5.0 mg/dL.

C. 6.0 mg/dL.

D. greater than 7.0 mg/dL.

13-9 *The most common cause of urinary tract obstruction is*

A. edema resulting from trauma.

B. a tumor.

C. ureterolithiasis.

D. a vascular problem.

13-10 *What is the first step in the treatment of uric acid kidney stones?*

A. Encouraging hydration

B. Alkalinizing the urine

C. Prescribing allopurinol (Zyloprim)

D. Reducing protein intake

13-11 *Which of the following is the likeliest outcome in clients with chronic kidney disease (CKD)?*

A. End-stage renal disease (ESRD)

B. Dialysis

C. Hypertension

D. Death

13-12 *The aging process begins to affect the kidneys with a progressive loss of nephron units by age*

A. 40 years.

B. 50 years.

C. 60 years.

D. 70 years.

13-13 *In the older adult, which physiological change does not affect pharmacokinetics?*

A. Decreased creatine clearance

B. Decreased lean muscle mass

C. Increased total body fat

D. Increased serum albumin level

13-14 *Which of the following groups is most prone to developing nephrolithiasis?*

A. White men

B. White women

C. Black men

D. Black women

13-15 *Who is at a higher risk for developing nephrolithiasis?*

A. Jean, who exercises every day and drinks copious amounts of water

B. Bill, who runs every day and takes excessive amounts of vitamin C

C. Mary Ann, who watches her weight and eats a low-sodium diet

D. Harvey, a "couch potato" who drinks a lot of no-sodium soda

13-16 *Which diagnostic finding(s) may lead to a diagnosis of nephrolithiasis?*

A. Urinary uric acid output of less than 750 mg/24 hours

B. Urinary pH greater than 5.5

C. Urinary calcium output of greater than 300 mg/24 hours

D. Serum calcium of 8 mg/dL

13-17 *What condition may result from clients taking NSAIDs on a long-term basis?*

A. Hemodynamically induced acute renal failure

B. Diabetes insipidus

C. Neurogenic bladder

D. Hypokalemia

13-18 *Jessica, age 79, has been on dialysis for 6 years due to CKD. She has been on an oral iron preparation and now asks you if she should think about switching to the new intravenous (IV) iron preparation. How do you respond?*

A. "If it ain't broke, don't fix it."

B. "There are more side effects with IV administration than oral administration."

C. "You have many more problems than iron deficiency anemia. Let's not worry about that."

D. "Let's try it. It corrects iron deficiency faster, more safely, and better than oral iron."

13-19 *Which of the following drugs is not associated with acute renal failure?*

A. Angiotensin-converting enzyme (ACE) inhibitors

B. Cimetidine (Tagamet)

C. NSAIDs

D. Erythromycin (E-Mycin)

13-20 *Janet has stress urinary incontinence and has been doing Kegel exercises with some success. What other simple action might help in relieving some of the problem?*

A. Stopping smoking

B. Limiting fluids

C. Taking a daily multivitamin

D. Beginning lifting 2-lb weights

13-21 *The most common factor predisposing a woman to a urinary tract infection is*

A. the use of an oral contraceptive.

B. the use of a diaphragm.

C. urinary stasis.

D. calculi.

13-22 *Sally, age 24, has frequent urinary tract infections. You are teaching her about measures to prevent them. You know she has misunderstood your directions when she tells you that she'll*

A. void after intercourse.

B. avoid bubble baths.

C. wear underwear with pantyhose.

D. drink 2–4 glasses of water per day.

13-23 *Which type of hematuria in an older adult is an ominous sign?*

A. Painless, gross hematuria

B. Flank pain with hematuria

C. Hematuria following trauma

D. Intermittent hematuria

13-24 *The most common cause of nephrotic syndrome is*

A. systemic lupus erythematosus.

B. diabetes mellitus.

C. routine use of NSAIDs.

D. glomerulosclerosis.

13-25 *Sam, age 42, has had persistent proteinuria on the previous two office visits. Which action is warranted next?*

A. Schedule extensive blood work.

B. Order an intravenous pyelogram.

C. Admit Sam to the hospital.

D. Have Sam collect one urine specimen on first arising and then another 2 hours later.

13-26 *Which finding in urinary sediment is indicative of pyelonephritis and interstitial nephritis?*

A. Hyaline casts

B. Granular casts

C. Red blood cell casts

D. White blood cell casts

13-27 *Which type of kidney stone is the most common?*

A. Calcium oxalate

B. Uric acid

C. Calcium phosphate

D. Cystine

13-28 *Transient urinary incontinence in women may be caused by*

A. hypertrophy of the vaginal or urethral walls.

B. diarrhea.

C. use of anticholinergic agents.

D. hypoglycemia.

13-29 *In clients receiving dialysis, which is the most common cause of end-stage renal disease in the United States?*

A. Diabetic nephropathy

B. Chronic renal failure secondary to vascular disorders

C. Acute tubular necrosis

D. Kidney trauma

13-30 *About 80% of all cases of dysuria are caused by ascending bacterial infection of the urinary tract by which organism?*

A. *Klebsiella*

B. *Proteus*

C. *Escherichia coli*

D. *Staphylococcus saprophyticus*

13-31 *Leslie, age 13, says that her mother has polycystic kidney disease and asks about her chances of developing it. How do you respond?*

A. "It is hereditary, but if you develop it, a cure is possible."

B. "It is hereditary and, unfortunately, incurable, but there are many measures we can use in dealing with it."

C. "It is not hereditary, but you may develop it anyway."

D. "It is hereditary, but skips generations."

13-32 *Which history is commonly found in a client with glomerulonephritis?*

A. Beta-hemolytic streptococcal infection

B. Frequent urinary tract infections

C. Kidney stones

D. Hypotension

13-33 *Which diuretic acts by inhibiting sodium chloride reabsorption in the thick ascending limb of the loop of Henle?*

A. Furosemide (Lasix)

B. Mannitol (Osmitrol)

C. Hydrochlorothiazide (Hydrodiuril)

D. Acetazolamide (Diamox)

13-34 *Which category of diuretic has the following side effects: hyperkalemia, headache, hyponatremia, nausea, diarrhea, urticaria, and menstrual disturbances?*

A. Osmotic diuretic

B. Loop diuretic

C. Potassium-sparing diuretic

D. Thiazide diuretic

13-35 *Which of the following diagnostic studies for the evaluation of renal function assesses for the lack of erythropoietin?*

A. Urine creatinine clearance

B. Blood urea nitrogen

C. Serum albumin

D. Serum hemoglobin and hematocrit

13-36 *Which of the following in the urinary sediment signifies an allergic reaction in the kidney?*

A. Leukocytes

B. Eosinophils

C. Crystals

D. Erythrocytes

13-37 *Which of the following radiological studies provides direct imaging in several planes conducive to detecting renal cystic disease, inflammatory processes, and renal cell carcinoma?*

A. Cystoscopy

B. Ultrasonography

C. Computed tomography

D. Magnetic resonance imaging

13-38 *Which diagnostic procedure can visualize the renal outline and identify lower rib fractures?*

A. Intravenous pyelogram

B. Renal angiography

C. Computed tomography

D. A kidneys, ureters, and bladder film

13-39 *Why is the right kidney slightly lower than the left kidney?*

A. The spleen pushes the left kidney upward.

B. The liver pushes the right kidney downward.

C. The diaphragm displaces the left kidney.

D. The right kidney is structurally larger than the left kidney.

13-40 *Which nephrotoxic agent should be avoided in clients with chronic renal failure (CRF)?*

A. NSAIDs

B. Kayexalate

C. Calcium carbonate

D. Erythropoietin

13-41 *Rita, age 16, has a 3-day history of red urine. You want her to go home for a few days and then return for some lab work. In teaching her what to avoid, you know she's misunderstood the directions when she tells you she shouldn't ingest any*

A. blackberries.

B. ibuprofen.

C. red food color.

D. watermelon.

13-42 *Which type of bloody urine is characteristic of bleeding from the upper urinary tract?*

A. Grossly bloody urine

B. Urine with blood clots

C. Brown, smoky, or tea-colored urine

D. Blood noted at the beginning or end of the stream

13-43 *Cloudy urine is usually indicative of which of the following conditions?*

A. Diabetes

B. Proteinuria

C. Malignancy

D. Urinary tract infection (UTI)

13-44 *Who is at risk of developing a prerenal type of acute renal failure?*

A. Joey, age 2, who is dehydrated from gastroenteritis

B. Tommy, age 3, who accidentally took an overdose of acetaminophen (Tylenol)

C. Justine, age 5, who nearly drowned in a swimming pool

D. Buddy, age 12, who was born with one kidney and just injured the other in a football game

13-45 *Why do middle-aged men not incur as many urinary tract infections as middle-aged women?*

A. Women are more prone to urinary stasis than men.

B. Men have the bacteriostatic effect of prostatic fluid and a longer urethra.

C. Women have a higher urine pH.

D. Men take more baths than women.

13-46 *Alice, age 29, is having an intravenous pyelogram (IVP). In teaching her about the procedure, you tell her that an IVP*

A. takes about 30 minutes and uses x-rays to show the structures of the kidney, ureters, and bladder after injection of a dye that is rapidly excreted in the urine.

B. involves first filling the bladder with a dye solution, then taking x-rays of the filled bladder and of the bladder and urethra during urination.

C. involves the use of radioisotopes.

D. is the same as a renal arteriogram.

13-47 *Thiazide diuretics are used for the treatment of which type of renal calculi?*

A. Calcium phosphate and/or oxalate stones

B. Struvite stones

C. Uric acid stones

D. Cystine stones

13-48 *Jim has had several episodes of kidney stones. The last stone he passed was examined and found to be an oxalate stone. You tell him to avoid foods high in oxalate such as*

A. beans and lentils, chocolate and cocoa, dried fruits, canned or smoked fish except tuna, flour, milk, and milk products.

B. cheese, cranberries, eggs, grapes, meat and poultry, plums and prunes, tomatoes, and whole grains.

C. asparagus, beer, beets, cabbage, celery, chocolate and cocoa, fruits, green beans, nuts, tea, colas, and tomatoes.

D. goose, organ meats, sardines, herring, and venison and to have a moderate intake of beef, chicken, crab, pork, salmon, and veal.

13-49 *Jake is having a urinary diversion procedure performed because of a urinary tract tumor. He states that*

he heard about a Koch pouch and asks you what it is. You respond,

A. "It is a cutaneous ureterostomy in which one or both of the ureters create a stoma on the skin surface."

B. "It is an ileal conduit in which the ileum is formed into a pouch with an open stoma and the ureters are inserted into the pouch."

C. "It is a continent internal ileal reservoir in which nipple valves are formed on the skin. The filling pressure closes the valves, preventing leakage and reflux."

D. "It is a ureterosigmoidostomy in which the ureters are inserted into the sigmoid colon. Urine empties into the rectum and is expelled with defecation."

13-50 *Which medication is used primarily in the treatment of acute postoperative and postpartum urinary retention and for neurogenic bladder atony with urinary retention?*

A. Bethanechol chloride (Urecholine)

B. Neostigmine (Prostigmin)

C. Propantheline bromide (Pro-Banthine)

D. Oxybutynin (Ditropan)

13-51 *Mary Lou, who has stress urinary incontinence, is desperate for some relief and asks for your help. She already takes several pills a day and does not really want to take any more, but she wants to do something about her problem. What do you suggest?*

A. Propantheline bromide (Pro-Banthine)

B. Dicyclomine hydrochloride (Bentyl)

C. Estrogen vaginal cream

D. Imipramine hydrochloride (Tofranil)

13-52 *Eric, age 5, has enuresis. The probable cause is*

A. anatomical disease.

B. neurological disease.

C. a psychological problem.

D. maturational delay.

13-53 *Which of the following does not cause urine to appear reddish in color?*

A. Cascara sagrada

B. Phenazopyridine (Pyridium)

C. Phenytoin (Dilantin)

D. Multivitamins

13-54   *Urine specific gravity is increased in clients with*

A. dehydration.

B. diabetes insipidus.

C. chronic renal failure.

D. overhydration.

13-55   *What amount of urine in a 24-hour period in an adult represents oliguria?*

A. No urine output

B. Urine output less than 50 mL/day

C. Urine output less than 100 mL/day

D. Urine output less than 500 mL/day

13-56   *After a renal biopsy, the client should be instructed*

A. that there may be some blood in the urine for the next several days.

B. to avoid strenuous activities for at least 2 weeks.

C. to drink 3–4 glasses of water per day.

D. to measure urine output for the first week.

13-57   *A 24-hour urine test for vanillylmandelic acid and catecholamines is done to diagnose*

A. a renal tumor.

B. hypertension secondary to pheochromocytoma.

C. renal artery stenosis.

D. hydronephrosis.

13-58   *Which statement is true regarding acute tubular necrosis (ATN)?*

A. It is a slow, progressive disease.

B. Creatinine clearance is greatly increased.

C. Peritoneal dialysis or hemodialysis should be reserved for severe cases.

D. The removal of the offending agent may allow renal function to return gradually to normal.

13-59   *Which of the following conditions does not cause flank pain?*

A. Pyelonephritis

B. Ureterolithiasis

C. Vascular occlusion of the kidney (renal vein thrombosis)

D. Renal cysts

13-60   *Urine that appears brownish in color may result from which of the following?*

A. Beets

B. Bile

C. Rifampin (Rifadin)

D. Phenazopyridine (Pyridium)

13-61   *In an assessment of renal function, what is the maximum amount of urine in a 24-hour period that a client would produce for a diagnosis of anuria to be considered?*

A. No urine output at all

B. Less than 100 mL

C. 100–150 mL

D. 151–200 mL

13-62   *What is the most common cause of death in dialysis clients?*

A. Infection

B. Bleeding from the access site

C. Cardiovascular failure

D. Sepsis

13-63   *An acidic urine pH favors precipitation of which type of kidney stone?*

A. Cystine stones

B. Calcium phosphate stones

C. Struvite stones

D. Magnesium stones

13-64   *The most common metabolic condition that predisposes to the formation of kidney stones is*

A. idiopathic hypercalciuria.

B. hyperuricosuria.

C. hyperoxaluria.

D. a low urinary citrate excretion.

13-65   *Which of the following renal hormones regulates intrarenal blood flow by vasodilation or vasoconstriction?*

A. Renin

B. Prostaglandins

C. Bradykinins

D. Erythropoietin

13-66 *Which type of white blood cell may be present in the urine and activated by antigens and antigen-induced hypersensitivity reactions?*

A. Lymphocytes

B. Monocytes

C. Basophils

D. Eosinophils

13-67 *Which group of persons experience more rapid age-related decreases in glomerular filtration rate (GFR) than do Caucasians?*

A. African Americans

B. Asians

C. Europeans

D. Native Americans

13-68 *Which class of antihypertensive drugs is contraindicated in clients with renal artery stenosis?*

A. Calcium channel blockers

B. Beta blockers

C. ACE inhibitors

D. Cardiac glycosides

13-69 *A urinary tract infection is best detected by performing*

A. a nitrite dipstick test.

B. a urinalysis.

C. a urine culture.

D. urine sensitivity.

13-70 *The most frequent reason why a person would come to your office complaining of burning on urination is*

A. prostatitis.

B. urethritis.

C. a urinary tract infection.

D. a sexually transmitted disease.

13-71 *A factor contributing to stress incontinence is*

A. a decreased estrogen level.

B. bladder irritation from a urinary tract infection.

C. prostatic hypertrophy.

D. a spinal cord lesion or trauma above S2.

13-72 *Postmenopausal women tend to have more recurrent urinary tract infections because of*

A. frequent urination.

B. estrogen depletion–related changes.

C. an increase in lactobacilli.

D. a decrease in *Escherichia coli.*

13-73 *The clinical presentation of a client with urolithiasis would include*

A. a gradual onset of nagging pain.

B. marked leukocytes in the urine.

C. a fever of 101°F or above.

D. pain starting in the flank and localizing in the costovertebral angle.

13-74 *Extracorporeal shock wave lithotripsy is not recommended for which type of kidney stones?*

A. Oxalate stones

B. Uric acid stones

C. Struvite stones

D. Cystine stones

13-75 *General recommendations for the prevention of kidney stones, regardless of the type of stone the client has, include*

A. drinking 3–4 L of mineral water per day.

B. reducing protein in the diet.

C. increasing vitamin C in the diet.

D. decreasing fiber in the diet.

13-76 *The inability to empty the bladder, resulting in overdistention and frequent loss of small amounts of urine, describes which type of urinary incontinence?*

A. Stress incontinence

B. Urge incontinence

C. Overflow incontinence

D. Reflex incontinence

13-77 *Decreased bladder capacity; bladder irritation from a urinary tract infection, tumor, stones, or irritants such as caffeine and alcohol; and central nervous system disorders or spinal cord lesions are all contributing factors to*

A. stress urinary incontinence.

B. urge urinary incontinence.

C. overflow urinary incontinence.

D. reflex urinary incontinence.

13-78 *You explain to Yolanda that pelvic floor (Kegel) exercises help to restore and maintain continence by improving pelvic muscle strength, increasing urethral pressure, and decreasing abnormal detrusor muscle contractions. These exercises are used for her diagnosis of*

A. stool incontinence.

B. full-bladder incontinence.

C. cystitis-related incontinence.

D. stress incontinence.

13-79 *Which of the following drugs is an analgesic used to treat dysuria?*

A. Hyoscyamine (Levsin)

B. Oxybutynin (Ditropan)

C. Propantheline (Pro-Banthine)

D. Phenazopyridine (Pyridium)

13-80 *Which of the following changes in laboratory values is associated with kidney disease?*

A. Serum creatinine greater than 4 mg/dL

B. Serum albumin 0.5–1.0 mg/dL

C. Serum sodium greater than 150 mEq/L

D. Serum calcium greater than 6.0 mEq/L

13-81 *What is the most common cause of end-stage renal disease (ESRD)?*

A. Hypertensive nephropathy

B. Glomerulonephritis (GN)

C. Diabetic nephropathy

D. Acute tubular necrosis

13-82 *Which of the following is defined as a pathophysiological process that occurs when there is a primary excess in the extracellular fluid of bicarbonate as a result of a loss of acid or the addition of excess bicarbonate?*

A. Metabolic acidosis

B. Metabolic alkalosis

C. Respiratory acidosis

D. Respiratory alkalosis

13-83 *Excessive alcohol ingestion can cause*

A. metabolic acidosis.

B. metabolic alkalosis.

C. respiratory acidosis.

D. respiratory alkalosis.

13-84 *Clinical manifestations of metabolic alkalosis include*

A. tetany.

B. nausea and vomiting.

C. weakness.

D. bradycardia.

13-85 *Sara, age 82, was unable to breathe for several minutes after choking on a piece of meat. A successful Heimlich maneuver was done and her arterial blood gases now are pH 7.39, $PaCO_2$, 48, PaO_2, 92, and HCO_3 24. What do you suspect?*

A. Respiratory alkalosis.

B. Respiratory acidosis

C. Metabolic alkalosis

D. Metabolic acidosis

13-86 *Maury has renal failure and his arterial blood gas readings show a decreased pH, normal PCO_2, and decreased HCO_3. What do you suspect?*

A. Respiratory acidosis

B. Respiratory alkalosis

C. Metabolic acidosis

D. Metabolic alkalosis

13-87 *The kidneys excrete increased amounts of HCO_3 to lower the pH as a mode of compensation for which acid-base disturbance?*

A. Respiratory acidosis

B. Respiratory alkalosis

C. Metabolic acidosis

D. Metabolic alkalosis

13-88 *Before using the radial artery to draw blood for arterial blood gas (ABG) testing, which test should be performed?*

A. The ABG test

B. The Thomas test

C. The Weber test

D. The Allen test

13-89 *Which of the following accounts for half of the bladder tumors among men and one-third in women?*

A. Cigarette smoke, both active and passive inhalation

B. Chemicals from plastic and rubber

C. Chronic use of phenacetin-containing analgesic agents

D. Working long hours and not voiding often

13-90 *Marvin, age 59, is going to have a total cystectomy to remove his bladder tumor. He states that when the surgeon was talking to him, he was not really listening, and he asks you about the incidence of impotence after such a surgery. How do you respond?*

A. "You'll have to talk to the surgeon; every case is unique."

B. "This surgery requires the removal of the prostate and seminal vessels, which does result in impotence. Let's talk about it."

C. "I'm not sure if this will be the case, but if it is, how would you feel about it?"

D. "How does your wife feel about the possibility?"

13-91 *Most calcium phosphate kidney stones are caused by*

A. a high dietary calcium intake.

B. a high phosphorus dietary intake.

C. primary hyperparathyroidism.

D. hyperthyroidism.

13-92 *The most frequent sign of bladder cancer is*

A. hematuria.

B. flank pain.

C. nocturia.

D. dysuria.

13-93 *Marie, age 16, fell off her bicycle and sustained a contusion of her left kidney. The treatment of choice is*

A. surgery.

B. urethral catheterization.

C. conservative therapy.

D. to continue normal activity because it is only a contusion.

13-94 *Jill, who has had urinary incontinence for several months, wants to have an evaluation to determine if*

any therapy will be beneficial. After having an initial pelvic examination, she has a postvoid residual catheterization. A residual volume of more than how many milliliters is abnormal?

A. 10 mL

B. 30 mL

C. 50 mL

D. 100 mL

13-95 *Urine tends to become colonized when indwelling urinary catheters are left in place for more than*

A. 24 hours.

B. 36 hours.

C. 48 hours.

D. 72 hours.

13-96 *Samuel wants his son circumcised, but it is noted that the baby has hypospadias. What do you tell Samuel?*

A. "Your son should be circumcised as soon as possible."

B. "Wait until your son is 1 month old; then he can be circumcised."

C. "We first have to check to see where the opening is; then we can determine if your son can be circumcised or not."

D. "Your son should not be circumcised."

13-97 *Doug, age 6, appears with abdominal distention and pain, an abdominal mass on the right side, fever, and slight hematuria. There is no precipitating event. What do you suspect?*

A. A urinary tract infection

B. Appendicitis

C. Wilms' tumor

D. An intestinal obstruction

13-98 *Martha, age 42, states that she has intercourse only about once a month, but immediately afterward she usually gets a urinary tract infection. She is frustrated with having to come to the office frequently to have an examination with a urine test. She says that she is ready to "kick her husband out of bed." How do you respond?*

A. "By taking a low-dose antibiotic every day, you can prevent a urinary tract infection."

B. "Take 200 mg of ofloxacin with a large glass of water after intercourse."

C. "I'll write you a prescription for a 3-day pack of antibiotics with several refills to take when you need it."

D. "Yes, not having sexual intercourse will resolve the problem."

13-99 *The best index of kidney function is*

A. a midstream urinalysis.

B. serum creatinine levels.

C. urine protein level.

D. glomerular filtration rate (GFR).

13-100 *The most common cause of sepsis in older adults is*

A. urinary stasis.

B. a urinary tract infection.

C. a kidney stone.

D. a common cold

13-101 *What is the percussion tone heard over a distended bladder?*

A. Dullness

B. Resonance

C. Hyperresonance

D. Tympany

13-102 *The increased presence of which of the following in a urinalysis indicates the presence of bacteria or protein, which is seen in severe renal disease and could also indicate urinary calculi?*

A. Crystals

B. Casts

C. Nitrates

D. Ketones

13-103 *Which of the following renal exams identifies the size of the kidneys or obstruction in the kidneys or the lower urinary tract and may detect tumors or cysts?*

A. Computed tomography (CT)

B. Voiding cystourethrography (VCUG)

C. Renal arteriogram

D. Ultrasonography (US)

13-104 *Samuel, age 67, is a diabetic with worsening renal function. He has frequent hypoglycemic episodes,*

which he believes means that his diabetes is getting "better." How do you respond?

A. "You've watched your diet for all these years and as a result, your body is using less insulin."

B. "I'll have to change your oral hyperglycemic agents as it seems your body is making more insulin."

C. "Because your kidneys are not functioning well, your insulin is not being metabolized and excreted as it should, so you need less of it."

D. "You're right; it seems like your diabetes is improving."

13-105 *Your client is on a low-protein diet for ESRD. Because of this, which of the following is essential that he include in his diet?*

A. A phosphate binder

B. Supplemental iron

C. Potassium supplements

D. Vitamin and mineral supplements

13-106 *Martha has been on peritoneal dialysis and is going to the OR for placement of an AV fistula to begin hemodialysis. How do you respond when she asks you what this is?*

A. "This is where an artery and a vein are sewn together internally."

B. "This is where a tubing is connecting an artery and a vein underneath the skin."

C. "This is where a catheter is tunneled underneath the skin with a little cuff on the outside."

D. "You'll have an exterior loop of tubing connecting an artery and a vein."

13-107 *The best test to determine microalbuminuria to assist in the diagnosis of diabetic nephropathy is*

A. a dipstick strip done during a routine urinalysis in the office.

B. a 24-hour urine collection.

C. an early morning spot urine collection.

D. a serum albumin test.

Answers

13-1 Answer D

Clinical manifestations of renal tumors include microscopic or gross hematuria, a palpable abdominal mass, fever, flank pain, fatigue, weight loss, and anemia or polycythemia.

13-2   Answer A

Cardiovascular failure and hypovolemia are the two major causes of prerenal acute renal failure. Vascular disease, glomerulonephritis, interstitial nephritis, and acute tubular necrosis are causes of intrarenal acute renal failure. Extrarenal obstruction, intrarenal obstruction, and bladder rupture are causes of postrenal acute renal failure. There is no such thing as perirenal failure.

13-3   Answer C

If a client with acute renal failure (ARF) excretes 400 mL of urine on Tuesday, the amount of fluid intake (both oral and intravenous) the client should have on Wednesday is 900 mL. A client with ARF is initially managed conservatively by fluid and dietary management. The permitted daily intake is calculated by allowing 500 mL for insensible losses (respiration, perspiration, bowel losses) and adding the amount excreted as urine in the previous 24 hours. The client excreted 400 mL as urine, so adding 500 mL for insensible loss equals 900 mL total intake for the next 24 hours.

13-4   Answer C

Dietary management for the client in acute renal failure (ARF) includes limiting protein intake to 0.7–1.0 g/kg of body weight per day to minimize the degree of azotemia. Carbohydrate intake is increased to maintain adequate calorie intake and provide a protein-sparing effect. Dietary sodium intake is decreased to assist in preventing fluid retention. Unless serum potassium levels are low, there should be no change in potassium intake.

13-5   Answer A

Goodpasture's syndrome is characterized by glomerulonephritis and pulmonary hemorrhage resulting from immune complex damage to the glomerular and alveolar basement membranes. Nephrotic syndrome is characterized by massive proteinuria, hypoalbuminemia, hyperlipidemia, and edema. Lupus nephritis is an inflammatory autoimmune disorder affecting the connective tissue of the body with inflammatory lesions involving the supportive tissues of the glomerulus. Chronic glomerulonephritis is typically the end stage of other glomerular disorders such as rapidly progressive glomerulonephritis, lupus nephritis, or diabetic nephropathy.

13-6   Answer C

The most common cause of chronic renal failure (CRF) is diabetic nephropathy. Diabetic nephropathy makes up about 34% of all cases of CRF, followed by hypertension (29%), glomerulonephritis (11%), and other urological diseases (6%).

13-7   Answer D

Hypotension is the most frequent complication seen during hemodialysis. It is related to many factors, such as changes in serum osmolality, rapid removal of fluid from the vascular compartment, and vasodilation. Bleeding is the next most common complication because of both altered platelet function associated with uremia and the use of heparin during dialysis. Infection may either occur locally, at the site of the arteriovenous fistula, or be systemic. Dialysis dementia is a progressive, potentially fatal neurological complication that affects clients on long-term hemodialysis.

13-8   Answer D

When a client has an elevated serum uric acid level (greater than 7.0 mg/dL), the following should be considered as possible causes: the use of diuretics, chronic renal failure (CRF), a high-protein diet, gout, leukemia, and lymphoma. To specifically look for CRF, a serum creatinine level and a 24-hour urinary uric acid test need to be performed.

13-9   Answer C

Ureterolithiasis—a stone in the ureter—is the most common cause of urinary tract obstruction. Pain with ureteral obstruction is compounded by the stretching of the renal capsule by edema and swelling. Edema does not usually cause complete obstruction. Although a tumor may cause an obstruction, it is not as common as an obstruction caused by ureterolithiasis. Vascular problems may aggravate or potentiate a problem leading to an obstruction but not be the actual cause.

13-10   Answer A

Encouraging hydration is the first step in the treatment of uric acid kidney stones. Additional steps include alkalinizing the urine with potassium citrate (Urocit-K) to keep the urine pH above 6.5. Reducing protein intake to 56 g/day will also help. As a last resort, allopurinol (Zyloprim) may be added. Usually clients with uric acid kidney stones will have a normal serum uric acid level but an elevated urine uric acid concentration.

13-11   Answer D

Clients with chronic kidney disease (CKD) are more likely to die from the disease than to start dialysis or progress to end-stage renal disease (ESRD), as most people would think is the likeliest outcome. It is now evident that CKD is a major risk factor for death from cardiovascular disease (CVD) and that this risk increases with worsening CKD. Clinicians need to focus their attention on preventing CKD progression, maximizing CVD risk reduction, and aggressively treating comorbidities associated with CKD. These comorbid conditions include anemia, volume overload, abnormal calcium phosphate homeostasis, hypertension, dyslipidemia, and metabolic syndrome, many of which predispose to CVD.

13-12   Answer A

The aging process begins to affect the kidneys with a progressive loss of nephron units by age 40. The kidneys lose about 20% of their mass between ages 40 and 80.

13-13   Answer D

Pharmacokinetics refers to the absorption, distribution, metabolism, and elimination of drugs and their metabolites. It is affected by the following physiological changes in the older adult: decreased creatine clearance, decreased lean muscle mass, increased total body fat, decreased hepatic blood flow, decreased renal blood flow, decreased serum albumin level, and decreased total body water. Serum albumin levels typically decrease, not increase, in the older adult.

13-14   Answer A

White men are most prone to developing nephrolithiasis. The incidence of nephrolithiasis (stone in the kidney) is four times higher in men than women, with white men having three times more attacks than black men, except for struvite stones, which occur more often in black men.

13-15   Answer B

Bill is at a higher risk for developing nephrolithiasis because of his intake of excessive amounts of

vitamin C. Other risk factors for nephrolithiasis include use of certain medications, such as vitamin D supplements, calcium, corticosteroids, and acetazolamide (Diamox); a diet high in oxalate or sodium; a low fluid intake; and a history of chronic diarrhea, peptic ulcer disease, gout, recurrent urinary tract infection, skeletal fractures, jejunoileal bypass, or renal tubular acidosis.

13-16   Answer C

A urinary calcium output greater than 300 mg in 24 hours (hypercalciuria) may lead to a diagnosis of nephrolithiasis. The following disorders and diagnostic findings may also lead to a diagnosis of nephrolithiasis: hyperuricosuria (urinary uric acid output greater than 750 mg in 24 hours), hyperoxaluria (urinary oxalate output greater than 40 mg in 24 hours), hypocitraturia (urinary citrate output less than 320 mg/day), gouty diathesis (urinary pH less than 5.5 and gouty arthritis), and hypomagnesuria (urinary magnesium output less than 50 mg in 24 hours). Serum calcium of 8 mg/dL is within normal range.

13-17   Answer A

For clients taking NSAIDs on a long-term basis, hemodynamically induced acute renal failure; acute interstitial nephropathy, with or without nephrotic syndrome; salt and water retention; papillary necrosis and chronic renal injury; hyperkalemia; vasculitis; and glomerulitis may be found.

13-18   Answer D

Ferumoxytol, a semisynthetic iron oxide formulated with mannitol and administered IV, corrects iron deficiency anemia in clients with CKD more quickly and more safely than do oral iron preparations. Oral iron does not raise hemoglobin that much because clients with CKD, whether or not they're on dialysis, don't absorb iron well. About 25%–50% of clients with CKD taking oral iron do not tolerate it well in the doses needed and have resulting gastrointestinal (GI) side effects. In one study, twice the number of clients taking oral iron had adverse side effects compared with those taking the IV drug.

13-19   Answer D

Erythromycin (E-Mycin) is not associated with acute renal failure (ARF). It is one of the safest antibiotics, even in pregnancy. NSAIDs and ACE inhibitors can cause the prerenal type of ARF by causing a decreased intrarenal arteriolar resistance. Cimetidine (Tagamet) can cause an elevation in serum creatinine levels without a change in glomerular filtration. Although this is not a problem in clients with normal renal function, there is a more profound effect on serum creatinine concentrations in clients with borderline renal dysfunction.

13-20 Answer A

If Janet stops smoking, her stress urinary incontinence may improve. Studies have shown that clients who smoke increase their risk of stress incontinence by 28% despite increased urethral sphincter tone. Limiting fluids, which may result in dehydration, may cause further problems. Although taking a multivitamin is good, it will not help with stress incontinence. In postmenopausal women not on hormone replacement therapy, using an estrogen vaginal cream has been shown to be effective. Lifting weights will not help with the urinary sphincter muscles. Kegel exercises have proved effective.

13-21 Answer C

Urinary stasis is the most common factor predisposing a woman to a urinary tract infection (UTI). It is followed by calculi and the presence of catheters, stents, and other foreign bodies. The use of an oral contraceptive (if the male partner is not using a condom) also predisposes a woman to a UTI because sexual intercourse increases the likelihood of developing a UTI. The use of a diaphragm also increases the risk of a UTI because of the properties of the spermicidal agents used in conjunction with the diaphragm.

13-22 Answer D

Clients with frequent urinary tract infections (UTIs) and, in fact, all persons should drink 8–10 glasses of water per day to help distribute the body's own antibodies. Other measures that should be taught to women prone to developing UTIs include voiding after intercourse, avoiding bubble baths, wearing underwear with pantyhose, and using methods of contraception other than diaphragms with spermicidal agents.

13-23 Answer A

Painless, gross hematuria in an older adult is an ominous sign. It is usually the result of a malignancy (prostate cancer, transitional cell cancer, or renal cell carcinoma). Flank pain with hematuria is commonly caused by the presence of a kidney stone in the upper collecting system of the affected kidney. Hematuria after trauma is quite common. Isolated asymptomatic hematuria is often found on a routine screening urinalysis with no apparent source determined by history and physical examination. The possibility of occult malignancy or other potentially serious etiology increases with age, and if the client is older than 40, he or she should be evaluated for urological tumor. Clients younger than 40 should be monitored at least monthly for 3 months and if the hematuria persists, then a more aggressive workup is indicated.

13-24 Answer B

Diabetes mellitus is the most common cause of nephrotic syndrome. Systemic lupus erythematosus, the routine use of NSAIDs, glomerulosclerosis, and diabetes mellitus are all causes of proteinuria.

13-25 Answer D

Before beginning an extensive workup for proteinuria, the syndrome of postural proteinuria should be ruled out. In this benign condition, which occurs in healthy, otherwise asymptomatic clients, urine collected first thing in the morning does not show any protein. If protein is present in the urine after the client has been ambulating for several hours, the syndrome of postural proteinuria is confirmed. The prognosis is excellent because clients with postural proteinuria do not develop renal disease with any greater frequency than that seen in the general population.

13-26 Answer D

White blood cell casts are seen in pyelonephritis and interstitial nephritis. Hyaline casts may be present in normal urine; granular casts may be present in a wide variety of renal disorders; and red blood cell casts indicate glomerular bleeding that is strongly suggestive of glomerulonephritis.

13-27 Answer A

The most common type of kidney stones are calcium oxalate stones. They make up about 75% of all kidney stones and are usually less than 2 cm in diameter. Uric acid stones, which are radiolucent, make up about 5% of all stones. Calcium phosphate stones, which occur with renal tubular acidosis, make up about 5% of all stones. Cystine stones, which are hexagonal crystals, are the result of an autosomal recessive genetic trait and make up less than 1% of all kidney stones. There are actually seven types of stones made of different types of crystals: calcium oxalate, calcium phosphate, a combination of calcium oxalate and calcium phosphate, magnesium ammonium phosphate (struvite or infection stones), uric acid, cystine, and miscellaneous types such as occur with drug metabolites.

13-28   Answer C

The use of anticholinergic agents may be responsible for transient urinary incontinence in women. Etiologies for transient urinary incontinence may be stated using a DIAPERS mnemonic: D for drugs, such as hypnotics, sedatives, anticholinergic agents, diuretics, and adrenergic agents, and delirium or altered mental status; I for infection; A for atrophy of the vagina or urethra; P for psychological disorders such as functional depression; E for endocrine disorders, such as hyperglycemia or hypercalcemia; R for restricted mobility; and S for stool impaction.

13-29   Answer A

In clients in the United States receiving dialysis, diabetic nephropathy (Kimmelstiel-Wilson syndrome) is the most common cause of end-stage renal disease (about 25%). Both type 1 and type 2 diabetes are implicated, indicating the need for good diabetes control throughout clients' life spans. Most clients with acute tubular necrosis recover with conservative management (fluid monitoring, protein restriction, drug adjustments, and dietary and potassium control). Dialysis may become necessary; however, it is usually temporary. In clients with major renal vascular occlusive disease, vascular repair or percutaneous angioplasty has been shown to slow the progression of the disease. Kidney trauma is not an end-stage renal disease.

13-30   Answer C

In women, approximately 80%–90% of cases of uncomplicated UTI are the result of the gram-negative rod bacteria *Escherichia coli*. The second most common cause (5%–20%) of uncomplicated bacterial infection is the gram-positive coccus *Staphylococcus saprophyticus*, although this agent is rare in complicated UTI. Other gram-negative rods identified as causative pathogens in a smaller number of cases, but particularly in complicated UTI, are *Proteus mirabilis*, *Klebsiella*, *Enterobacter*, *Serratia*,

and *Pseudomonas*. In addition, the gram-positive coccus *Enterococcus* has been identified.

13-31   Answer B

Polycystic kidney disease is a hereditary, incurable renal disease in which multiple outpouchings (cysts) of the nephrons occur in both kidneys. The cysts may be filled with urine, serous fluid, blood, or a combination of these. As the cysts enlarge, they distort and compress surrounding renal tissue and blood vessels, causing ischemia and necrosis. Eventually, too few normal nephrons remain to support the client and end-stage renal disease slowly develops.

13-32   Answer A

Clients with glomerulonephritis commonly have a history of beta-hemolytic streptococcal infections, as well as a history of systemic lupus erythematosus or other autoimmune diseases. Glomerulonephritis is usually caused by an immunological response.

13-33   Answer A

Loop diuretics, such as furosemide (Lasix), bumetanide (Bumex), and ethacrynic acid (Edecrin), all act to inhibit sodium chloride reabsorption in the thick ascending limb of the loop of Henle. Mannitol (Osmitrol) is an osmotic diuretic, hydrochlorothiazide (Hydrodiuril) is a thiazide diuretic, and acetazolamide (Diamox) is a carbonic anhydrase inhibitor; these diuretics exert their effects through different mechanisms.

13-34   Answer C

Potassium-sparing diuretics, such as spironolactone (Aldactone) and triamtere (Dyrenium), have the following side effects: hyperkalemia, headache, hyponatremia, nausea, diarrhea, urticaria, and menstrual disturbances. Osmotic diuretics may precipitate congestive heart failure, high doses of loop diuretics may cause hearing loss, and thiazide diuretics may cause hypokalemia and hyperglycemia.

13-35   Answer D

Serum hemoglobin and hematocrit testing assesses bleeding or the lack of erythropoietin. A urine creatinine clearance rate measurement is a very specific indicator of renal function and is used to evaluate the glomerular filtration rate. Blood urea nitrogen level measures the nitrogen portion of urea, a product formed in the liver from protein metabolism.

Serum albumin measurement is used to assist in the diagnosis of nephrotic syndrome.

13-36   Answer B

Eosinophils in the urinary sediment signify an allergic reaction in the kidney. Leukocytes are present in an infection and interstitial nephritis. Crystals are present in diseases of stone formation or following ethylene glycol intoxication. Erythrocytes are present in large amounts in active glomerulonephritis, interstitial nephritis, and infections.

13-37   Answer D

Magnetic resonance imaging provides direct imaging in several planes conducive to detecting renal cystic disease, inflammatory processes, and renal cell carcinoma. Cystoscopy detects bladder or urethral pathological processes. Ultrasonography identifies hydronephrosis and fluid collections. Computed tomography identifies tumors and other pathological conditions that create variations in body density.

13-38   Answer D

A kidneys, ureters, and bladder film can visualize the renal outline and identify lower rib fractures. An intravenous pyelogram compares the kidneys and shows distortion of the calyces and incomplete filling. Renal angiography provides information on the integrity of the renal vasculature. Computed tomography can determine the extent of injury in three dimensions.

13-39   Answer B

The liver on the right side displaces the right kidney slightly downward.

13-40   Answer A

All nephrotoxic agents such as NSAIDs and radiocontrast dye should be avoided in clients with CRF. Low-dose Kayexalate (sodium polystyrene sulfonate) 5 mg PO one to three times a day with meals may be used as a potassium binder for hyperkalemia. Given the kidney's reduced ability to synthesize activated vitamin D in CRF and the propensity for subsequent hypocalcemia and renal osteodystrophy, oral 1.25-dihydroxyvitamin D (calcitrol 0.25 mg every day) and calcium carbonate (600 mg twice a day) supplements should be given, along with a renal-specific multivitamin

(Nephrocaps). Anemia should be treated with erythropoietin (80–120 U/kg SC per week).

13-41   Answer D

Eating watermelon will not cause the urine to change color. Ingesting blackberries or beets, taking ibuprofen or phenazopyridine (Pyridium), and eating foods with red food color all may cause the urine to be pink, red, burgundy, or cola colored.

13-42   Answer C

Brown, smoky, or tea-colored urine indicates blood coming from the upper urinary tract. The color is the result of the acidic urine changing the hemoglobin to hematin, which has a brown color. Grossly bloody urine and urine with blood clots come from the lower urinary tract. Blood noted at the beginning or end of the stream also indicates lower tract bleeding, whereas blood throughout the stream may suggest upper urinary tract bleeding.

13-43   Answer D

The appearance of urine may indicate ingestion of certain products and/or lead to possible common differential diagnoses. For the following urine colors, the following may apply: Cloudy urine may indicate UTI, hematuria, bilirubin, and mucus. For colorless urine, the differential diagnoses would be diabetes insipidus, diuretic agents, and fluid overload. For dark urine, they are hematuria, malignancy, stones, and acidic urine. For pink/red urine, they are hematuria, hemoglobin, myoglobin, beets, and food coloring. For orange/yellow urine, the differentials are phenazopyridine, rifampin, and bile pigments. For brown/black urine, they are myoglobin, bile pigments, melanin, cascara, and iron preparations. For green urine, they are bile pigments, methylene blue, indigo, carmine. For foamy urine, they are bile salts and proteinuria.

13-44   Answer A

The prerenal classification (problems occurring prior to reaching the kidney) of acute renal failure (ARF) may be caused by dehydration secondary to gastroenteritis, malnutrition, or diarrhea, as well as by hemorrhage, hypovolemia, shock, and heart failure. Therefore, Joey, who is dehydrated, is at risk for developing a prerenal type of ARF. The renal classification (within the kidney) of ARF may be caused by nephrotoxins such as acetaminophen (Tylenol), near drowning (especially in fresh water), acute glomerulonephritis, severe infections, and diseases of the kidney and blood vessels; this applies to Tommy and Justine. Postrenal causes of ARF include obstructions caused by tumor, hematoma, stones, renal vein thrombosis, or trauma to a solitary kidney or collecting system (Buddy).

13-45   Answer B

Middle-aged men do not incur as many urinary tract infections as middle-aged women because men have the bacteriostatic effect of prostatic fluid and a longer urethra. However, prostatic hypertrophy commonly associated with aging increases the risk of cystitis for older men. Men and women are equally prone to urinary stasis and have the same urinary pH.

13-46   Answer A

The intravenous pyelogram is an examination that takes about 30 minutes and uses x-rays to show the structures of the kidney, ureters, and bladder after injection of a dye that is rapidly excreted in the urine. In a voiding cystourethrogram, the bladder is filled with dye solution and then x-rays of the filled bladder and of the bladder and urethra during urination are taken. Radioisotope studies provide information regarding renal anatomy; blood flow; and glomerular, tubular, and collecting system function. Renal arteriography or venography is indicated in children only when it is necessary to define vascular abnormalities such as renal artery stenosis before a surgical intervention. Usually other less invasive measures are used.

13-47   Answer A

Thiazide diuretics, along with phosphates and calcium-binding agents, are used for calcium phosphate and oxalate stones. Antibiotic therapy is used for the urinary tract infections that occur with struvite stones; allopurinol is used for uric acid stones; and penicillamine and sodium bicarbonate are used for cystine stones.

13-48   Answer C

Foods high in oxalate that a client with oxalate kidney stones should avoid include asparagus, beer, beets, cabbage, celery, chocolate and cocoa, fruits, green beans, nuts, tea, colas, and tomatoes. Foods high in calcium are beans and lentils, chocolate and cocoa, dried fruits, canned or smoked fish except tuna, flour, milk, and milk products. Acid ash foods

to avoid with calcium phosphate or oxalate stones and struvite stones include cheese, cranberries, eggs, grapes, meat and poultry, plums and prunes, tomatoes, and whole grains. A low-purine diet is often effective in reducing stones formed from excess uric acid. This diet is achieved by limiting intake of purine-rich foods such as organ meats, red meats, seafood (especially sardines, anchovies, and scallops), poultry, legumes, whole grains, and alcohol (which decreases uric acid clearance).

13-49   Answer C

A Koch pouch is a continent internal ileal reservoir or continent ileal bladder conduit in which a pouch is created to be an ileal conduit. Nipple valves are formed on the skin by intussuscepting tissue backward into the reservoir to connect the pouch to the skin and the ureters to the pouch. The filling pressure closes valves, preventing leakage and reflux.

13-50   Answer A

Cholinergic drugs such as bethanechol chloride (Urecholine) are used primarily in the treatment of acute postoperative and postpartum urinary retention and for neurogenic bladder atony with urinary retention. Anticholinesterase agents such as neostigmine (Prostigmin) and pyridostigmine (Mestinon) are used primarily in the treatment of myasthenia gravis, but they are also useful in the treatment of urinary retention because they stimulate contraction of the detrusor muscle. Anticholinergic agents such as propantheline bromide (Pro-Banthine), dicyclomine (Bentyl), flavoxate hydrochloride (Urispas), and oxybutynin (Ditropan) act to relax the detrusor muscle and increase contraction of the internal sphincter. They serve to increase the bladder capacity of clients with spastic or hyperreflexive neurogenic bladder.

13-51   Answer C

Propantheline bromide (Pro-Banthine), dicyclomine hydrochloride (Bentyl), and imipramine hydrochloride (Tofranil) all help urinary incontinence. However, if the client does not like taking pills, the best (and least invasive) agent to suggest is estrogen vaginal cream. One type of stress urinary incontinence is anatomical incontinence, which may be caused by hormone deprivation and atrophic vaginitis. Using estrogen replacement cream to correct the vaginal dryness will also improve bladder outlet function.

13-52   Answer D

Most children with voiding disturbances do not have an anatomical or neurological disease nor a psychological problem causing their enuresis. Although the cause of primary nocturnal enuresis has not been clearly established, it appears to be related to maturational delay of mechanisms involved in sleep and arousal or to a delay in the development of increased bladder capacity. Most children can be helped through parental involvement, such as restricting fluids after dinner, encouraging bladder training, awakening the child during the night to void, and using electronic devices that establish a conditioned reflex response to waken the child the moment urination starts. (Such devices are only mildly successful.) Imipramine (Tofranil) is effective (50 mg PO at bedtime), as well as desmopressin acetate (DDAVP) nasal spray (one spray in each nostril at bedtime).

13-53   Answer D

Multivitamins do not cause urine to appear reddish in color. Cascara sagrada, a stimulant laxative, may cause urine color to be red in alkaline urine and yellow-brown in acid urine; phenazopyridine (Pyridium), a urinary tract analgesic, will cause urine to appear orange to red; and phenytoin (Dilantin), an anticonvulsant, may cause urine to appear pink, red, or red-brown.

13-54   Answer A

Urine specific gravity is increased in clients who are dehydrated; in those who have a pituitary tumor that causes the release of excessive amounts of antidiuretic hormone; and in those with decreased renal blood flow, glycosuria, or proteinuria. The specific gravity of urine is decreased in clients who are overhydrated and in those who have diabetes insipidus or chronic renal failure.

13-55   Answer D

While many sources differ, oliguria (diminished urination) in an adult is typically defined as less than 500 mL urine output per day. Anuria, although defined as "without urine," is an output of less than 100 mL per day. The body makes 1 mL of urine per minute, or 1440 mL per day. In the hospital, the least acceptable amount of urine is 30 mL per hour, but we actually produce 60 mL per hour.

13-56   Answer B

After a renal biopsy, the client should be instructed to avoid strenuous activities for at least 2 weeks. These activities include heavy lifting, contact sports, or any other activity that will cause jolting of the kidney. The client should also be warned that he or she may notice some blood in the urine for the first 24 hours following the procedure and should be instructed to drink large amounts of fluid, such as 8–10 glasses of water per day, to prevent clot formation and urine retention. Caution should be used in an oliguric client in renal failure who might develop pulmonary edema with increased fluid intake.

13-57   Answer B

A 24-hour urine test for vanillylmandelic acid (VMA) and catecholamines is done to diagnose hypertension secondary to pheochromocytoma. A pheochromocytoma is an adrenal tumor that frequently secretes abnormally high levels of epinephrine and norepinephrine, resulting in episodic or persistent hypertension from arterial vasoconstriction. A renal tumor would be diagnosed by an intravenous pyelogram (IVP). To test for renal artery stenosis, duplex ultrasound, captopril renal scintigraphy, and magnetic resonance angiography (MRA) are used. Nuclear medicine and radiological tests will assess and measure kidney function and structure to determine the amount of hydronephrosis present.

13-58   Answer D

In many cases of ATN, which is often caused by nephrotoxic agents, the removal of the offending agent will allow renal function to return gradually to normal. In the meantime, supportive measures should be provided, often in the form of peritoneal dialysis or hemodialysis. Because most cases of ATN are reversible, it is essential for diagnosis and aggressive management to begin early. ATN is characterized by altered renal ability to conserve sodium. Clinically, ATN is seen as a urinary sodium level greater than 20 mEq/L. Laboratory serum sodium levels vary in ATN, depending on the state of hydration. Oliguria is usually associated with postischemic ATN, whereas either oliguria or nonoliguria may be associated with nephrotoxic ATN. Creatinine clearance is severely decreased and plasma creatinine rises about 0.5–1 mg/dL per day in ATN. The clinical course of ATN is often divided into three phases: initial injury, maintenance, and recovery. The maintenance phase is expressed as either oliguric or nonoliguric. Nonoliguric ATN has a better outcome.

13-59   Answer D

Renal cysts are usually asymptomatic and usually do not cause flank pain. Pyelonephritis, ureterolithiasis, and vascular occlusion of the kidney (renal vein thrombosis) all usually cause flank pain.

13-60   Answer B

Bile produces urine that is brownish in color. Beets, rifampin (Rifadin), and phenazopyridine (Pyridium) can cause reddish or reddish-orange urine.

13-61   Answer B

Anuria refers to a 24-hour urine volume of less than 100 mL. It indicates a severe reduction in urine volume commonly associated with obstruction, renal cortical necrosis, or severe acute tubular necrosis. It is important to make the distinction between oliguria (less than 500 mL in a 24-hour period) and anuria so that the appropriate treatment may be initiated early.

13-62   Answer C

The most common cause of death in dialysis clients is cardiovascular failure, with hypotension and diabetes as predisposing factors. Sepsis is the next leading cause of death, followed by bleeding complications, cerebrovascular accidents, pericardial effusion with tamponade, and trauma. The mortality in dialysis clients remains significant, about 15% in the first year.

13-63   Answer A

An acidic urine pH favors precipitation of organic stones: uric acid and cystine stones. An alkaline urine pH favors the precipitation of inorganic stones: calcium phosphate and magnesium ammonium phosphate (struvite) stones.

13-64   Answer A

The most common metabolic condition that predisposes clients to the formation of kidney stones is idiopathic hypercalciuria. Idiopathic hypercalciuria is present in approximately 50% of stone-forming

clients, followed by a low urinary citrate excretion at a slightly lower percentage. Hyperuricosuria is present in approximately 30% of stone-forming clients and hyperoxaluria in approximately 15% of all stone-forming clients.

13-65   Answer B

All of the answer options are renal hormones. Prostaglandins regulate intrarenal blood flow by vasodilation or vasoconstriction. Renin raises blood pressure as a result of angiotensin (local vasoconstriction) and aldosterone (volume expansion) secretion. Bradykinins increase blood flow (vasodilation) and vascular permeability. Erythropoietin stimulates bone marrow to make red blood cells.

13-66   Answer D

Eosinophils are present in the urine in interstitial nephritis, urinary tract infections, and acute tubular necrosis (ATN). They are not present in normal urine but are activated by antigens and antigen-induced hypersensitivity reactions. Normally only a few white blood cells are found in urine. Increased numbers of leukocytes in the urine generally indicate either renal or genitourinary tract disease.

13-67   Answer A

The GFR is affected more in older African Americans than in Caucasians. Sodium is not excreted as well by the kidneys in hypertensive African Americans who have high sodium intake, and the kidneys have approximately 20% less blood flow as a result of anatomical changes in small renal vessels. End-stage renal disease (ESRD) is three to four times more common in African Americans, Native Americans, and Mexican Americans than in Caucasians.

13-68   Answer C

ACE inhibitors are the antihypertensive drugs contraindicated in clients with renal artery stenosis. In bilateral renal artery stenosis or stenosis to a solitary kidney, the renal perfusion pressure and the glomerular filtration rate depend on the local renin-angiotensin system. When the system is blocked by an ACE inhibitor, a marked decrease in the efferent arterial pressure with subsequent decrease in renal perfusion pressure results, causing a diminished GFR.

13-69   Answer C

A urine culture is still the "gold standard" for detecting a urinary tract infection.

13-70   Answer C

Urinary tract infections (UTIs) are the most common cause of burning on urination. UTIs cause approximately 7 million episodes of acute cystitis per year.

13-71   Answer A

A decreased estrogen level contributes to stress incontinence. Bladder irritation from a urinary tract infection contributes to urge incontinence; prostatic hypertrophy contributes to overflow incontinence; and spinal cord lesion or trauma contributes to reflex incontinence.

13-72   Answer B

Postmenopausal women tend to have more recurrent urinary tract infections because of postvoid residual urine secondary to anatomical changes such as a dropped bladder or uterus; estrogen depletion–related changes such as a dry, thin vaginal lining; a decrease in lactobacilli; and an increase in the colonization of the vagina by *Escherichia coli*.

13-73   Answer D

The clinical presentation of a client with urolithiasis includes pain that typically starts in the flank and may localize at the costovertebral angle. The pain may radiate to the lower abdomen, groin, or perineum and is often associated with nausea and vomiting. Fever is unlikely unless there is a coexisting urinary tract infection. Hematuria may be present, but the urine should not have any leukocytes unless an infection is also present. Because the question is asked only about a client with urolithiasis and did not mention any infection, an assumption of an infection being present should not be made.

13-74   Answer C

Extracorporeal shock wave lithotripsy is not recommended for struvite stones because bacteria or endotoxins inside the stone may be systemically dispersed during the procedure. Appropriate antibiotics are required.

13-75   Answer B

General recommendations for the prevention of kidney stones, regardless of the type of stone the client has, include reducing protein in the diet because protein enhances calcium, urate, and oxalate excretion; drinking 3–4 L of water per day with the avoidance of nonsoftened and mineral water; avoiding vitamin C supplements because they stimulate oxalate excretion; increasing fiber to decrease calcium absorption; restricting sodium to 2.5 g/day to decrease excretion of urinary calcium; restricting the consumption of oxalate-containing foods; limiting calcium intake to 800–1000 mg/day; and restricting alcohol to no more than one to two drinks per day.

13-76   Answer C

Overflow incontinence is the inability to empty the bladder, resulting in overdistention and frequent loss of small amounts of urine. Stress incontinence is the loss of urine associated with increased intra-abdominal pressure such as occurs with sneezing, coughing, and lifting; the quantity of urine lost is usually small. Urge incontinence is the inability to inhibit urine flow long enough to reach the toilet after the urge sensation. Reflex incontinence is the involuntary loss of a moderate volume of urine without stimulus or warning. It may occur during the day or night.

13-77   Answer B

Decreased bladder capacity; bladder irritation from a urinary tract infection, tumor, or stones; irritants such as caffeine and alcohol; central nervous system disorders; and spinal cord lesions contribute to urge urinary incontinence. Contributing factors of stress urinary incontinence include multiple pregnancies; decreased estrogen levels; a short urethra; weakness of the abdominal wall; prostate surgery; and increased intra-abdominal pressure as a result of tumor, ascites, or obesity. For overflow urinary incontinence, contributing factors include spinal cord injuries below S2; diabetic neuropathy; prostatic hypertrophy; fecal impaction; and drugs, especially those with an anticholinergic effect. For reflex urinary incontinence, contributing factors include a spinal cord lesion or trauma above S2, history of a cerebrovascular accident, neurological disorders such as Parkinson's or Alzheimer's disease, and multiple sclerosis.

13-78   Answer D

Kegel exercises are essential for the advanced-practice nurse (APN) to teach clients with stress incontinence to improve their quality of life. Pelvic floor (Kegel) exercises help to restore and maintain continence by improving pelvic muscle strength, increasing urethral pressure, decreasing abnormal detrusor muscle contraction, and decreasing pressure within the bladder. Kegel exercises are recommended for women with urinary stress incontinence, for some men who have urinary incontinence after prostate surgery, and for people who have fecal incontinence.

13-79   Answer D

Phenazopyridine (Pyridium) is the only analgesic listed. For the first few days of a UTI, all of the drugs listed may be prescribed, in addition to antibiotics, to decrease the pain and discomfort of a UTI. Use of these agents should not be prolonged, however, given their significant side effect profile. Analgesics such as phenazopyridine (Pyridium) may be prescribed, but this alters the color of urine to orange and may cause urinary leakage secondary to anesthetization of the urethra and sphincter. Anticholinergics, including atropine (Donnatal), hyoscyamine (Levsin, Cystospaz), propantheline (Pro-Banthine), or oxybutynin (Ditropan), produce an antispasmodic effect, relieving pain. However, anticholinergics may also contribute to urinary retention (especially in the elderly), which is a clear risk factor for UTI, and should thus be used with caution.

13-80   Answer A

A serum creatinine level greater than 4 mg/dL is associated with kidney disease and is indicative of severe impairment of renal function. A decreased serum level of albumin occurs in nephrotic syndrome. Serum sodium is decreased in nephrotic syndrome and serum calcium is decreased in renal failure. Normal values are as follows:
Serum creatinine: 0.5–1.0 mg/dL
Serum albumin: 3.3–4.5 g/dL
Serum sodium: 135–145 mEq/L
Serum calcium: 4.5–5.5 mEq/L

13-81   Answer C

Diabetic nephropathy is the most common cause of ESRD. Hypertensive nephropathy is the second most commonly occurring cause of renal failure, and glomerulonephritis (GN) is the third most common cause.

13-82   Answer B

Metabolic alkalosis is a pathophysiological process that occurs when there is a primary excess of bicarbonate in the extracellular fluid because of loss of acid (hydrogen ions) or the addition of excess bicarbonate. Metabolic acidosis results from an accumulation in the blood of keto acids (derived from fat metabolism) at the expense of bicarbonate. Respiratory acidosis occurs with a reduction of alveolar ventilation, resulting in an accumulation of carbonic acid. Respiratory alkalosis occurs with an increase of alveolar ventilation, resulting in a decrease of carbonic acid.

13-83   Answer A

Excessive alcohol ingestion can cause metabolic acidosis because alcohol results in excess acid levels in the blood.

13-84   Answer A

Clinical manifestations of metabolic alkalosis include tetany, hypotension, tachycardia, confusion, decreasing level of consciousness, hyperreflexia, dysrhythmias, seizures, and respiratory failure. Nausea and vomiting, weakness, and bradycardia are manifestations of metabolic acidosis.

13-85   Answer B

The arterial blood gas values of pH 7.39, PaO_2 92, and HCO_3 24 are within normal range. However, the $PaCO_2$ level of 48 is elevated, which would indicate acute respiratory acidosis.

13-86   Answer C

A decreased pH, normal PCO_2, and decreased HCO_3 indicated metabolic acidosis. Renal failure, diabetes, shock, and intestinal fistulas all cause metabolic acidosis because of an increased production of metabolic acids from diabetic ketoacidosis, impaired excretion of metabolic acids from renal failure, an increased bicarbonate loss from loss of intestinal secretions and increased renal losses, or an increased chloride level from abnormal renal function.

13-87   Answer B

The kidneys excrete increased amounts of HCO_3 to lower the pH as a mode of compensation for respiratory alkalosis. In respiratory acidosis, renal compensatory mechanisms elevate the bicarbonate level, and eventually the pH approaches normal. Signs of compensation in metabolic acidosis are hyperventilation (causing increased intake of oxygen and increased blowing off of carbon dioxide), decreased $PaCO_2$, and increased amounts of ammonia in the urine. The compensatory response to metabolic alkalosis is retention of carbon dioxide.

13-88   Answer D

Before using the radial artery to draw blood for measurement of arterial blood gas values, the Allen test should be performed to evaluate the presence of the ulnar artery. To perform the Allen test, first cause the hand to blanch by obliterating both the radial and ulnar pulses. Then, release the pressure over the ulnar artery only. If the flow is adequate, flushing will immediately be seen. The Allen test is then considered positive and the radial artery may be used to draw the blood. ABGs are arterial blood gases. The Thomas test assesses hip motion, and the Weber test assesses hearing.

13-89   Answer A

Cigarette smoke, from both active and passive inhalation, is a significant risk factor for urinary tract neoplasms and may account for half of the incidence of bladder tumors among men and a third among women. Other factors implicated in the formation of urinary tract neoplasms include chemicals and dyes used in the plastics, rubber, and cable industries; the chronic use of phenacetin-containing analgesic agents; and substances in the environment of textile workers, leather finishers, spray painters, hairdressers, and petroleum workers. The breakdown products of these chemicals and those from cigarette smoke are stored in the bladder and excreted in the urine, which causes a local influence on abnormal cell development. Working long hours with inability to void may often result in a bladder infection, not a neoplasm.

13-90   Answer B

With a total cystectomy in a man, the prostate and seminal vessels are also removed, resulting in impotence. With Marvin, it is important to state the facts, then explore his feelings. Referring to the surgeon when you know the answer is an evasive tactic. Asking Marvin how his wife feels negates his own feelings.

13-91   Answer C

Most calcium phosphate stones are caused by primary hyperparathyroidism. Treatment involves surgical excision of the parathyroid adenoma. If the surgery is not successful or is impossible, treatment involves hydration and the administration of orthophosphate. The client is then observed for hypertension and sodium and water retention.

13-92   Answer A

The most frequent sign of bladder cancer is hematuria. With gross hematuria, an intravenous pyelogram should be performed to detect bladder cancer as early as possible. Flank pain is usually a sign of glomerulonephritis or kidney stones; nocturia is the number one symptom of benign prostatic hypertrophy; and dysuria is present with a urinary tract infection.

13-93   Answer C

The treatment of choice for a contusion of the kidney after trauma is conservative therapy, including bedrest and observation. With these injuries, bleeding is typically minor and self-limiting. Treatment of major renal injuries is usually surgical to stop hemorrhaging. A urethral catheterization will be done to assess the characteristics of the urine (quantity and color), but this is a procedure to assess the condition, not to treat the kidney contusion.

13-94   Answer B

A postvoid residual catheterization volume of more than 30 mL is abnormal.

13-95   Answer D

Urine tends to become colonized with bacteria when indwelling urinary catheters are left in place for more than 72 hours. If catheters are left in place only temporarily and removed quickly when the client can void, infection will usually not result. Antibacterial coverage is warranted if catheters are left in place for 5–10 days.

13-96   Answer D

A circumcision should never be done on a baby with hypospadias because the surgeon who may ultimately correct hypospadias may need the prepuce to repair the defect. Surgical correction should be undertaken by the time the child enters the first grade.

13-97 Answer C

A child with Wilms' tumor commonly has abdominal distention or an abdominal mass. There may also be fever, abdominal pain, or hematuria. This kidney tumor requires surgical removal, followed by chemotherapy. Radiation therapy is not necessary.

13-98 Answer B

Clients who recognize an association between a urinary tract infection and recent sexual intercourse can be instructed to take a single small dose of an antibiotic, such as ofloxacin (Floxin), with a large glass of water after intercourse.

13-99 Answer D

The best index of kidney function is the glomerular filtration rate (GFR). In the past, kidney function used to be assessed by serum creatinine level. Both diet and muscle mass influence generation of creatinine, however, making it an inaccurate indicator of renal function. Lower serum creatinine levels are typically observed with older age, female gender, vegetarian diet, and muscle-wasting states, while higher values are associated with muscular habitus and a high-protein diet. Serum creatinine levels can underestimate kidney disease. The National Kidney Foundation defines chronic kidney disease (CKD) as the presence of kidney damage and/or reduced GFR for 3 or more months. The most precise method to measure the GFR is to measure iothalamate or insulin clearance. This is the gold standard for investigational studies, but it is not practical in clinical practice. The 24-hour urine creatinine clearance test is an alternative in clinical practice, and that measurement is required for the calculation of the GFR. Clients often have difficulty conducting this 24-hour test. Recently, the Modification of Diet in Renal Disease (MDRD) equation has been recommended by the National Kidney Foundation to better estimate the GFR. Besides serum creatinine, the MDRD GFR requires input of client age, gender, and ethnicity.

13-100 Answer B

The most common cause of sepsis in the older adult is a urinary tract infection (UTI). An older adult who is ill with hypothermia (below normal body temperature) or high fever, has a change in mental status and a documented UTI, or has a suspected UTI and sepsis should be treated vigorously with adequate hydration, immediate use of potent antibiotics, and support of blood pressure. Urinary stasis may precipitate a UTI, and kidney stones may accompany one, along with genitourinary problems, but a UTI alone is the most common cause of sepsis in the older adult.

13-101 Answer A

A distended bladder sounds dull when percussed. You should not be able to percuss the bladder above the level of the symphysis pubis after the client has voided. Tympany indicates the presence of gas in organs.

13-102 Answer B

The presence of casts in a urinalysis in increased amounts indicates the presence of bacteria or protein, which is seen in severe renal disease and could also indicate urinary calculi. The presence of ketones reflects incomplete metabolism of fatty acids, as in diabetic ketoacidosis, prolonged fasting, and anorexia nervosa. The presence of normal or abnormal crystals may indicate that the specimen has been allowed to stand. The presence of nitrates suggests bacteria, usually *Escherichia coli*.

13-103 Answer D

A renal ultrasound identifies the size of the kidneys or obstruction in the kidneys or the lower urinary tract and may detect tumors or cysts. A CT scan measures the size of the kidneys and may evaluate the contour to assess for masses or obstruction. A VCUG outlines the bladder's contour and evaluates abnormal bladder emptying and incontinence. A renal arteriogram identifies vascular abnormalities within each kidney and adjacent aorta.

13-104 Answer C

Clients with worsening kidney function may have frequent hypoglycemic episodes and have a decreased need for insulin or oral antihyperglycemic agents. The clinician must explain to the client that the kidneys metabolize and excrete insulin and when renal function declines, the insulin is available for a longer period of time and thus less of it is needed. As in this case, the end result is that many clients think that their diabetes is improving. It usually means that ESRD is approaching.

13-105   Answer B

Anemia is a chronic problem in clients with ESRD. Because of the limited iron content of low-protein diets and decreased erythropoietin production by the kidneys, supplemental iron is needed in the diet. Most clients with renal failure also require daily vitamin and mineral supplementation, but this question specified that the client was on a low-protein diet, thus making one think of iron. Potassium is usually restricted because hyperkalemia can cause dangerous cardiac dysrhythmias. Control of phosphate levels is begun early in CRF to avoid osteodystrophy.

13-106   Answer A

An AV fistula is an internal anastomosis of an artery to a vein. An AV graft is a synthetic vessel tubing tunneled beneath the skin, connecting an artery and a vein.

A dual-lumen hemodialysis catheter is an extended-use catheter, surgically tunneled under the skin with a barrier cuff. An AV shunt is an external loop of tubing connecting an artery and a vein. Each section of tubing is sutured into a vessel and brought through a skin stab wound.

13-107   Answer C

Microalbuminuria is the earliest indicator of impaired renal function. The best way to determine microalbuminuria to assist in the diagnosis of diabetic nephropathy is a timed overnight urine collection or albumin-creatinine ratio in an early morning spot urine collected upon awakening. At least two of three timed overnight or early morning spot urine collections over a period of 3 to 6 months should be abnormal prior to making a diagnosis of microalbuminuria. The urine dipstick is not sensitive enough and a 24-hour urine collection, while being inconvenient, also shows a wide variety of albumin excretion due to factors such as sustained erect posture, protein intake, and exercise. These all tend to increase albumin excretion rates.

Bibliography

Bloom, RD, and Bress, J: Chronic kidney disease: A primary-care guide. *The Clinical Advisor* 10(4):31–38, April 2007.

Brown, K: *Management Guidelines for Women's Health Nurse Practitioners.* FA Davis, Philadelphia, 2002.

Dillon, PM: *Nursing Health Assessment—A Critical Thinking, Case Studies Approach,* ed 2. FA Davis, Philadelphia, 2007.

Dunphy, LM: *Management Guidelines for Nurse Practitioners Working With Adults,* ed 2. FA Davis, Philadelphia, 2004.

Dunphy, LM, et al: *Primary Care: The Art and Science of Advanced Practice Nursing,* ed 2. FA Davis, Philadelphia, 2007.

VanLeeuwen, AM, Kranpitz, TR, and Smith, L: *Davis's Comprehensive Handbook of Laboratory and Diagnostic Tests With Nursing Implications,* ed 2. FA Davis, Philadelphia, 2006.

How well did you do?

85% and above, congratulations! This score shows application of test-taking principles and adequate content knowledge.

75%–85%, keep working! Review test-taking principles and try again.

65%–75%, hang in there! Spend some time reviewing concepts and test-taking principles and try the test again.

Chapter 16: *Musculoskeletal Problems*

ALLISON M. JEDSON
LYNNE M. DUNPHY
JILL E. WINLAND-BROWN

Questions

16-1 *Colchicine may be used to terminate an acute attack of gouty arthritis, as well as to prevent recurrent episodes. The mechanism of action is to*

A. interrupt the cycle of urate crystal deposition and inflammatory response.

B. increase serum uric acid levels.

C. potentiate the excretion of uric acid.

D. inhibit the tubular reabsorption of urate, promoting the excretion of uric acid.

16-2 *Jim, age 64, has rheumatoid arthritis (RA). Which of the following drugs would be of the least benefit?*

A. Disease-modifying antirheumatic drugs (DMARDs)

B. Acetaminophen (Tylenol)

C. NSAIDs

D. Glucocorticoids

16-3 *For your client with a knee injury, you order an NSAID to be taken on a routine basis for the next 2 weeks. Your teaching should include which of the following?*

A. "You may take this medication on an empty stomach as long as you eat within 2–3 hours of taking it."

B. "If one pill does not seem to help, you can double the dose for subsequent doses."

C. "If you notice nausea/vomiting or black or bloody stools, take the next dose with a glass of milk or a full meal."

D. "If you have additional pain, an occasional acetaminophen (Tylenol) is permitted in between the usual doses of the NSAID."

16-4 *Jessie, age 49, states that she thinks she has rheumatoid arthritis. Before any diagnostic tests are ordered, you complete a physical examination and make a tentative diagnosis of osteoarthritis rather than rheumatoid arthritis. Which clinical manifestation ruled out rheumatoid arthritis?*

A. Fatigue

B. Affected joints are swollen, cool, and bony hard on palpation

C. Decreased range of motion

D. Stiffness

16-5 *Marsha, age 34, presents with symptoms resembling both fibromyalgia and chronic fatigue syndrome, which have many similarities. Which of the following is more characteristic of fibromyalgia than of chronic fatigue syndrome?*

A. Musculoskeletal pain

B. Difficulty sleeping

C. Depression

D. Fatigue

16-6 *Steve, age 32, fell off a roof while shingling it. He is complaining of pain in his left hip and leg area. Other than an x-ray, what would make you suspect a fractured pelvis?*

A. A clicking sensation when moving the hips

B. A positive pelvic tilt test

C. Hematuria

D. Absence of distal reflexes

16-7 *Stan, age 34, fractured his femur when his horse tripped over a jump. With this type of injury, you know that Stan is at risk for fat emboli. Early assessment findings for this complication include*

A. fever, tachycardia, rapid respirations, and neurological manifestations.

B. neurological manifestations, temperature elevation, bradycardia, and pallor.

C. hostility; combativeness; substernal pain; and weak, thready pulse.

D. lethargy, hypothermia, paresthesia, and absent peripheral pulses.

16-8 *Manny, age 52, is a postal worker who drives a truck every day. He presents with lower back pain and has decreased sensation to a pinprick in the lateral leg and web of the great toe. This indicates discogenic disease in the dermatomal pattern of which area?*

A. L3/L4 (L4 root involvement)

B. L4/L5 (L5 root involvement)

C. L5/S1 (S1 root involvement)

D. None of the above

16-9 *You are driving home from work and stop at the scene of a motorcycle accident that must have just occurred because there are no rescue vehicles at the scene. The driver is lying at the side of the road unconscious with an obvious open fracture of his femur. Which of the following actions should take priority?*

A. Stop the bleeding from the wound.

B. Determine if there has been a cervical fracture.

C. Establish an airway.

D. Palpate the peripheral pulses.

16-10 *You are assessing Mike, age 16, after a football injury to his right knee. You elicit a positive anterior/ posterior drawer sign. This test indicates an injury to the*

A. lateral meniscus.

B. cruciate ligament.

C. medial meniscus.

D. posterior meniscus.

16-11 *When grading muscle strength on a scale of 1–5, a grade of 4 indicates*

A. full range of motion (ROM) against gravity with full resistance.

B. full ROM against gravity with some resistance.

C. full ROM with gravity.

D. full ROM with gravity eliminated (passive motion).

16-12 *In assessing your client, you place the tips of your first two fingers in front of each ear and ask him to open and close his mouth. Then you drop your fingers into the depressed area over the joint and note for smooth motion of the mandible. With this action, you are assessing for*

A. maxillomandibular integrity.

B. well-positioned permanent teeth or well-fitting dentures.

C. temporomandibular joint syndrome.

D. mastoid inflammation.

16-13 *If any limitation or any increase in range of motion occurs when assessing the musculoskeletal system, the angles of the bones should be measured by using*

A. Phalen's tool.

B. skeletometry.

C. the Thomas joint measure.

D. a goniometer.

16-14 *During your assessment of your client's foot, you note that the foot is in alignment with the long axis of the lower leg and that weight-bearing falls on the middle of the foot, from the heel, along the midfoot, to between the second and third toes. What do you diagnose?*

A. A normal foot

B. Hallux valgus

C. Talipes equinovarus

D. Hammertoes

16-15 *In assessing an infant for developmental dysplasia of the hip (DDH), the practitioner places the infant supine, flexes the knees by holding the thumbs on the inner midthighs, with fingers outside on the hips touching the greater trochanters, stabilizes one hip and abduct and gently pulls anteriorly on the other thigh. If this external rotation feels smooth with no sound present, there is no hip dislocation. This is*

A. the Allis test.

B. Lasègue's sign.

C. the McMurray test.

D. Ortolani maneuver.

16-16 *When teaching Alice, age 67, to use a cane because of osteoarthritis of her left knee, an important point to stress is to tell her to*

A. carry the cane in the ipsilateral hand.

B. advance the cane with the ipsilateral leg.

C. make sure that the cane length equals the height of the iliac crest.

D. use the cane to aid in joint protection and safety.

16-17 *To diagnose fibromyalgia, there must be tenderness on digital palpation in at least 11 of 18 (nine pairs) tender-point sites, which would include*

A. the occiput, low cervical, trapezius, and supraspinatus.

B. the proximal interphalangeal (PIP), metacarpophalangeal (MCP) joints of the hands and the metatarsophalangeal (MTP) and PIP joints of the foot.

C. the facet joints of the cervical, thoracic, and lumbar spine.

D. the radial and ulnar styloids and the medial and lateral maleoli.

16-18 *Alan, age 46, presents with a tender, red, swollen knee. You rule out septic arthritis and diagnose gout by confirming*

A. an elevated WBC.

B. hyperuricemia.

C. a significant response to a dose of ceftriaxone (Rocephin).

D. a positive antinuclear antibody test.

16-19 *First-line drug therapy for acute low back pain includes the use of*

A. NSAIDs.

B. muscle relaxants.

C. opioids.

D. a combination of the above.

16-20 *Jim, age 22, a stock boy, has an acute episode of low back pain. You order an NSAID and tell him which of the following?*

A. Maintain moderate bedrest for 3–4 days.

B. Call the office for narcotic medication if there is no relief with the NSAID after 24–48 hours.

C. Begin lower back strengthening exercises depending on pain tolerance.

D. Wear a Boston brace at night.

16-21 *Mrs. Matthews has rheumatoid arthritis. On reviewing an x-ray of her hip, you notice that there is a marked absence of articular cartilage. What mechanism is responsible for this?*

A. Antigen-antibody formation

B. Lymphocyte response

C. Immune complex formation

D. Lysosomal degradation

16-22 *Mrs. Kelly, age 80, has a curvature of the spine. This is likely to indicate which age-related change?*

A. Lordosis

B. Dorsal kyphosis

C. Scoliosis

D. Kyphoscoliosis

16-23 *Mr. McKinsey was recently given a diagnosis of degenerative joint disease. Which assessment test would you use to check for effusion on his knee?*

A. Thomas test

B. Tinel's sign

C. Bulge test

D. Phalen's test

16-24 *During a sports preparticipation physical examination, when you ask the client to rise up on his toes and raise his heels, you are observing for*

A. calf symmetry and leg strength.

B. hip, knee, and ankle symmetry.

C. hip, knee, and ankle motion.

D. scoliosis, hip motion, and hamstring tightness.

16-25 *A clinical manifestation of symmetric neurogenic pain may indicate*

A. radiculopathy.

B. reflex sympathetic dystrophy.

C. entrapment neuropathy.

D. peripheral neuropathy.

16-26 *Which test is used to diagnose an Achilles tendon rupture?*

A. Boutonnière test

B. Lachman test

C. Thompson test

D. Drawer test

16-27 *James, age 17, has been complaining of a painful knob below his right knee that has prevented him from actively participating in sports. He has recently been given a diagnosis of Osgood-Schlatter disease and asks you about his treatment options. You tell him that the initial treatment is*

A. relative rest; he could benefit from hamstring stretching, heel cord stretching, and quadriceps stretching exercises.

B. immobilization; a long-leg knee immobilizer is recommended.

C. surgical intervention; removal of the bony fragments is necessary.

D. bedrest for 1 week.

16-28 *Trevor, age 4, has an apparent hypertrophy of the calf muscles, which seem doughy on palpation. His mother is concerned because Trevor is unable to raise himself from the floor without bracing his knees with his hands. What do you suspect?*

A. Duchenne's muscular dystrophy

B. Cerebral palsy

C. Legg-Calvé-Perthes disease

D. Multiple sclerosis

16-29 *The C5 myotome innervates*

A. wrist extension.

B. elbow extension.

C. shoulder abduction and elbow flexion.

D. ulnar deviation at the wrist along with finger flexion and abduction.

16-30 *Janine, age 69, has a class III case of rheumatoid arthritis. According to the American Rheumatism Association, her function would be*

A. adequate for normal activities despite a handicap of discomfort or limited motion of one or more joints.

B. largely or wholly incapacitated, bedridden, or confined to a wheelchair permitting little or no self-care.

C. completely able to carry on all usual duties without handicaps.

D. adequate to perform only few or none of the duties of usual occupation or self-care.

16-31 *Carol, age 62, has swollen, bony proximal interphalangeal joints. You describe these as*

A. Heberden's nodes.

B. Bouchard's nodes.

C. Osler's nodes.

D. Murphy's nodes.

16-32 *In analyzing synovial fluid, a yellow-green color may indicate which of the following?*

A. Trauma

B. Gout

C. A bacterial infection

D. Rheumatoid arthritis

16-33 *Which test assesses for thoracic outlet syndrome by having the client abduct his or her arms 90°*

externally rotated with the elbows flexed 90°, and then having the client open and close his or her hands for 3 minutes?

A. Neer test

B. Speeds test

C. Hawkins test

D. Roos test

16-34 *How can you differentiate between a ganglion cyst and a neoplasm?*

A. A neoplasm is more painful.

B. Ganglia transilluminate.

C. Ganglia cause more swelling.

D. A neoplasm may fluctuate in size.

16-35 *When wrist and finger extension causes pain over the extensor carpi radialis brevis tendon, the extensor carpi radialis longus tendon, and the extensor digitorum communis, you would suspect*

A. tennis elbow.

B. golfer's elbow.

C. de Quervain's disease.

D. intersection syndrome.

16-36 *Sandy, age 49, presents with loss of anal sphincter tone, impaired micturition, incontinence, and progressive loss of strength in the legs. You suspect cauda equina syndrome. What is your next action?*

A. Order physical therapy.

B. Order a lumbar/sacral x-ray.

C. Order extensive lab work.

D. Refer to a neurosurgeon.

16-37 *Heidi, age 29, is a nurse who has an acute episode of back pain. You have determined that it is a simple "mechanical" backache and order*

A. bedrest for 2 days.

B. muscle relaxants.

C. "let pain be your guide" and continue activities.

D. back-strengthening exercises.

16-38 *RoseMarie has a 15-year-old son who wants to play sports; however, she is very leery because she has heard of so many accidents. Which one of the following* sports does the American Academy of Pediatrics list as a limited contact/impact sport?

A. Field hockey

B. Soccer

C. Basketball

D. Lacrosse

16-39 *Steve, age 15, has only one testicle. When he asks you if he can play on the soccer team at school, how do you respond?*

A. "No, you'd be taking too much of a chance of injuring your remaining testicle."

B. "You can play any noncontact sport; however, soccer is too strenuous."

C. "As long as you can protect the remaining testicle, go for it."

D. "It should have no bearing on any activity."

16-40 *Which test is routinely recommended for a preparticipation sports physical?*

A. A complete blood count

B. A chest x-ray

C. An electrocardiogram

D. A Snellen test

16-41 *Which of the following statements concerning developmental dysplasia of the hip (DDH) is correct?*

A. It is often associated with being the firstborn female child.

B. It results from an orthopedic malformation in utero.

C. It has no genetic predisposition.

D. It is more common in males.

16-42 *Which of the following is a modifiable risk factor for osteoporosis?*

A. Low alcohol intake

B. Low caffeine intake

C. Smoking

D. Excessive exercise

16-43 *Sam, age 50, presents with Paget's disease that has been stable for several years. Recently, his serum alkaline phosphatase level has been steadily rising. You determine that it is time to start him on*

A. NSAIDs.

B. corticosteroids.

C. bisphosphonates.

D. calcitonin.

16-44 *John, age 17, works as a stock boy at the local supermarket. He is in the office for a routine visit. You notice that he had an episode of low back pain 6 months ago from improperly lifting heavy boxes. In discussing proper body mechanics with him to prevent future injuries, you tell him,*

A. "Bend your knees and face the object straight on."

B. "Hold boxes away from your body at arm's length."

C. "Bend and twist simultaneously as you lift."

D. "Keep your feet firmly together."

16-45 *Dan, age 49, developed osteomyelitis of the femur after a motorcycle accident. Which of the following statements about the clinical manifestations of osteomyelitis is correct?*

A. Integumentary effects include swelling, erythema, and warmth at the involved site.

B. There is a low-grade fever with intermittent chills.

C. Musculoskeletal effects include tenderness of the entire leg.

D. Cardiovascular effects include bradycardia.

16-46 *You are assessing Maya, a 69-year-old Asian woman, for the first time. You are trying to differentiate between scoliosis and kyphosis. Kyphosis involves*

A. asymmetry of the shoulders, scapulae, and waist creases.

B. a lateral curvature and vertebral rotation on posteroanterior x-rays.

C. one leg may appear shorter than the other.

D. a posterior rounding at the thoracic level.

16-47 *Mr. Miller is a 72-year-old African American with insulin-dependent diabetes mellitus. He has been a chronic smoker for 50 years. He has been told recently that he must have an above-the-knee amputation because of a gangrenous foot. He has lost the will to live and states, "They shoot horses, don't they?" How do you respond?*

A. "You should be thankful they can save your life, if not your leg."

B. "Your wife needs you; you must think of her at this time."

C. "How do you feel this surgery will affect you?"

D. "I will stay with you before, during, and after the surgery because I know that this is a difficult time for you."

16-48 *Emily, age 21, presents today with another muscle strain from one of her many sports activities. You think that she was probably never taught about health promotion and maintenance regarding physical activity. What information do you include in your teaching?*

A. "After an activity, if any part hurts, apply ice for 20 minutes."

B. "You must first get in shape with a rigorous schedule of weight training and then you can participate in any activity once you are physically fit."

C. "After any strenuous activity, you must completely rest your muscles before beginning your next activity."

D. "Stretching and warm-up exercises are an important part of any exercise routine."

16-49 *Alexander, age 18, sprained his ankle playing ice hockey. He is confused as to whether to apply heat or cold. What do you tell him?*

A. "Use continuous heat for the first 12 hours, then use heat or cold to your own preference."

B. "Use continuous cold for the first 12 hours, then use heat or cold to your own preference."

C. "Apply cold for 20 minutes, then take it off for 30–45 minutes; repeat for the first 24–48 hours while awake."

D. "Alternate between cold and heat for 20 minutes each for the first 24–48 hours."

16-50 *Joyce, age 87, broke her wrist after falling off a curb. She just had a plaster cast applied to her wrist. In instructing her family on allowing the cast to dry properly, tell them to*

A. continuously elevate Joyce's arm on a pillow.

B. change the position of Joyce's arm every hour.

C. position a fan near Joyce during the night to ensure even drying of the cast.

D. put a blanket over the cast to absorb the dampness.

16-51 *A Baker's cyst is*

A. an inflammation of the bursa.

B. a form of tendinitis.

C. the buildup of synovial fluid behind the knee.

D. the result of a "swollen" ligament.

16-52 *The straight-leg-raising maneuver can be used to diagnose*

A. nerve root compression.

B. a fractured hip.

C. an anterior cruciate ligament tear.

D. tendinitis.

16-53 *Ginny, age 48, has rheumatoid arthritis and gets achy and stiff after sitting through a long movie. This is referred to as*

A. longevity stiffness.

B. gelling.

C. intermittent arthritis.

D. molding.

16-54 *AnneMarie states that she has a maternal history of rheumatoid disease but that she has never been affected. Today she presents with complaints of dryness of the eyes and mouth. What do you suspect?*

A. Rheumatoid arthritis

B. Systemic lupus erythematosus

C. Sjögren's syndrome

D. Rosacea

16-55 *Sandra, a computer programmer, has just been given a new diagnosis of carpal tunnel syndrome. Your next step is to*

A. refer her to a hand surgeon.

B. take a more complete history.

C. try neutral position wrist splinting and order an oral NSAID.

D. order a nerve conduction study such as an electromyography (EMG).

16-56 *In a client with osteomalacia, you would expect levels of*

A. serum calcium to be elevated.

B. alkaline phosphatase to be elevated.

C. creatinine excretion to be elevated.

D. serum phosphorus to be elevated.

16-57 *Anna, age 42, is pregnant and was just given a diagnosis of carpal tunnel syndrome. She is worried that* *this will affect her in caring for the baby. What do you tell her?*

A. "Don't worry, we'll find a brace that is very malleable."

B. "After childbirth, your carpal tunnel syndrome may resolve."

C. "If we do surgery now, you'll be recovered by the time the baby arrives."

D. "You should prepare yourself for the probability of being unable to care for your baby."

16-58 *You suspect adolescent idiopathic scoliosis in Victoria, age 15, who is in her growth spurt. You perform the Adams forward-bending test and note a right-sided rib hump. What is this indicative of?*

A. Right lumbar shifting

B. Right thoracic curvature

C. Right truncal shift

D. Spondylolysis

16-59 *Lois, age 52, who has just been given a diagnosis of sarcoidosis, has joint symptoms including arthralgias and arthritis. Your next plan of action would be to*

A. order a bone scan.

B. obtain a tissue biopsy.

C. begin a course of glucocorticoids.

D. obtain an electrocardiogram.

16-60 *Jeffrey, age 16, was involved in a motor vehicle accident. He walks into the office with an obvious facial fracture, then collapses. What should your first action be?*

A. Call his parents for permission to treat.

B. Assess for an adequate airway.

C. Obtain head and maxillofacial CT.

D. Assess for a septal hematoma.

16-61 *Which of the following would be considered a common cause of sudden death in athletes younger than age 30?*

A. Bronchospasm from exercise-induced asthma

B. Hypertrophic cardiomyopathy

C. Compartment syndrome

D. Meningitis

16-62 *Matthew, age 52, is a chef who just severed two of his fingers with a meat cutter. You would recommend that he*

A. wrap the severed fingers tightly in a dry towel for transport to the ER with him.

B. leave the severed fingers at the scene as fingers cannot be reattached.

C. immediately freeze the severed fingers for reattachment in the near future.

D. pack the fingers in a saline-soaked dressing and seal in a plastic bag.

16-63 *What part of the body is affected by Dupuytren's contracture?*

A. The fourth and fifth fingers

B. The great toe

C. The tibia

D. The penis

16-64 *You have just completed a workup on Michael, age 13, and confirmed Osgood-Schlatter disease. You should*

A. refer for early surgical correction.

B. recommend quadriceps-strengthening exercises.

C. advise him to discontinue all sports activities until his growth plates have completely fused.

D. tell Michael that he can resume his usual activities immediately without concern and should begin aggressive exercises to increase muscle bulk and strength.

16-65 *Mary, age 72, has severe osteoarthritis of her right knee. She obtains much relief from corticosteroid injections. When she asks you how often she can have them, how do you respond?*

A. Only once a year in the same joint

B. No more than twice a year in the same joint

C. No more than three to four times a year in the same joint

D. No more than five to six times a year in the same joint

16-66 *Sean, age 48, has asymptomatic hyperuricemia. What is your initial therapy?*

A. NSAIDs

B. Dietary counseling

C. Colchicine

D. Allopurinol (Zyloprim)

16-67 *To aid in the diagnosis of meniscus damage, which test should you perform?*

A. Bulge test

B. Lachman test

C. Drawer test

D. Apley's compression test

16-68 *Which of the following can assist in the diagnosis of myasthenia gravis?*

A. Repetitive nerve stimulation

B. The presence of cogwheel rigidity

C. Chvostek's sign

D. Trousseau's sign

16-69 *A common cause of in-toeing in childhood is*

A. internal tibial torsion.

B. femoral retroversion.

C. external tibial torsion.

D. flat feet.

16-70 *Tara, the mother of a 2-year-old, is concerned because her daughter walks on her toes all the time. What do you tell her?*

A. "Toe walking is considered normal until age 3."

B. "Don't worry, she'll outgrow it."

C. "Toe walking is normal until she starts kindergarten."

D. "We should do further testing now."

16-71 *Shane, age 26, has a cast on his right arm because of an in-line skating accident. Twelve hours after the cast was applied, he complains of severe pain even though he recently took his pain medication. His fingers are pink, yet he states that they are tingling and feel slightly numb. What do you suspect?*

A. Compartment syndrome

B. Phlebitis

C. Osteomyelitis

D. Muscle contraction

16-72 *Mike, a golf pro, has had chronic back pain for many years. His workup reveals that it is not the result of a degenerative disk problem. His back "goes out" about*

twice per year, and he is out of work for about a week each time. Which of the following should you advise him to do?

A. Consider changing careers to a less physical job.

B. Begin a planned exercise program to strengthen back muscles.

C. Make an appointment with a neurosurgeon for a surgical consultation.

D. Start on a daily low-dose narcotic to take away the pain.

16-73 *Your client has just been told that he has a primary bone tumor. He was so upset when he heard this that he focused only on the word "malignant" and not on the prognosis or type of tumor. Which of the following tumors is malignant?*

A. Osteochondroma

B. Chondroma

C. Osteosarcoma

D. Giant-cell tumor

16-74 *Paul has a malignant fibrosarcoma of the femur. He recently had surgery and is now on radiation therapy. You want to order a test to determine the extent of the tumor invasion of the surrounding tissues and the response of the bone tumor to the radiation. Which of the following tests should you order?*

A. An x-ray

B. A magnetic resonance imaging (MRI) scan

C. A computed tomography (CT) scan

D. A needle biopsy

16-75 *Mickey is on a chemotherapeutic antibiotic for a musculoskeletal neoplasm. Which drug do you think he is taking?*

A. Cyclophosphamide (Cytoxan)

B. Doxorubicin (Adriamycin)

C. Methotrexate (Rheumatrex)

D. Cisplatin (Platinol)

16-76 *Jane, age 64, comes in for a visit. She has a cast on her right arm and tells you that she has a comminuted fracture of her radius. When she asks what that means, you tell her that in a comminuted fracture the*

A. bony fragments are in many pieces.

B. broken ends of the bone protrude through the soft tissues and skin.

C. bone breaks cleanly but does not penetrate the skin.

D. bone is crushed.

16-77 *Grating of the bones or entrance of air into an open fracture is manifested as*

A. swelling.

B. ecchymosis.

C. crepitus.

D. pain and tenderness.

16-78 *There are many precursors of deep venous thrombosis, such as decreased blood flow, injury to the blood vessel wall, and altered blood coagulation. Which one is the result of blood loss whereby the body attempts to maintain homeostasis by increasing the production of platelets and clotting factors?*

A. Altered blood coagulation

B. Decreased blood flow

C. Injury to the blood vessel wall

D. None of the above

16-79 *When Maxwell, age 12, slid into home plate while playing baseball, he injured his ankle. You are trying to differentiate between a sprain and a strain. You know that a sprain*

A. is an injury to the ligaments that attach to bones in a joint.

B. is an injury to the tendons that attach to the muscles in a joint.

C. is an injury resulting in extensive tears of the muscles.

D. does not result in joint instability.

16-80 *Jill, age 49, has recently begun a rigorous weight-lifting regimen. She presents in your office with a shoulder dislocation. Which of the following clinical manifestations make you suspect an anterior shoulder dislocation over a posterior dislocation?*

A. Inability to shrug the shoulder

B. Absence of pain

C. Inability to rotate the shoulder externally

D. Shortening of the arm

16-81 *What is the type of joint that is freely movable, such as the shoulder joint, called?*

A. A synarthrosis joint

B. An amphiarthrosis joint

C. A diarthrosis joint

D. None of the above

16-82 *Jennifer says that she has heard that caffeine can cause osteoporosis and asks you why. How do you respond?*

A. "Caffeine has no effect on osteoporosis."

B. "A high caffeine intake has a diuretic effect that may cause calcium to be excreted more rapidly."

C. "Caffeine affects bone metabolism by altering intestinal absorption of calcium and assimilation of calcium into the bone matrix."

D. "Caffeine increases bone resorption."

16-83 *Karen, who is postmenopausal, is taking 1500 mg of calcium but does not understand why she also needs to take vitamin D. You tell her that*

A. a deficiency of vitamin D results in an inadequate mineralization of bone matrix.

B. all vitamins need to be supplemented.

C. vitamin D increases intestinal absorption of dietary calcium and mobilizes calcium from the bone.

D. vitamin D binds with calcium to allow active transport into the cells.

16-84 *The American College of Obstetricians and Gynecologists' guidelines for exercise during pregnancy and after delivery include which of the following?*

A. Women should try to exercise moderately for at least 30 minutes on most, if not all, days of the week.

B. Exercise in the supine position is the position of choice.

C. Anaerobic exercise during pregnancy is preferred over aerobic exercise.

D. Exercise should be discontinued upon discovery of pregnancy and be resumed after delivery.

16-85 *What pathophysiology associated with transient pain after exercising usually begins a few hours post exercise with soreness and may last up to a week?*

A. Increased lactic acid production, muscle breakdown, and minor inflammation

B. Mild musculotendinous inflammation

C. Major musculotendinous inflammation, periostitis, and bone microtrauma

D. Breakdown in soft tissue and stress fracture

16-86   Greg, age 26, runs marathons and frequently complains of painful contractions of his calf muscles after running. You attribute this to

A. hypercalcemia.

B. hyponatremia.

C. heat exhaustion.

D. dehydration.

16-87   Jake, age 16, comes into the office with a human bite on his fist. What is the first course of action?

A. Debride and irrigate the wound thoroughly.

B. Initiate broad-spectrum antibiotics.

C. Leave the wound open for drainage.

D. Administer a tetanus injection.

16-88   When you elicit a painful Finkelstein's sign, you are testing for

A. carpal tunnel syndrome.

B. bursitis of the shoulder.

C. de Quervain's tenosynovitis.

D. tennis elbow.

16-89   A coccygeal fracture is treated with

A. traction.

B. surgical repair.

C. analgesia and by use of a "donut" cushion when sitting.

D. bedrest.

16-90   Martin, age 58, presents with urethritis, conjunctivitis, and asymmetric joint stiffness, primarily in the knees, ankles, and feet. Which condition do you suspect?

A. Syphilis

B. Gonorrhea

C. HIV

D. Reactive arthritis

16-91   You correctly perform the obturator test when you raise the client's leg with knee flexed and internally rotate the leg. A positive obturator test is indicative of

A. avascular necrosis (AVN) of the femoral head.

B. cholecystitis.

C. hip bursitis.

D. appendicitis.

16-92   To plan for a community education program, the nurse practitioner needs to know that persons at highest risk for developing thoracic outlet syndrome are

A. bicycle riders.

B. dancers.

C. computer programmers.

D. swimming instructors.

16-93   Which muscle enzyme is elevated in polymyositis?

A. Aldolase A

B. Aspartate aminotransferase

C. Creatine kinase

D. Lactate dehydrogenase

16-94   Management of fibromyalgia would include

A. giving psychotropic drugs, such as amitriptyline (Elavil), in a low dose at bedtime.

B. instructing clients to keep as busy as possible to keep their minds off the symptoms.

C. using high doses of NSAIDs.

D. avoiding exercise.

16-95   Bone mass measurement for which of the following female clients should be taken to assess whether they are at high risk for osteoporosis?

A. All women age 65 and older regardless of risk factors

B. All women age 65 and older with two or more risk factors

C. All women in their 30s for baseline

D. All premenopausal women who present with fractures

16-96   In assessing the skeletal muscles, you turn the forearm so that the palm is up. This is called

A. supination.

B. pronation.

C. abduction.

D. eversion.

16-97   What is the largest joint in the body?

A. The hip

B. The shoulder

C. The knee

D. The elbow

16-98 *Lillian, age 70, was told that she has osteoporosis. When she asks you what this is, you respond that osteoporosis*

A. develops when loss of bone matrix (resorption) occurs more rapidly than new bone growth (deposition).

B. is a degenerative joint disease characterized by degeneration and loss of articular cartilage in synovial joints.

C. is a chronic, systemic inflammatory disorder characterized by persistent synovitis of multiple joints.

D. is a metabolic bone disorder characterized by inadequate mineralization of bone matrix.

16-99 *Black men have a relatively low incidence of osteoporosis because they have*

A. increased bone resorption.

B. higher bone mass.

C. wide and thick long bones.

D. decreased bone deposition.

16-100 *Which of the following tests assesses the patency of the radial and ulnar arteries?*

A. Allen test

B. Finkelstein's test

C. Phalen's test

D. Tinel's sign

16-101 *Daniel, who is 45 and of northern European ancestry, has a dysfunctional and disfiguring condition affecting the palmar tissue between the skin and the distal palm and fourth and fifth fingers. What do you suspect?*

A. Hallux valgus

B. De Quervain's tenosynovitis

C. Dupuytren's contracture

D. Hallux rigidus

16-102 *June, a 59-year-old cashier, presents with back pain with no precipitating event. Pain is over her lower back and muscles without sciatica, and it is aggravated by sitting, standing, and certain movements. It is alleviated*

with rest. Palpation localizes the pain, and muscle spasms are felt. There was an insidious onset with progressive improvement. What is your initial diagnosis?

A. Ankylosing spondylitis

B. Musculoskeletal strain

C. Spondylolisthesis

D. Herniated disk

16-103 *You suspect a herniated disk on Sarah, age 72. You elevate her affected leg when she is in the supine position and it elicits back pain and sciatic nerve pain, which indicates a positive test. This is known as which test or sign?*

A. Femoral stretch test

B. Cross straight-leg-raising test

C. Doorbell sign

D. Straight-leg-raising test

16-104 *Beth, age 49, comes in with low back pain. An x-ray of the lumbar/sacral spine is within normal limits. Which of the following diagnoses do you explore further?*

A. Scoliosis

B. Osteoarthritis

C. Spinal stenosis

D. Herniated nucleus pulposus

16-105 *Which of the following is true regarding scoliosis?*

A. Functional scoliosis is flexible; it is apparent with standing and disappears with forward bending.

B. Functional scoliosis is fixed; the curvature shows both on standing and bending forward.

C. Structural scoliosis is fixed; the curvature shows both on standing and bending forward.

D. Functional scoliosis is permanent, whereas structural scoliosis can result from outside influences such as leg length discrepancy or muscle spasms.

16-106 *What is stiffness or fixation of a joint called?*

A. Contracture

B. Ankylosis

C. Dislocation

D. Subluxation

16-107 Which of the following statements is true regarding vertebrae?

A. All people have only 24 vertebrae (cervical, thoracic, lumbar).

B. Due to differences in race or gender, select groups may have 23 or 25 vertebrae (cervical, thoracic, lumbar).

C. It is common to have fewer than 23 vertebrae (cervical, thoracic, lumbar).

D. It is common to have more than 25 vertebrae (cervical, thoracic, lumbar).

16-108 Which of the following statements is true regarding range of motion (ROM) of a joint?

A. The normal active range of motion of a joint is greater than the passive range of motion of the same joint.

B. If there is a limitation of active range of motion, you should not attempt passive range of motion to avoid further injury to the joint.

C. Active and passive range of motion of a joint should be equal, full, and cause only mild discomfort.

D. Active and passive range of motion of a joint should be equal, full, and pain free.

16-109 Margaret, a 55-year-old female, presents to you for evaluation of left hand and wrist pain and swelling after a slip and fall on the ice yesterday. On examination, you note tenderness at her "anatomical snuffbox." You know this probably indicates

A. ulnar styloid fracture.

B. scaphoid fracture.

C. hamate fracture.

D. radial head fracture.

16-110 The knee is an example of a

A. spheroidal joint.

B. hinge joint.

C. condylar joint.

D. fibrous joint.

16-111 Christian, a 22-year-old carpenter who is right-hand dominant, comes to you for follow-up from the ER where he was seen for right forearm pain. He states he was diagnosed with right forearm tendinitis and wants you to explain this diagnosis to him. You explain that he has inflammation of one or more tendons, which are

A. the ropelike bundles of collagen fibrils that connect bone to bone.

B. the collagen fibers that connect muscle to bone.

C. the pouches of synovial fluid that cushion bone and other joint structures.

D. the fibrocartilaginous disks that separate bony surfaces.

16-112 Ethan, a 10-year-old boy, jumps off a 2-foot wall, twisting his foot and ankle upon landing. His ankle x-ray demonstrates a fracture of the distal tibia over the articular surface into the epiphysis and physis. Based on the Salter-Harris classification for growth plate injuries, you know this is a

A. Salter-Harris II.

B. Salter-Harris III.

C. Salter-Harris IV.

D. Salter-Harris V.

16-113 Anne, a 67-year-old female who sustained a fall on an outstretched hand, presents holding her arm against her chest with her elbow flexed. Based on the specific location of her pain, you suspect a radial head fracture. Your best initial assessment strategy to assess for radial head fracture would be

A. to palpate for tenderness, swelling, and crepitus just distal to the lateral epicondyle.

B. to palpate for tenderness, swelling, and crepitus along the radial wrist.

C. to palpate for tenderness in the "anatomical snuffbox."

D. to order an x-ray of the wrist.

16-114 A 13-year-old obese (BMI >95%) boy reports low-grade left knee pain for the past 2 months. He denies antecedent trauma but admits to frequent "horseplay" with his friends. The pain has progressively worsened, and he is now unable to bear weight at all on his left leg. His current complaints include left groin, thigh, and medial knee pain and tenderness. His examination demonstrates negative drawer, Lachman, and McMurray tests; left hip with decreased internal rotation and abduction; and knee flexion causing external hip rotation. Based on the above scenario, you suspect

A. left meniscal tear.

B. left anterior cruciate ligament (ACL) tear.

C. slipped capital femoral epiphysis (SCFE).

D. Osgood-Schlatter disease.

Answers

16-1 Answer A

The mechanism of action of colchicine is to interrupt the cycle of urate crystal deposition and inflammatory response. Used to treat an acute attack of gout, colchicine does not alter serum uric acid levels. Colchicine is generally used as a second-line therapy in gout when NSAIDs or corticosteroids are contraindicated or ineffective. Allopurinol (Zyloprim) acts on purine metabolism to reduce the production of uric acid and decrease serum and urinary concentrations of uric acid. It is useful for prevention of gout but not in the treatment of acute gout.

16-2 Answer B

The client with rheumatoid arthritis (RA) benefits from DMARDs, NSAIDs, and steroids because they all treat the disease of RA, as well as the pain. Acetaminophen (Tylenol) is a pain reliever but does not have anti-inflammatory effects. Acetaminophen is not considered a treatment option for the disease of RA and is likely even ineffective as a pain reliever for the pain associated with RA.

16-3 Answer D

When teaching clients about NSAIDs, tell them not to take these drugs on an empty stomach but to take them with food or milk and to stop the medication and call immediately if they notice any nausea/vomiting, coffee-ground emesis, black stools, or blood in the stool. If the client is having additional pain, acetaminophen (Tylenol) may be taken in conjunction with an NSAID because it is not an NSAID and will not potentiate gastric bleeding. Clients should be taught to never take more than the prescribed dose of an NSAID due to the likelihood of increasing the chances of gastrointestinal (GI) damage and kidney damage.

16-4 Answer B

In osteoarthritis, the affected joints are swollen, cool, and bony hard on palpation. With rheumatoid arthritis, the affected joints appear red, hot, and swollen and are boggy and tender on palpation.

Fatigue, decreased range of motion, and joint stiffness are common to both diseases.

16-5 Answer A

Musculoskeletal pain is not characteristic of chronic fatigue syndrome; rather, it is characteristic of fibromyalgia. The musculoskeletal pain, usually an achy muscle pain that may be localized or involve the entire body, is usually gradual in onset, although the onset may be sudden, occasionally after a viral illness. Fatigue is a more significant feature of chronic fatigue syndrome. With both disorders, difficulty sleeping and depression occur.

16-6 Answer C

To determine if a client has a fractured pelvis, a test for hematuria will usually prove positive. A fracture of the pelvis usually results in hypovolemia caused by a generally significant associated blood loss. Surrounding blood vessels rupture and result in a large retroperitoneal hematoma with shock. Pelvic fractures also commonly injure the urinary bladder or urethra. A client with a fracture in several locations of the pelvis may need a pneumatic antishock garment to control the blood loss and stabilize the pelvis. Only x-ray studies will confirm the diagnosis.

16-7 Answer A

Fat emboli are a serious and potentially fatal complication after a long-bone fracture. They usually occur within 72 hours after the injury. Fat emboli commonly lodge in the lung and produce sudden-onset respiratory problems resulting in hypoxemia. Symptoms include fever, tachycardia, rapid respirations, and neurological manifestations.

16-8 Answer B

If a client presents with lower back pain and has decreased sensation to a pinprick in the lateral leg and web of the great toe, this indicates a dermatomal pattern of discogenic disease in the L4/L5 area (L5 root involvement). L3/L4 (L4 nerve root) innervates the sensory function of the distal thigh to medial calf to the arch of the foot. L5/S1 (S1 nerve root) innervates the sensory function of the lateral lower leg/calf to the fifth toe.

16-9 Answer C

Follow the ABCs of first aid: airway, breathing, circulation. Establishing the airway is the first priority, followed by breathing, then circulation.

Stopping the bleeding from the wound, assessing if there has been a cervical fracture, and palpating the peripheral pulses are all important actions, but if the client is not breathing, the other actions will not be necessary.

16-10   Answer B

A positive anterior or posterior drawer sign indicates an injury to the anterior or posterior cruciate ligaments, respectively. The drawer test, or Lachman test, are both utilized to assess for cruciate ligament injury. Meniscus tears are also a common cause of knee joint pain or injury with the medial meniscus being injured more frequently than the lateral meniscus. The most consistent physical finding of a meniscal tear is tenderness to palpation along the joint line. To examine for a meniscal tear, perform the McMurray test by fully flexing the knee with leg externally rotated for medial meniscus and internally rotated for lateral meniscus. Then firmly extend the leg. A painful cartilage click is considered a positive McMurray test for meniscal injury. There is no posterior meniscus.

16-11   Answer B

In grading muscle strength on a scale of 1–5, a grade of 4 indicates full range of motion (ROM) against gravity with some resistance. A grade of 5 is full ROM against gravity with full resistance. A grade of 3 is full ROM with gravity. A grade of 2 is full ROM with gravity eliminated (passive motion). A grade of 1 indicates slight muscle contraction. A grade of 0 indicates no muscle contraction.

16-12   Answer C

In assessing your client, place the tips of your first two fingers in front of each ear and ask him to open and close his mouth. Then drop your fingers into the depressed area over the temporomandibular joint (TMJ) and note for smooth motion of the mandible. With this action, you are assessing for TMJ syndrome. Clicking or popping noises, decreased range of motion, pain, or swelling may indicate TMJ syndrome. However, an audible and palpable snap or click does occur in many normal people as they open their mouths. In rare cases, this may indicate osteoarthritis.

16-13   Answer D

If any limitation or increase in ROM occurs when assessing the musculoskeletal system, the angles of the bones should be measured by using a goniometer, which gives precise measurements of joint ROM. Phalen's test is used to diagnose carpal tunnel syndrome; it is not a tool. Skeletometry does not exist. The Thomas test is for evaluation of hip range of motion.

16-14   Answer A

If you note during your assessment of your client's foot that the foot is in alignment with the long axis of the lower leg and that weight-bearing falls on the middle of the foot, from the heel, along the midfoot, to between the second and third toes, you would diagnose a normal foot. Hallux valgus is a common deformity in which a lateral or outward deviation of the toe with medial prominence of the head of the first metatarsal is present. A hammertoe deformity is common in hallux valgus and is a deformity in the second, third, fourth, or fifth toes that includes hyperextension of the metatarsophalangeal joint and flexion of the proximal interphalangeal joint. Talipes equinovarus (clubfoot) is a congenital defect; it presents as a rigid and fixed malposition of the foot, including inversion, forefoot adduction, and the foot pointing downward.

16-15   Answer D

In performing Ortolani's maneuver to assess for developmental dysplasia of the hip (formerly referred to as congenital hip dislocation), the practitioner places the infant supine, flexes the knees, and places thumbs on medial proximal thighs and fingers on greater trochanters. Stabilize one thigh while the other thigh is gently abducted. If this movement results in a palpable 'clunk' (the hip moving back into the socket) there is dislocation of that hip. If the movement is smooth and silent, there is no hip dislocation. The Allis test is also used to check for hip dislocation or dysplasia by comparing leg lengths by checking knee heights while both knees are flexed and feet are flat on the table. Lasègue's sign is straight leg raising, which helps to confirm the presence of a herniated nucleus pulposus. The McMurray test is performed to evaluate for a torn meniscus.

16-16   Answer B

When teaching clients about using a cane, tell them to advance the cane with the ipsilateral (affected) leg. The cane should be carried in the contralateral hand and the cane length should equal the height of the greater trochanter. The use of assistive devices is an important strategy to protect the joints, as well as provide safety, but clients must be taught the proper use of all devices.

16-17   Answer A

To diagnose fibromyalgia, there must be tenderness on digital palpation in at least 11 of 18 (nine pairs) tender-point sites, including the occiput, low cervical, trapezius, supraspinatus, second rib, lateral epicondyle, gluteal, greater trochanter, and knee. PIP, MCP, and MTP joint tenderness occurs primarily in rheumatoid arthritis. Facet joints of the spine are often tender in facet arthritis. Tenderness over the bony prominences of the wrist and ankle would be specific to injury at those areas.

16-18   Answer B

To diagnose gout, there should be a negative joint culture and hyperuricemia. A septic joint would likely cause an elevated white blood count (WBC) and a positive bacterial joint culture. Rocephin (Ceftriaxone) is an antibiotic used in the treatment of bacterial infections such as a septic arthritis. A positive antinuclear antibody test may indicate systemic lupus erythematosus or scleroderma.

16-19   Answer A

First-line drug therapy for acute low back pain includes the use of NSAIDs. NSAIDs, as well as aspirin and acetaminophen (Tylenol), have been shown to be as effective as muscle relaxants and opioids for the control of acute low back pain but without the potential for dependence and abuse. Muscle relaxants have not been shown to be any more effective than NSAIDs, and combination therapy has no more effect than NSAIDs used alone.

16-20   Answer C

Years ago, muscle relaxants and bedrest were the treatments of choice for low back pain. Studies have now shown that resuming normal activity within the limits imposed by the pain has as good an effect as, if not better than, 2 days of bedrest. Exercise should begin as soon as possible after the acute injury and is directed at building endurance and stamina with consideration given to one's pain tolerance. NSAIDs, not narcotics, are generally the first-line medication treatment of low back pain without the risk of opioid dependency. A Boston brace may be used in the treatment of scoliosis.

16-21   Answer D

Lysosomal degradation results when leukocytes produce lysosomal enzymes that destroy articular cartilage in rheumatoid arthritis. The collagen fibers and the protein polysaccharides of articular cartilage are broken down by the enzymes. Immune complexes initiate the inflammatory process that brings leukocytes to the cartilage. Immune complexes are formed by the combination of immunoglobulin G with rheumatoid factors that are the result of antigen-antibody formation.

16-22   Answer B

Dorsal kyphosis, an exaggerated convexity of the thoracic curvature, typically accompanies the aging process. Lordosis occurs when the normal lumbar concavity is further accentuated, such as with pregnancy or obesity. Scoliosis, which is more prevalent in adolescent girls, is a lateral S-shaped or C-shaped curvature of the thoracic and/or lumbar spine and can also involve vertebral rotation.

16-23   Answer C

The bulge test assesses for an effusion of the knee. If effusion is present, a bulge will appear to the sides of or below the patella when the practitioner compresses the area above the patella. The Thomas test is used to assess for hip problems. Both Tinel's sign and Phalen's test assess for carpal tunnel syndrome.

16-24   Answer A

To observe for calf symmetry and leg strength, the practitioner asks the client to rise up on the toes and raise the heels. Simple inspection and observation while the client is standing with feet together is required to assess for hip, knee, and ankle symmetry. The "duck walk" of four steps away from the examiner with buttocks on heels would be used to observe for hip, knee, and ankle motion. Standing with the knees straight and then touching the toes is to check for scoliosis, hip motion, and hamstring tightness.

16-25   Answer D

Symmetric neurogenic pain (burning, numbness, tingling) will include peripheral neuropathy and myelopathy. Asymmetric neurogenic pain will include radiculopathy, reflex sympathetic dystrophy, and entrapment neuropathy. A claudication pain pattern will be present in peripheral vascular disease, giant-cell arteritis (with jaw pain), and lumbar spinal stenosis. These conditions all include the clinical manifestations of neurogenic pain.

16-26   Answer C

The Thompson test is used to diagnose an Achilles tendon rupture. With an Achilles tendon rupture, there is local swelling and bruising and a weak push-off. The Thompson test is positive when the gastrocnemius muscle belly is firmly squeezed and the foot does not plantarflex. Boutonnière deformity, not test, usually results from an injury at the proximal interphalangeal joint, involving the extensor slip that attaches to the middle phalanx. It can also develop in inflammatory disorders such as rheumatoid arthritis. The Lachman test assesses for an anterior cruciate ligament (ACL) tear. The knee is flexed 30°, the examiner places one hand on the distal femur and the other on the proximal tibia, and an anterior force is applied to the proximal tibia. An intact ACL should prevent forward movement of the tibia. Any perceived contralateral difference is usually significant. The anterior drawer test is also used to assess for an ACL tear, but it is much less reliable than the Lachman test.

16-27   Answer A

Osgood-Schlatter disease is an overuse injury that results from excessive tension and pull of the patellar tendon on the tibial tuberosity. Treating the client conservatively while an adolescent will avoid potential problems as an active adult. Initially, relative rest should be used with hamstring stretching, heel cord stretching, and quadriceps stretching exercises. If the problem persists, a long-leg knee immobilizer may be used. Surgical intervention is rarely required, but if so, only in an adult after bone growth is complete.

16-28   Answer A

Duchenne's muscular dystrophy, inherited in a sex-linked recessive pattern, afflicts boys, with the onset usually occurring around ages 3–5. The inability of the child to raise himself without supporting his knees because of weakness beginning primarily in the calf muscles, quadriceps, and hip extensor muscles is characteristic. Cerebral palsy affects motor function along with occasionally affecting intellect, emotional behavior, speech, sight, hearing, and touch. Damage occurs to the upper motor neurons during the prenatal or neonatal period.

Legg-Calvé-Perthes disease is avascular necrosis of the capital femoral epiphysis. A limp would be present. Multiple sclerosis usually appears in the client around ages 20–40. The most common symptoms involve visual, sensory, and gait disturbances.

16-29   Answer C

In reviewing myotomes, the C5 myotome innervates shoulder abduction (deltoid) and elbow flexion (biceps). Wrist extension results from the muscles and their corresponding nerves at C6; elbow extension from C7; and ulnar deviation at the wrist along with finger flexion and abduction from C8.

16-30   Answer D

The American Rheumatism Association has identified functional classes from I–IV depending on the client's ability to accomplish activities of daily living. Because Janine is a class III, her function would be adequate to perform only few or none of the duties of usual occupation or self-care. Class I refers to the client who can carry on all usual duties without handicaps. Class II refers to the client whose function is adequate for normal activities despite a handicap of discomfort or limited motion at one or more joints. Class IV refers to the client who is largely or wholly incapacitated, bedridden, or confined to a wheelchair, permitting little or no self-care.

16-31   Answer B

Swollen, bony proximal interphalangeal joints are Bouchard's nodes. Bony enlargements of the distal interphalangeal joints are Heberden's nodes. Both suggest osteoarthritis. Osler's nodes are painful, raised lesions of the fingers, toes, or feet that occur with bacterial endocarditis. There are no Murphy's nodes.

16-32   Answer D

Synovial fluid that is turbid and yellow-green on analysis indicates an inflammation, such as one that occurs in rheumatoid arthritis. Normal synovial fluid is clear and light yellow or straw colored. With trauma, the color would be turbid and red or xanthrochromic. With osteoarthritis, it is clear and yellow or straw colored. With gout, synovial fluid is turbid and yellow/milky white in color. With a septic infection such as a bacterial infection or TB, the fluid is turbid and gray-green or greenish-yellow.

16-33   Answer D

The Roos test suggests thoracic outlet syndrome if pain or paresthesias are present when the client positions his or her shoulders in abduction and external rotation of 90° with the elbows flexed to 90°. The client then opens and closes his or her hands for 3 minutes. The Neer test suggests inflammation or injury to the structures in the subacromial space when pain is experienced when the client is seated and maximal forced flexion of the shoulder is imposed with the forearm pronated. The Speeds test suggests tendinitis of the long head of the biceps when there is pain at the bicipital groove with forward elevation of the shoulders plus resistance. The Hawkins test assesses for inflammation or injury to the structures in the subacromial space when pain is elicited with forced internal rotation of the shoulder.

16-34   Answer B

Ganglia can be distinguished from neoplasms by their ability to transilluminate. Large ganglia and neoplasms may both restrict joint motion. Painless swelling is usually the main feature of ganglia. Ganglia may fluctuate in size depending on the individual's activity level and often will spontaneously resolve.

16-35   Answer A

With tennis elbow, wrist and finger extension causes pain over the extensor carpi radialis brevis tendon, the extensor carpi radialis longus tendon, and the extensor digitorum communis. With golfer's elbow, pain is experienced on wrist flexion over the flexor carpi radialis, the flexor carpi ulnaris, and the pronator teres tendons. With de Quervain's disease, pain is experienced on thumb extension over the abductor pollicis longus and the extensor pollicis brevis tendons. With intersection syndrome, pain is experienced with a grip and wrist extension over the extensor carpi radialis brevis and the extensor carpi radialis longus tendons.

16-36   Answer D

A prompt referral to a neurosurgeon is required when a diagnosis of cauda equina syndrome is suspected. Cauda equina syndrome is a widespread neurological disorder in which there is loss of anal sphincter tone; impaired micturition and incontinence; saddle anesthesia at the anus, perineum, or genitals; and motor weakness or sensory loss in both legs. An x-ray is not helpful in the diagnosis of cauda equina, and precious time should not be wasted in a client with suspected cauda equina. An MRI can be a useful diagnostic tool, but prompt evaluation by a neurosurgeon is an essential first step to prevent permanent neurological damage.

16-37   Answer C

Faster symptomatic recovery has been seen in clients with a simple "mechanical" backache who continue normal activities as much as they can with "pain being their guide" than in clients who use traditional medical treatments, such as bedrest and use of NSAIDs. Muscle relaxants should be ordered only if muscle spasms are actually present, although acetaminophen (Tylenol) and NSAIDs have also been shown to help the muscle spasms adequately. Back-strengthening exercises should be started within 6 weeks of the onset of pain.

16-38   Answer C

Basketball is listed as a limited contact/impact sport by the American Academy of Pediatrics Committee on Sports Medicine. Field hockey, soccer, and lacrosse all involve high-speed running and have the potential for collision and serious injury and therefore are classified as contact/ collision sports.

16-39   Answer C

For the client with only one testicle, as long as the remaining testicle can be protected, the client can participate in any sport.

16-40   Answer D

Other than a gross eye examination (most commonly performed using a Snellen eye chart) and vital signs, no specific tests are routinely recommended for a preparticipation sports physical.

16-41   Answer A

Developmental dysplasia of the hip (DDH), previously referred to as congenital hip dislocation, occurs in approximately 1% of live births and is more common in females than males. Factors related to development of DDH include being the firstborn female child, a family history of congenital dislocation of the hip, and breech presentation. Orthopedic malformation in utero is not considered a developmental cause.

16-42   Answer C

Modifiable risk factors for osteoporosis include smoking, high caffeine intake, high alcohol intake, sedentary lifestyle, calcium deficiency, and estrogen deficiency. Over the course of their lives, women tend to lose up to one-third of their original bone mass, ultimately affecting 80% of their skeletal system. It is essential that modifiable risk factors be modified because there are many that cannot, including increasing age, race (incidence is greater in white women), gender, pale complexion, and long-term glucocorticoid therapy.

16-43   Answer C

NSAIDs are helpful for clients with Paget's disease who have mild symptoms and pain. However, once the serum alkaline phosphatase level rises, which indicates that the disease has progressed, bisphosphonates, which decrease bone resorption by inhibiting osteoclast activity, are the treatment of choice. Calcitonin (Calcimar) also inhibits osteoclastic bone resorption but is not as powerful as the bisphosphonates and does not suppress the disease activity for as long after cessation. Corticosteroids do inhibit bone metabolism but are limited by the side effects of long-term therapy with high doses.

16-44   Answer A

In discussing proper body mechanics with John to prevent future injuries, you tell him to bend his knees and face the object straight on, to hold boxes close to his body and not at arm's length, and to spread his feet about shoulder-width apart. Using legs and arms, facing objects straight on, and keeping a wide stance provides a broad base of support and allows for use of supporting muscles, relieving stress on the back muscles. Never bend and twist simultaneously, but rather keep the spine straight to minimize injury.

16-45   Answer A

The clinical manifestations of osteomyelitis include the integumentary effects of swelling, erythema, and warmth at the involved site, as well as drainage and ulceration through the skin and lymph node involvement, especially in the involved extremity. The client with osteomyelitis may also have tachycardia, localized tenderness, and a high fever with chills.

16-46   Answer D

Kyphosis involves a posterior rounding at the thoracic level and a kyphotic curve of more than 45°

on x-ray. There may be moderate pain with kyphosis. Scoliosis involves asymmetry of the shoulders, scapulae, and waist creases; a lateral curvature and vertebral rotation on the posteroanterior x-rays; and one leg may appear shorter than the other.

16-47   Answer C

Exploring Mr. Miller's feelings and getting more clarification of how the surgery will affect him will allow you to know him better and be better able to assist him in dealing with the situation.

16-48   Answer D

Health promotion and maintenance information regarding physical activity that should be included in client teaching includes reminding the client that stretching and warm-up exercises are an important part of any exercise routine. After proper stretching and warm-up exercises, muscles should not hurt after most sports activities if engaged in on a regular basis. If the activity is new, a muscle group may be slightly sore, in which case ice applied to the area may help relieve the discomfort. Any rigorous exercise should be avoided until one is in proper physical condition. This is usually obtained after a conservative, lengthy program of physical fitness activities. After any strenuous activity, a cool-down period should be employed.

16-49   Answer C

Tell a client who has sprained his ankle to apply cold for 20 minutes, then take it off for 30–45 minutes, and repeat that procedure for the first 24–48 hours while awake. Cold will cause vasoconstriction and decrease edema, preventing any further bleeding into the tissues. Ice has been proven to speed recovery in ankle sprains; however, ice should never be applied continuously because it could hinder proper circulation and cause frostbite. Therefore, always recommend a protective padding between the ice and the skin. Applying heat may increase swelling and subsequently slow recovery. After any sprain, use the principles of RICE: R for rest, I for ice, C for compression, and E for elevation.

16-50   Answer B

Instructions to the client and family on how to allow a cast to dry properly should include advising them to change the position of the extremity with the cast every hour. In this case, Joyce's arm should be repositioned frequently to prevent indentations in the cast itself (caused by continuous placement on a pillow) and to ensure drying on all the surfaces of the cast. Elevating her arm will prevent edema, but elevation is not needed continuously. A fan will dry only the outside of the cast. A blanket will prevent drying of the cast.

16-51 Answer C

A Baker's cyst, also called popliteal cyst, is the buildup of synovial fluid behind the knee. It usually results from inflammation resulting from knee arthritis or a cartilage (especially meniscal) tear and consists of local pain, inability to extend the knee, and symptoms related to compression of surrounding structures. The latter symptoms may mimic venous thrombophlebitis.

16-52 Answer A

The straight-leg-raising maneuver can be used to diagnose nerve root compression by eliciting radiating pain down the leg in the affected dermatomal distribution. The leg is straight and lifted by the heel. The leg may also be brought across the body to increase the sensitivity of this maneuver. Leg shortening and external rotation may be present with a fractured hip. Extending the knee would elicit pain if an anterior cruciate ligament tear were present. Pressure over an affected tendon would elicit pain if tendinitis were present.

16-53 Answer B

Gelling refers to the achiness and stiffness that occur in clients with rheumatoid arthritis after a period of inactivity.

16-54 Answer C

Sjögren's syndrome, which affects the salivary and lacrimal glands, causes clients to have dry eyes and mouths. It is an inflammatory disease of the exocrine glands and may be an isolated entity or may be associated with other rheumatic disease, such as rheumatoid arthritis (RA) or systemic lupus erythematosus (SLE). Because AnneMarie has no other symptoms of RA or SLE, Sjögren's syndrome should be considered first. Rosacea is a chronic facial skin disorder with a vascular component.

16-55 Answer C

For the client who has just been given a diagnosis of carpal tunnel syndrome, your next step is to try neutral position wrist splinting and order an oral NSAID. For symptoms of less than 10 months' duration, conservative treatment should be tried first. Taking a more complete history is not essential at this point because a diagnosis has already been made. Nerve conduction studies (i.e., electromyography [EMG]) confirm focal median nerve conduction delay within the carpal canal and also provide information about disease severity. For refractory cases, median nerve decompression may be accomplished by surgery, but complete recovery is not possible if atrophy is pronounced.

16-56 Answer B

The alkaline phosphatase level is moderately elevated in osteomalacia. Serum calcium and phosphorus, urinary calcium, and creatinine excretion levels are all low in osteomalacia.

16-57 Answer B

Pregnant women have an increased incidence of carpal tunnel syndrome (CTS) but often have their carpal tunnel syndrome resolve after delivery. Although repetitive use of the hand can lead to carpal tunnel syndrome, certain medical conditions such as diabetes, obesity, and thyroid disease also increase the likelihood of CTS. Often, the cause of CTS is unknown.

16-58 Answer B

When you have a client bend forward to assess the spine (the Adams forward-bending test) and you note a right-sided rib hump, this is indicative of a right thoracic curve. Adolescent idiopathic scoliosis is a lateral spinal curvature of greater than 10° when no pathological cause has been determined. Management consists of the three Os: observation, orthosis, and operation. Spondylolysis is a bony defect of the pars interarticularis.

16-59 Answer C

Sarcoidosis is the result of an exaggerated immune system response to a class of antigens or self-antigens. Fifty percent of clients experience joint symptoms, including myopathy and polyarthritis, and glucocorticoids are prescribed to suppress the immune process, thus relieving symptoms. About 25% show some form of cardiac dysfunction, although it is often not recognized clinically.

16-60   Answer B

The primary concern in the management of facial fractures is to ensure an adequate and stable airway. Displaced soft tissues, blood, secretions, or other foreign material may obstruct the airway and cause asphyxia. Septal hematomas are more commonly seen in children than in adults, but the first priority is to maintain an adequate airway. Once his airway is established and he is stabilized, permission to treat Jeffrey can be obtained from his parents. Head and maxillofacial CT would then be obtained.

16-61   Answer B

Although exercise-induced asthma is common among athletes, it is not a common cause of sudden death. Cardiac conditions are responsible for the three most common causes of sudden death in athletes younger than age 30 and include hypertrophic cardiomyopathy, idiopathic left ventricular hypertrophy, and coronary artery anomalies. Compartment syndrome and meningitis can occur in both athletes and nonathletes, but, by definition, they are not causative of sudden death.

16-62   Answer D

If a client has severed his fingers, the fingers should be wrapped in a saline-soaked dressing, placed in a plastic bag, and transported to the emergency room along with the client. The fingers should be cooled on ice, not frozen or kept at body temperature. Severed fingers can be reattached after 1–2 days or more, if properly stored.

16-63   Answer A

Dupuytren's contracture manifests itself by nodular thickening of the connective tissue of one or both hands, usually affecting the fourth and fifth fingers. There is tenderness with the inability to extend the fingers. Peyronie's disease is a connective tissue disorder that results in painful curvature of the erect penis.

16-64   Answer B

Osgood-Schlatter is usually a benign, self-limited knee condition in adolescent boys and girls. Treatment consists of ice, analgesics, NSAIDs, and temporary avoidance of pain-producing activities. Conservative treatment includes quadriceps-stretching exercises to decrease tension on the tibial tubercle. Surgical correction for Osgood-Schlatter

disease is not recommended until all other options have been tried and have failed.

16-65   Answer C

Intra-articular corticosteroid injections provide much needed pain relief in weight-bearing joints of clients with osteoarthritis; however, they should be limited to no more than three to four in the same joint per year because of potential damage to the cartilage if given more frequently.

16-66   Answer B

Asymptomatic hyperuricemia does not require any therapy because most people never develop symptoms. Although diet plays a minor role, dietary counseling to avoid foods high in purine and alcoholic beverages may be helpful to prevent future gout attacks. An acute attack of gout may be treated with colchicine or an NSAID. Allopurinol (Zyloprim) decreases uric acid production and might be prescribed to clients after multiple gouty attacks but should not be given as treatment for an acute gouty attack.

16-67   Answer D

To aid in the diagnosis of meniscus damage such as a torn meniscus, you should perform Apley's compression test. With the client in the prone position, the suspected knee is flexed to 90° and then downward pressure is exerted on the foot so that the tibia is firmly opposed to the femur. The leg is then rotated externally and internally. If the knee locks and there is pain or clicking with this maneuver, it is a positive Apley's sign, indicating the presence of a loose body, such as a torn cartilage, trapped in the joint articulation. The bulge test assesses for effusions in the knee joint. The Lachman test is an indicator of injury to the anterior cruciate ligament. The drawer test assesses for stability of the anterior and posterior cruciate ligaments.

16-68   Answer A

Repetitive nerve stimulation (RNS) is the most frequently used electrodiagnostic test for myasthenia gravis. The nerve to be studied is electrically stimulated and the compound muscle action potential (CMAP) is recorded with surface electrodes over the muscle. Serological tests such as serum anti-AChR antibodies are also usually included along with electrodiagnostic testing. Cogwheel rigidity is present in Parkinson's disease. Chvostek's and Trousseau's signs are indications of tetany.

16-69   Answer A

Internal tibial torsion is the most common overall cause of in-toeing. External tibial torsion is the most common overall cause of out-toeing. Femoral retroversion is a common cause of out-toeing, whereas femoral anteversion is a cause of in-toeing. Flat feet often causes out-toeing.

16-70   Answer A

Toe walking is considered normal until age 3 years. Constant toe walking after that age is considered abnormal and requires further investigation for neuromuscular disorders.

16-71   Answer A

Compartment syndrome occurs when external pressure constricts the structures within a compartment, compromising tissue perfusion. The pressure causes compressed nerves, muscles, and blood vessels. Cellular acidosis results, followed by edema, further increasing compartment pressures. This usually develops within the first 48 hours of injury. When assessing for compartment syndrome, remembering the five Ps—pain, pulselessness, pallor, paresthesias, and paralysis—can be helpful, but they are not true diagnostic criteria. Phlebitis usually involves the lower extremities. Osteomyelitis might be considered if the fracture were an open one and bacteria entered through the open wound, but it would not develop this soon after the injury. Osteomyelitis can occur at any age, but children younger than age 12 and adults older than age 50 are the usual victims. A muscle contraction is a normal physiological function and would not result in these symptoms.

16-72   Answer B

In this case, Mike may benefit from a regular planned exercise program to strengthen back muscles and attempt to reduce the probability of future episodes of back pain. Surgery is recommended only for clients with low back pain caused by degenerative disk disorders, and then only when severe neurological involvement has occurred. Surgery benefits only approximately 1% of persons with low back problems. Suggesting a career change should be considered only in cases of disability or inability to safely continue one's current

employment. Narcotic pain medications are not considered first-line treatment for mechanical back pain.

16-73   Answer C

An osteosarcoma is the most common malignant tumor that occurs in the long bones and the knee. An osteochondroma is the most common benign tumor and usually occurs in the pelvis, scapula, and ribs. A chondroma occurs in the hands, feet, ribs, spine, sternum, or long bones. A giant-cell tumor is a tumor of the bone marrow cells in the shaft of the long bones, such as the femur, tibia, radius, and humerus.

16-74   Answer B

For Paul, who has a malignant fibrosarcoma of the femur, a magnetic resonance imaging scan will determine the extent of the tumor invasion on the surrounding tissues and the response of the bone tumor to the radiation. It will also determine response to chemotherapy and will detect recurrent disease. A conventional x-ray will show the location of the tumor and the extent of bone involvement. Metastatic bone destruction has a characteristic "moth-eaten" pattern in which the growth has a poorly defined margin that cannot be separated from normal bone. A computed tomography scan will evaluate the extent of the tumor invasion into bone, soft tissues, and neurovascular structures. A needle biopsy, usually performed at the time of surgery, will determine the type of tumor.

16-75   Answer B

The only antibiotic listed is Doxorubicin (Adriamycin). All of the other medications are chemotherapeutic agents that may be used for musculoskeletal neoplasms. Cyclophosphamide (Cytoxan) is an alkylating agent, methotrexate (Rheumatrex) is an antimetabolite, and cisplatin (Platinol) is a synthetic agent.

16-76   Answer A

A comminuted fracture occurs when the bony fragments are in many pieces. An open fracture occurs when the broken ends of the bone protrude through soft tissues and skin. A closed fracture occurs when the bone breaks cleanly but does not penetrate the skin. A compression fracture occurs when the bone is crushed.

16-77 Answer C

Grating of the bones or entrance of air into an open fracture is manifested as crepitus. The extremity should not be manipulated to elicit crepitus because it may cause additional damage. Swelling is manifested by edema from localization of serous fluid and bleeding. Ecchymosis results from extravasation of blood into the subcutaneous tissue. Pain and tenderness result from muscle spasm, direct tissue trauma, nerve pressure, or movement of the fractured bone.

16-78 Answer A

One of the precursors of deep vein thrombosis is altered blood coagulation, which may result from active blood loss. The body then attempts to compensate by increasing the production of platelets and clotting factors. Decreased blood flow is common in clients with a fracture and those who are immobilized and not as active. Venous flow can be decreased by 50% in bedridden persons. Injury to the blood vessel wall may occur as a direct result of force, such as from a fracture, or may occur during surgery.

16-79 Answer A

A sprain is defined as an injury to the ligaments that connect bone to bone in a joint that results from a twisting motion and may cause joint instability. A strain is defined as an injury to the muscles and/or the tendons that attach muscles to bones.

16-80 Answer A

Clinical manifestations of an anterior shoulder dislocation, which is far more common than a posterior dislocation, include the inability to shrug the shoulder, pain, and lengthening of the arm. The inability to rotate the shoulder externally is a clinical manifestation of a posterior shoulder dislocation, along with the inability to elevate the arm.

16-81 Answer C

The type of joint that is freely movable, such as the shoulder joint, is called a diarthrosis joint. Diarthrosis joints include the joints of the limbs, shoulders, and hips. Synarthrosis joints are immovable and include skull sutures, epiphyseal plates, ribs, and the manubrium of the sternum. Amphiarthrosis joints are slightly movable joints, such as the vertebral joints and the joint of the pubic symphysis.

16-82 Answer B

The effect of caffeine in causing osteoporosis is controversial, but it is postulated to result from caffeine's diuretic effect that causes calcium to be excreted more rapidly.

16-83 Answer C

Advise clients taking calcium supplements that they also need to take vitamin D because vitamin D raises serum calcium levels by increasing the intestinal absorption of dietary calcium and mobilizing calcium from the bone. Vitamin D deficiency results in an inadequate mineralization of bone matrix (rickets), more commonly seen in children.

16-84 Answer A

The guidelines from the American College of Obstetricians and Gynecologists for exercise during pregnancy and after delivery include the following: Women can and should try to exercise moderately for at least 30 minutes on most, if not all, days. Exercise in the supine position should be avoided after the first trimester because this position is associated with a decreased cardiac output. Because of decreased oxygen available for aerobic exercise during pregnancy, the intensity of the workout should be based on maternal symptoms.

16-85 Answer A

The pathophysiology associated with transient pain after exercising that usually lasts a few hours with postexercise soreness and may last up to a week is increased lactic acid production, muscle breakdown, and minor inflammation. Longer-lasting pain late in an activity or immediately after is often caused by mild musculotendinous inflammation. When there is pain in the beginning or middle of the activity, there might be major musculotendinous inflammation, periostitis, and bone microtrauma. When the pain begins before or early in the exercise, preventing or affecting the performance, it is often the result of breakdown in soft tissue or stress fracture.

16-86 Answer B

Painful contractions of muscles after exertion, such as heat cramps, may be related to hyponatremia or other electrolyte imbalances. Usually the gastrocnemius and hamstring muscles are involved. Treatment of heat cramps includes passive muscle stretching, cessation of activities, transfer to a cooler environment, and drinking cool liquids.

Sports drinks such as Gatorade that contain electrolytes may be beneficial. Heat exhaustion is a more serious condition, with symptoms ranging from nausea, vomiting, headache, loss of appetite, and dizziness to irritability, tachycardia, and hyperventilation. Hyperkalemia may cause muscular weakness, fatigue, and muscle cramps. Greg's dehydration is attributed to his hyponatremia and would be a good second-choice answer. Hypercalcemia may affect gastrointestinal, renal, and neurological function. Symptoms may include constipation, polyuria, and at times, nausea, vomiting, and anorexia.

16-87   Answer A

When a client has a human bite, the first immediate course of action must be to debride and irrigate the wound. Then, an x-ray should be taken to rule out osteomyelitis, fractures, and retained teeth from the offender. A wound culture would be required only for an older injury or a wound with evidence of infection. Broad-spectrum antibiotics such as IV ampicillin/sulbactam (Unasyn) and/or po Amoxicillin with clavulanic acid (Augmentin) should be started and the wound left open for drainage. Rabies is not a concern with human bites. Clients should then be evaluated for the need for a tetanus injection.

16-88   Answer C

Pain elicited when the Finkelstein's test is performed indicates de Quervain's tenosynovitis at the base of the thumb. The test is performed by flexion of the thumb across the palm, with ulnar deviation of the wrist. Gliding the inflamed tendons will produce pain, which is considered a positive Finkelstein's test. Tinel's sign and Phalen's test are used to diagnose carpal tunnel syndrome. The tennis elbow test evaluates for lateral epicondylitis. The client's elbow is stabilized in the examiner's hand and the thumb of that hand positioned on the client's lateral epicondyle. The client makes a fist, pronates the forearm, and radially deviates and extends the wrist while the examiner applies a resisting force at the wrist. This test is positive if pain is elicited in the area of the lateral epicondyle. There is no specific test for shoulder bursitis.

16-89   Answer C

A coccygeal fracture, usually incurred by a fall onto the sacrococcygeal area, is treated conservatively with analgesia and by using a "donut" cushion when sitting.

16-90   Answer D

Reactive arthritis (formerly Reiter's syndrome) is arthritis of the lower extremities and is more common in white men. Associated symptoms include the classic triad of conjunctivitis, nongonococcal urethritis, and arthritis. A common mnemonic is the client who "can't see, can't pee, and can't climb a tree."

16-91   Answer D

A positive obturator test, especially with a positive McBurney's point and a positive psoas sign, is indicative of appendicitis. Although internal rotation of the hip may cause hip discomfort in a client with hip bursitis and AVN of the femoral head, the obturator test elicits right lower quadrant (RLQ) abdominal pain, which is indicative of appendicitis.

16-92   Answer C

Thoracic outlet syndrome (TOS) results from a compression of nerves, blood vessels, or both, into the upper extremity arising from the head, neck, shoulders, upper extremities, and chest. Predisposing factors for thoracic outlet syndrome include a history of head and neck trauma, poor posture, chronic illness, and occupations that result in compression of the neurovascular structures supplying the upper extremity such as computer programming and piano playing.

16-93   Answer C

Increased levels of creatine kinase are found in polymyositis, traumatic injuries, and progressive muscular dystrophy. Aldolase A level is elevated in muscular dystrophy and dermatomyositis. Aspartate aminotransferase is found in skeletal muscle but mainly in heart and renal cells. Lactate dehydrogenase level is elevated in skeletal muscle necrosis, extensive cancer, and progressive muscular dystrophy.

16-94   Answer A

Management of fibromyalgia includes giving tricyclic antidepressants such as amitriptyline (Elavil) in a low dose at bedtime. Although clients with fibromyalgia are fatigued and have stiff joints and muscle pain, physical therapy, including exercise, is an important aspect of care. Injecting trigger points with local anesthetics and steroids can also be helpful. NSAIDs have not proven beneficial in the treatment of fibromyalgia, and NSAIDs are always associated with the risk of GI bleeding, especially in high doses.

16-95   Answer A

The National Osteoporosis Foundation guidelines indicate that bone mass density (BMD) testing should be performed on all women age 65 and older regardless of risk factors; on younger post-menopausal women with one or more risk factors (other than being white, postmenopausal, and female); and on postmenopausal women who present with fractures to confirm underlying disease and severity.

16-96   Answer A

Turning the forearm so that the palm is up is supination. Turning the forearm so that the palm is down is pronation. Abduction is moving a limb away from the midline of the body. Eversion is moving the sole of the foot outward at the ankle.

16-97   Answer C

The knee is the largest joint in the body, with the articulation of four bones, the femur, tibia, fibula, and patella, in one common articular cavity. It is a joint that not only permits flexion and extension but also some degree of rotation. The knee also has the body's largest synovial membrane.

16-98   Answer A

Osteoporosis develops when bone resorption occurs more rapidly than bone deposition. Osteoarthritis is a degenerative joint disease characterized by degeneration and loss of articular cartilage in synovial joints. Rheumatoid arthritis is a chronic, systemic inflammatory disorder characterized by persistent synovitis of multiple joints. Osteomalacia is a metabolic bone disorder characterized by inadequate mineralization of bone matrix, often caused by vitamin D deficiency.

16-99   Answer B

Black men have a relatively low incidence of osteoporosis because they have higher levels of bone mass and are protected by the bone-resorptive effects of parathyroid hormone. Osteoporosis has the highest incidence in white women.

16-100   Answer A

The Allen test assesses the patency of the radial and ulnar arteries in the arterial arch. Have the client make a fist and use your fingers to occlude both radial and ulnar arteries. Then, have the client open the hand and you release the radial pressure. Observe for rapid refill of color to the palm indicating patency of the radial artery. Repeat the same maneuver, releasing ulnar pressure to assess ulnar artery competency. Finkelstein's test assesses for de Quervain's tenosynovitis. Phalen's test and Tinel's sign assess for carpal tunnel syndrome.

16-101   Answer C

Dupuytren's contracture affects the palmar tissue between the skin and the distal palm and fingers, most often in the fourth and fifth fingers but also in the thumb-index finger web space. It is progressive and results in flexor contracture while not affecting the flexor tendons. Most frequently occurring in males between the ages of 40 and 60, it is common among persons of Northern European ancestry. It is dysfunctional and disfiguring. Although not actually painful, it may be tender. Surgery is recommended when the inability to straighten the fingers limits the client's hand function. Hallux valgus, commonly referred to as a bunion, is an osseous deformity at the MTP joint of the great toe with medial deviation of the toe. Hallux rigidus is a common condition of arthritis at the base of the great toe at the MTP joint, causing stiffness and decreased movement of the great toe.

16-102   Answer B

Pain over the lower back and spine, as well as the muscles, without sciatica is musculoskeletal strain. Often there is no precipitating event, and there is an insidious onset. It is aggravated by sitting, standing, and certain movements. Palpation localizes the pain, and muscle spasms may be felt. It is alleviated by rest, and there is progressive improvement. Ankylosing spondylitis is back pain and stiffness over several months where there is a systemic inflammatory condition of the vertebral column and sacroiliac joints. Painful ankylosed sacroiliac joints, reduced chest wall expansion, and excessive thoracic kyphosis are also present. It most frequently affects males between the ages of 20 and 30, causing chronic low back pain that is worse in the morning. There is relief with exercise and reduced mobility of the spine. A herniated disk is often preceded by years of recurrent episodes of localized back pain and there is usually leg pain that overshadows the back pain. With spondylolisthesis, there is a defect or fracture of the pars interarticularis with forward shifting of one vertebra on top of another. This can cause nerve irritation and damage if the vertebrae are pressing on a spinal nerve root.

16-103   Answer D

All of the tests listed as possible options are tests done to assess for a herniated disk. In the straight-leg-raising test, you elevate the affected leg when the client is in the supine position; back pain and sciatic nerve pain (radiating leg pain) indicate a herniated disk. In the cross straight-leg-raising test, elevation of the uninvolved leg produces sciatic pain down the contralateral leg. The doorbell sign is the development of sciatica when the spinous process over the protruded disk is deeply palpated. The femoral stretch test is done with the client prone and the leg extended and the knee flexed. Pain radiating to the anterior thigh indicates an L4 radiculopathy. Suspect a herniated disk.

16-104   Answer D

A plain x-ray film will not show a herniated nucleus pulposus nor a muscle strain. It will show spondylolisthesis, scoliosis, osteoarthritis, and spinal stenosis. Note that x-rays of the spine are not indicated in low back pain unless the cause of the pain is thought to have a bony origin or to be traumatic in nature or to rule out systemic disease.

16-105   Answer A

Scoliosis is a curve in the spine. It is prominent beginning between ages 8 and 10 years through adolescence and is more common in females than in males. Functional scoliosis is flexible; it is apparent with standing and disappears with forward bending. It is due to a problem that does not involve the spine such as leg length discrepancy or muscle spasm. Structural scoliosis is fixed; the curvature shows both on standing and bending forward. When the person is standing, note unequal shoulder elevation, unequal scapulae, obvious curvature, unequal elbow length, and unequal hip level.

16-106   Answer B

Ankylosis is stiffness or fixation of a joint. It often involves inflammation of the connective tissue, muscles, and the joint itself. A contracture is a shortening of a muscle leading to limited range of motion of a joint. This is often the result of scar formation from trauma, genetics, or chronic disease. Dislocation is one or more bones in a joint being

out of position. Subluxation is a partial dislocation of a joint.

16-107   Answer B

Although 24 vertebrae (cervical, thoracic, lumbar) are found in 85%–93% of all people, racial and gender differences reveal 23 or 25 vertebrae in select groups. There are usually 7 cervical, 12 thoracic, and 5 lumbar vertebrae. There are also 5 sacral and 3–4 coccygeal vertebrae.

16-108   Answer D

Both active range of motion (AROM) and passive range of motion (PROM) of a joint should normally be equal, full, and pain free. Active range of motion requires strength against gravity and passive range of motion is performed by the examiner without the effects of muscle contraction or gravity. Any pain or limitation with range of motion should be further investigated to determine the cause. If you note a limitation of active range of motion, you should gently attempt passive motion to further assess the joint.

16-109   Answer B

There is tenderness over the "anatomical snuffbox" in a scaphoid (aka navicular) fracture, the most common injury of the carpal bones. Poor blood supply puts the scaphoid bone at risk for avascular necrosis; therefore, wrist pain and tenderness in the anatomical snuffbox, even without history of antecedent trauma, warrants a wrist x-ray. A fracture of the hook of the hamate is an uncommon fracture seen in golfers and in players of other racket sports and involves pain and tenderness on the ulnar side of the palm. An ulnar styloid fracture would produce tenderness at the distal ulna. A radial head fracture would result in pain at the elbow joint where the radial head lies proximal to the distal humerus. Be sure not to confuse the radial head (proximal end of the radius) with the radial styloid (distal end of the radius at the wrist).

16-110   Answer C

In a condylar joint, such as the knee and temporomandibular joint, the articulating surfaces are convex or concave and are termed condyles. Spheroidal joints have a ball-and-socket configuration—a rounded convex surface articulating with a cuplike cavity, allowing a wide range of rotary movement, as in the shoulder and hip. Often the knee is mistakenly referred to as a hinge joint, but hinge joints are flat and uniplanar, allowing only a gliding motion in a single plane, as in flexion and extension of the interphalangeal joints. In fibrous joints, such as the sutures of the skull, intervening layers of fibrous tissue or cartilage hold the bones together. The bones are almost in direct contact, which allows no appreciable movement.

16-111 Answer B

Tendons are the collagen fibers that connect muscle to bone. Ligaments connect bone to bone in the joints. Bursae are the pouches of synovial fluid that reduce friction between bones, muscles, or tendons. Fibrocartilaginous disks separate bony surfaces such as those between the vertebrae in the spine.

16-112 Answer B

The Salter-Harris classification system of growth plate injuries divides most growth plate injuries into five categories based on the damage: Salter-Harris I is through the physis; Salter-Harris II is through the metaphysis and the physis; Salter-Harris III is through the epiphysis and the physis; Salter-Harris IV is through the metaphysis, epiphysis, and the physis; and a Salter-Harris V is a compression injury of the physis.

16-113 Answer A

The radial head is the proximal aspect of the radius, located in the elbow joint. Falling on an outstretched hand transfers a significant amount of force to the radial head. Often a fracture line cannot be seen on an x-ray, but presence of an anterior or posterior fat pad sign (or sail sign) indicates an occult radial head fracture. Tenderness, swelling, and crepitus at the radial wrist could indicate a distal radius fracture or fracture of the carpal bones. Tenderness in the "anatomical snuffbox" is used to assess for possible fracture of the scaphoid bone in the wrist. A wrist x-ray will demonstrate abnormalities of only the distal radius, ulna, or carpal bones. An elbow x-ray would assist in the diagnosis of a radial head fracture.

16-114 Answer C

Slipped capital femoral epiphysis (SCFE) is a displacement of the femoral head relative to the femoral neck that occurs through the physis (growth plate) of the femur. The vast majority of the clients are obese as the added weight increases shear stress across the physis. The mean age at diagnosis is 12 years for females and 13½ years for males. Surgery is often required via in situ pin fixation (single screw) to stabilize the growth plate to prevent further slippage and to avoid complications. There would be a positive McMurray sign and a positive Lachman and/or drawer test in meniscal or cruciate ligament tears, respectively. Osgood-Schlatter disease would result in swelling, pain, and tenderness at the tibial tubercle.

Bibliography

American Academy of Pediatrics Committee on Sports Medicine: Recommendations for participation in competitive sports. *Pediatrics* 81:5, 1988.

Bickley, L: *Bates' Guide to Physical Examination and History Taking*, ed 9. Lippincott Williams & Wilkins, Philadelphia, 2007.

Broderick, PA, et al: Exfoliative cytology interpretation of synovial fluid in joint disease. *Journal of Bone & Joint Surgery. American Volume* 58:3, 1976.

Carithers, JS, and Koch, BB: Evaluation and management of facial fractures. *American Family Physician* 55:8, 1997.

Chumbley, EM, O'Connor, FG, and Nirschl, RO: Evaluation of overuse elbow injuries. *American Family Physician* 61:3, 2000.

Dillon, PM: *Nursing Health Assessment—A Critical Thinking, Case Studies Approach.* FA Davis, Philadelphia, 2003.

Gibbons, WJ, et al: Subclinical cardiac dysfunction in sarcoidosis. *Chest* 100:44–50, 1991.

Grottkau, B: Top 5 orthopedic referrals from the PCP: An orthopedist's perspective. PRIMED East 2007. *Current Clinical Issues in Primary Care*, October 13, 2007.

Gutierrez, G: Management of radial head fracture. *American Family Physician*, May 1997.

Haasbeek, JF: Adolescent idiopathic scoliosis. *Postgraduate Medicine* 101:6, 1997.

Isasi, C, et al: Successful treatment of optic neuropathy on osteitis deformans. *Rheumatology* 41:8, 2002.

Jarvis, C: *Physical Examination and Health Assessment*, ed 4. WB Saunders, Philadelphia, 2004.

Jones, AK: Primary care management of acute low back pain. *Nurse Practitioner* 22:7, 1997.

National Osteoporosis Foundation: NOF Guidelines for BMD Testing, 2007. http://www.NOF.org, accessed 3/15/07.

Plank, LM, and Dunphy, LM: Musculoskeletal problems. In Dunphy, LM, and Winland-Brown, JE: *Primary Care: The Art and Science of Advanced Practice Nursing*, ed 2. FA Davis, Philadelphia, 2007.

Sass, P, and Hassan, G: Lower extremity abnormalities in children. *American Family Physician* 68:3, 2007.

Schlesinger, N, et al: Colchicine for acute gout. *Cochrane Database of Systematic Reviews* 4:CD006190.

Schneider, D, Hofmann, M, and Peterson, J: Diagnosis and treatment of Paget's disease of bone. *American Family Physician* 65:10, 2002.

Thompson, C, Kelsberg, G, and St. Anna, L: Heat or ice for acute ankle sprain? *Journal of Family Practice* 52:642–643, August 2003.

Wheeless, CR, Nunley, JA, and Urbaniak, JR (eds): *Wheeless' Textbook of Orthopaedics*. Data Trace Publishing, Brooklandville, MD, 2007.

Zitkus, BS: Sarcoidosis. *American Journal of Nursing* 97:10, 1997.

Zollo, AJ: *Medical Secrets*, ed 2. Hanley & Belfus, Philadelphia, 1997.

How well did you do?

85% and above, congratulations! This score shows application of test-taking principles and adequate content knowledge.

75%–85%, keep working! Review test-taking principles and try again.

65%–75%, hang in there! Spend some time reviewing concepts and test-taking principles and try the test again.

Chapter 17: *Endocrine and Metabolic Problems*

JILL E. WINLAND-BROWN

Questions

17-1 *The thyroid-stimulating hormone (TSH) test measures the*

A. total serum level of thyroxine.

B. serum level of T_3 and T_4.

C. pituitary's response to peripheral levels of thyroid hormone.

D. combined serum levels of T_3 and T_4.

17-2 *Which of the following is a sign of hypothyroidism?*

A. A thyroid bruit

B. Brittle hair

C. Gynecomastia

D. Warm, smooth, moist skin

17-3 *What does a low level of thyroid-stimulating hormone indicate?*

A. Hypothyroidism

B. Myxedema

C. Hyperthyroidism

D. Thyroid nodule

17-4 *When teaching Marcy how to use her new insulin pump, you tell her that she needs to monitor her blood glucose level*

A. at least once a day.

B. only occasionally because glycemic levels are maintained very steadily.

C. at least four times a day.

D. on an as-needed basis when she feels she needs to give herself an extra dose of insulin.

17-5 *Jim, a type 2 diabetic, overheard the nurse practitioner talking to the physician about putting him on "BIDS." He asks what this means. You respond,*

A. "BID (twice a day) sulfonylurea."

B. "Bedtime insulin, daytime sulfonylurea."

C. "Blood indicator daily sulfonylurea."

D. "Baby insulin dose several times daily."

17-6 *Diabetes and coronary artery disease (CAD) have a close interrelationship. Which of the following statements about the relationship between diabetes and CAD is true?*

A. Hyperinsulinemia decreases sympathetic tone and cardiac contractility by increasing plasma catecholamines, epinephrine, and norepinephrine.

B. An increase of glucose causes the distal nephrons of the kidneys to absorb less sodium, resulting in more fluid, expanding the intravascular volume and increasing the blood pressure.

C. Hyperinsulinemia causes a large number of vascular smooth muscle cells to be formed and deposited on the walls of vessels, eventually decreasing space for blood flow.

D. An increase in glucose stimulates more secretion of epinephrine, thus raising the blood pressure (BP).

17-7 *Morris has had type 1 diabetes for 10 years. Several recent urinalysis reports have shown microalbuminuria. Your next step would be to*

A. order a 24-hour urinalysis.

B. start him on an angiotensin-converting enzyme (ACE) inhibitor.

C. stress the importance of strict blood sugar control.

D. send him to a dietitian because he obviously has not been following his diet.

17-8 *Which of the following statements about primary hyperparathyroidism (PHPT) is true?*

A. PHPT is the most common cause of hypercalcemia.

B. Hypotension is one of the first clinical manifestations.

C. On a DEXA scan, a client with PHPT will have bone cysts as a common finding.

D. The history and physical examination are crucial elements in diagnosing PHPT.

17-9 *The Diabetes Control and Complications Trial recommends intensive management of diabetes for*

A. children younger than age 13.

B. older adults.

C. persons who already have a diagnosis of beginning nephropathy, neuropathy, or retinopathy.

D. individuals with a history of frequent severe hypoglycemia.

17-10 *Which is the only treatment option that is curative for primary hyperparathyroidism (PHPT)?*

A. Type II calcimimetic cinacalcet

B. Hormone therapy

C. Parathyroidectomy

D. Bisphosphonates

17-11 *Marty has pheochromocytoma. You instruct him to*

A. void in small amounts.

B. not exercise for more than 30 minutes at a time.

C. avoid sleeping in the prone position.

D. take steroids.

17-12 *What is the most common cause of chronic hypocalcemia?*

A. Alkalosis

B. Burn trauma

C. Hypoalbuminemia

D. Renal failure

17-13 *Sandy is being treated for chronic hypocalcemia. When her serum calcium level returns to normal, you assess her urinary calcium level and note that it is greater than 250 mg in a 24-hour sample. This indicates that*

A. her vitamin D dosage should be increased.

B. her vitamin D dosage should be decreased.

C. she needs to restrict foods high in calcium.

D. she needs to eat more foods high in calcium.

17-14 *Jeffrey, age 17, has gynecomastia. You should also assess him for*

A. obesity.

B. endocrine abnormalities.

C. testicular cancer.

D. tuberculosis.

17-15 *Which of the following medications can produce gynecomastia?*

A. Cimetidine (Tagamet)

B. Cholesterol-lowering medications

C. Beta blockers

D. Aspirin

17-16 *Kelley has a score of 8 on the Ferriman-Gallivey scale. This is diagnostic for*

A. gynecomastia.

B. hirsutism.

C. adrenal hyperplasia.

D. an ovarian cyst.

17-17 *Polydipsia occurs in diabetes as a result of a high serum glucose level, which*

A. interferes with the release of antidiuretic hormone.

B. has an osmotic effect on fluids and eventually triggers the thirst mechanism for compensation.

C. causes a dry mouth, increasing the client's thirst to the point of drinking compulsively.

D. disrupts fluid and electrolyte imbalance, increasing the thirst mechanism to compensate for fluid loss or gain.

17-18 *The most common cause of hyperthyroidism is*

A. Graves' disease.

B. a toxic uninodular goiter.

C. subacute thyroiditis.

D. a pituitary tumor.

17-19 *Which of the following statements is true about the ophthalmopathy in Graves' disease?*

A. Propranolol (Inderal) initially helps to control symptoms related to ophthalmopathy.

B. Treatment often includes diuretics and ophthalmic prednisone.

C. Radiation or surgical decompression should never be done until the eyes are no longer bulging.

D. Radioactive iodine may be effective.

17-20 *The most common worldwide cause of hypothyroidism is*

A. an autoimmune process.

B. Hashimoto's thyroiditis.

C. iodine deficiency.

D. iatrogenic hypothyroidism.

17-21 *The American Diabetes Association recommends which of the following quarterly blood tests to be performed on all clients with diabetes?*

A. Urine

B. Liver function

C. Glycohemoglobin

D. Serum glucose

17-22 *What percentage of cases of type 2 diabetes is associated with excess body weight?*

A. 20%

B. 40%

C. 60%

D. 80%

17-23 *Nancy, age 52, has been on a sulfonylurea medication for type 2 diabetes, but it is still not under good control. Your next step would be to*

A. stop the sulfonylurea and start metformin (Glumetza).

B. add insulin to the sulfonylurea regimen.

C. add metformin (Glumetza) to the sulfonylurea.

D. increase the dosage of the sulfonylurea.

17-24 *The three P's of diabetes include all of the following except*

A. polyuria.

B. polydipsia.

C. paresthesias.

D. polyphagia.

17-25 *You are counseling your client with diabetes about diet. You know she misunderstands when she tells you that*

A. "I can substitute two Oreo cookies for a fresh pear."

B. "I can have an occasional glass of chardonnay."

C. "I should monitor the amount of carbohydrates I eat at each meal."

D. "As long as I monitor my blood sugar and it's normal, I can eat anything."

17-26 *Peter, age 62, has diabetes and wants to start an exercise program. Which type of exercise would you not recommend?*

A. Swimming

B. Jogging

C. Tennis

D. Dancing

17-27 *Which class of antihypertensive agents is contraindicated for clients with diabetes?*

A. ACE inhibitors

B. Calcium channel blockers

C. Beta blockers

D. Alpha blockers

17-28 *Your diabetic client asks you about Lantus. You tell her that*

A. it may be administered SC at home, or IV in the hospital if need be.

B. the onset of action is 15 minutes.

C. Lantus stays in your system for 24 hours.

D. it can be mixed with any other insulin.

17-29 *Jenny, age 46, has hypertension that has been controlled with hydrochlorothiazide (Hydrodiuril) 50 mg every day for the past 3 years. She is 5 ft 8 in. tall and weighs 220 lb. Her fasting blood sugar (FBS) level is 300 mg/dL, serum cholesterol level is 250 mg/dL, serum potassium level is 3.4 mEq, and she has 4+ glycosuria. Your next course of action would be to*

A. discontinue her hydrochlorothiazide.

B. order a glucose tolerance test (GTT).

C. repeat her FBS test.

D. start insulin therapy.

17-30 *Harriet, age 62, has type 1 diabetes that is well controlled by insulin. Recently, she has been having marital difficulties that have left her emotionally upset. As a result of this stress, it is possible that she will*

A. have an insulin reaction more readily than usual.

B. have an increased blood sugar level.

C. need less daily insulin.

D. need more carbohydrates.

17-31   Jason, age 14, appears with tender discoid breast tissue enlargement (2–3 cm in diameter) beneath the areola. Your next action would be to

A. perform watchful waiting for 1 year.

B. order an ultrasound.

C. obtain laboratory tests.

D. refer Jason to an endocrinologist.

17-32   June stopped breastfeeding 2 years ago. Yesterday, when doing a breast self-examination, she noticed a small amount of yellowish liquid when she squeezed her nipples. She is concerned that this is one of the signs of breast cancer. You tell her,

A. "Let's get a mammogram to be on the safe side."

B. "Let's wait for a month and reassess."

C. "A small amount of breast milk can be expressed from the nipple in many parous women and is not a cause for concern."

D. "We should do an ultrasound."

17-33   Steve, age 42, has never been hypertensive but appears today in the office with a blood pressure of 162/100 mm Hg. He also complains of "attacks" of headache, perspiration, and palpitations with frequent attacks of nausea, pain, weakness, dyspnea, and visual disturbances. He has lost 10 lb over the past 2 months and seems very anxious today. Your next action would be to

A. start him on an antianxiety agent.

B. obtain a 24-hour urine test.

C. start him on a diuretic or beta blocker.

D. recheck his blood pressure in 1 week.

17-34   Leah has had diabetes for many years. When teaching her about foot care, you want to stress

A. that her calluses will protect her from infection.

B. the need to assess the bottom of her feet carefully after walking barefoot.

C. that painless ulceration might occur and feet should be examined with a mirror.

D. that mild pain is to be expected because of neuropathies.

17-35   Early-morning increases in blood glucose concentration that occur with no corresponding hypoglycemia during the night are referred to as

A. the Somogyi phenomenon.

B. insulin shock.

C. diabetic ketoacidosis.

D. the dawn phenomenon.

17-36   After a subtotal thyroidectomy, it is crucial to assess

A. heart tones.

B. for peripheral edema.

C. speaking ability.

D. skin turgor.

17-37   Which of the following serum laboratory findings are found in the client with Cushing's syndrome?

A. Increased cortisol, decreased sodium, and decreased potassium levels

B. Decreased cortisol, decreased potassium, and decreased glucose levels

C. Increased cortisol, increased sodium, and decreased potassium levels

D. Normal blood urea nitrogen, increased sodium, and decreased potassium levels

17-38   Joan has severe asthma and has been on high doses of oral corticosteroids for 2 years. She has been reading some home remedy books and stops all of her medications. What condition may she develop?

A. Myxedema crisis

B. Diabetes insipidus

C. Hypoparathyroidism

D. Addisonian crisis

17-39   Sara has diabetes and is now experiencing anhidrosis on the hands and feet, increased sweating on the face and trunk, dysphagia, anorexia, and heartburn. Which complication of diabetes do you suspect?

A. Macrocirculation changes

B. Microcirculation changes

C. Somatic neuropathies

D. Visceral neuropathies

17-40 *Pathological changes that occur with diabetic neuropathies include*

A. a thinning of the walls of the blood vessels that supply nerves.

B. the formation and accumulation of amino glycosol within the Schwann cells, which impairs nerve conduction.

C. demyelinization of the Schwann cells, which results in slowed nerve conduction.

D. increase of nutrients clogging the vessels that supply nerve endings.

17-41 *Clients with diabetes are more prone to cardiovascular disease than those without diabetes. This is probably because*

A. of their difficulty in metabolizing fats and proteins, the end products of which accumulate in the blood vessels.

B. they are usually overweight, which increases the workload on the heart and blood vessels.

C. most are older adults, who are more likely to have degenerative cardiovascular disease.

D. the high levels of glucose and fat that occur with poor control result in atherosclerotic changes in the blood vessels.

17-42 *Betty, age 40, has had insulin-dependent diabetes for 20 years and takes a combination of neutral protamine Hagedorn (NPH) and regular insulin every day. She comes to the office because she has developed a severe upper respiratory infection with chills, fever, and production of yellow sputum. Because of her acute infection, you know that Betty is likely to require*

A. a decrease in her daily insulin dosage.

B. an increase in her daily insulin dosage.

C. a high-caloric dietary intake and no insulin change.

D. a change in her insulin from NPH to Lente insulin.

17-43 *Ben, a client with insulin-dependent diabetes, is hospitalized with an admitting diagnosis of diabetic ketoacidosis. Which of the following signs and symptoms would be consistent with this condition?*

A. Hypoglycemia and glycosuria

B. Decreased respiratory rate with shallow respirations

C. Polydipsia and an increased blood pH

D. Ketonuria and polyuria

17-44 *Marie, age 50, has insulin-dependent diabetes mellitus and checks her blood glucose level several times every day. Her blood glucose level ranges from 250–280 mg/dL in the morning and is usually about 140 at lunch, about 120 at dinner, and about 100 at bedtime. In the morning she takes 30 units of neutral protamine Hagedorn (NPH) insulin and 4 units of regular insulin, and before dinner she takes 18 units of NPH insulin and 4 units of regular insulin. Although she has had her insulin dosage adjusted several times in the past month, it has had no effect on her high morning blood glucose level. What is your next course of action?*

A. Increase the evening NPH insulin dosage by 2 more units.

B. Have her check her blood glucose level between 2 a.m. and 4 a.m. for the next several days.

C. Increase the morning regular insulin dosage by 2 units.

D. Order a fasting blood sugar test.

17-45 *ACE inhibitors are given to clients with diabetes who have*

A. an elevated glycohemoglobin level.

B. insulin sensitivity.

C. persistent proteinuria.

D. an elevated serum creatinine level.

17-46 *When you inspect the integumentary system of clients with endocrine disorders, coarse hair may be an indicator of*

A. Addison's disease.

B. diabetes mellitus.

C. Cushing's syndrome.

D. hypothyroidism.

17-47 *Trousseau's sign assesses for*

A. hypocalcemia.

B. hyponatremia.

C. hypercalcemia.

D. hypermagnesemia.

17-48 *Martin, age 62, has acute nontransient abdominal pain that grows steadily worse in the epigastric area and radiates straight through to the back. The pain has lasted for days. He is also complaining of nausea, vomiting, sweating, weakness, and pallor. Physical examination reveals abdominal tenderness and distention and a low-grade fever. What do you suspect?*

A. Cholecystitis

B. Acute pancreatitis

C. Cirrhosis

D. Cushing's syndrome

17-49 *Scott has type 2 diabetes and asks if he needs to do self-monitoring of his blood glucose (SMBG) level. You tell him,*

A. "No, it is indicated only in type 1 diabetes."

B. "Yes, definitely; you should be performing SMBG at least on a daily basis."

C. "You should be doing SMBG at least three times a week."

D. "We'll just test your serum glucose each month and you'll be OK."

17-50 *Your insulin-resistant client is hesitant to begin injection therapy. He asks about Exubera, the inhaled human insulin. Which of the following statements is accurate?*

A. "This would be very appropriate because you're a smoker and you can inhale very well."

B. "You'll need to be on SC insulin for the first month of inhaled insulin while it gets into your system."

C. "It is very convenient with one inhalation after each meal."

D. "We'll need to start with baseline pulmonary function testing."

17-51 *The major risk factor for development of thyroid cancer is*

A. inadequate iodine intake.

B. presence of a goiter.

C. exposure to radiation.

D. smoking.

17-52 *Lynne has Cushing's syndrome. You would expect her to have or develop*

A. onychomycosis.

B. generalized increased pigmentation of the skin.

C. hair loss.

D. excitability and nervousness.

17-53 *Dena said that she read on her husband's hospital chart that he has podagra. She asks what this is. You tell her it is*

A. rheumatoid arthritis.

B. a fungal nail infection.

C. an ingrown toenail.

D. gout.

17-54 *What is the medication of choice for an initial acute attack of gout?*

A. An NSAID

B. Colchicine

C. A corticosteroid

D. Allopurinol (Zyloprim)

17-55 *Joy has gout. In teaching her about her disease, which food do you tell her is allowed on the diet?*

A. Asparagus

B. Beans

C. Broccoli

D. Mushrooms

17-56 *Mandy has type 2 diabetes. She says she heard that if she becomes pregnant, she must go on insulin therapy. How do you respond?*

A. "You're under good glycemic control now with your oral agents. As long as you stay in good control, you'll stay on the medication you are on now."

B. "Don't worry about it now; wait until you get pregnant."

C. "Yes, you should use insulin during your pregnancy. Then, after delivery, we'll try to get you back to your old routine of oral agents."

D. "You need to start on insulin therapy now before you get pregnant. You'll also need it throughout your pregnancy."

17-57 *Eunice, age 32, has type 2 diabetes. She said that she heard that she should take an aspirin a day after she reaches menopause for its cardioprotective action. She* does not have coronary artery disease, but her father does. How do you respond?

A. "You're right. Your hormones protect you against coronary artery diseases until menopause; then you should start on aspirin therapy."

B. "The American Diabetes Association recommends that you start on aspirin therapy now."

C. "Aspirin therapy is recommended only if you have a family history of coronary artery disease."

D. "If you maintain good glycemic control, you don't need aspirin therapy."

17-58 *Jeramiah, age 72, has gout and is obese. When teaching him about diet, which of the following do you tell him?*

A. "Beer and wine are OK because they have no effect on uric acid."

B. "Keeping your weight stable, even if you are a little overweight, is better than fluctuating."

C. "You must go on a very low caloric-restricted diet to effect immediate change."

D. "Fluid intake should exceed 3000 mL daily to prevent formation of uric acid kidney stones."

17-59 *A fetus with intrauterine growth retardation is prone to hypoglycemia at birth because of*

A. an imbalance in insulin-glucagon secretion resulting from hyperinsulinemia from islet cell hyperplasia.

B. few carbon stores in the form of glycogen and body fat.

C. an inborn error of metabolism: glycogen storage disease.

D. a complication of birth asphyxia.

17-60 *Susie has insulin-dependent diabetes mellitus. To forestall hypoglycemia, how much carbohydrate must she eat if she misses a regular meal?*

A. 5–15 g

B. 15–30 g

C. 30–35 g

D. More than 35 g

17-61 *Mindy is scheduled to have an oral glucose tolerance test. For 3 days before the test, she is instructed*

to discontinue many of her medications. Which one is it safe to continue taking?

A. Vitamin C

B. Aspirin

C. Calcium

D. Her oral contraceptive

17-62 *Sandra, who has diabetes, states that she heard that fiber is especially good to include in her diet. How do you respond?*

A. "Fiber is important in all diets."

B. "Too much fiber interferes with insulin, so only include a moderate amount in your diet."

C. "Fiber, especially soluble fiber, helps improve carbohydrate metabolism, so it is more important in the diet of persons with diabetes."

D. "You get just the amount of fiber you need with a normal diet."

17-63 *Sandra has diabetes and frequently develops vaginitis. You instruct her to*

A. wipe from back to front after voiding.

B. wear white nylon underwear.

C. wear pantyhose if wearing tight jeans.

D. avoid douching.

17-64 *Sadie, age 40, has just been given a diagnosis of Graves' disease. She has recently lost 25 lb, has palpitations, is very irritable, feels very warm, and has a noticeable bulge on her neck. The most likely cause of her increased thyroid function is*

A. hyperplasia of the thyroid.

B. an anterior pituitary tumor.

C. a thyroid carcinoma.

D. an autoimmune response.

17-65 *Marisa, age 16, is an active cheerleader who just became insulin dependent. She is worried that she will not fit in with her friends anymore because she does not think she can have all the same snacks they have. How do you respond?*

A. "As long as your snacks are low in fats and carbohydrates, you'll be fine."

B. "Any snacks that are sufficient in calories to maintain your normal weight are OK."

C. "Just be sure that your snacks are high in fats and proteins."

D. "Be sure to stick to snacks that are high in simple carbohydrates."

17-66 *Jay has had insulin-dependent diabetes for 10 years. He recently had a physical and was told he has some evidence of renal nephropathy. What is the first manifestation of this renal dysfunction?*

A. Proteinuria

B. Development of Kimmelstiel-Wilson nodules

C. Decreased blood urea nitrogen levels

D. Increased serum creatine levels

17-67 *Diane has had Cushing's disease for 20 years and has been taking hydrocortisone since then. Today, she appears with a thick trunk and thin extremities. She has a "moon face," a "buffalo hump," thin skin with visible capillaries, and a number of bruises that appear to be slow in healing. To what do you attribute these symptoms?*

A. Decreased adrenal androgen levels

B. Malfunctioning of the adrenal cortex

C. Excessive levels of circulating cortisol

D. Ectopic secretion of adrenocorticotropic hormone

17-68 *How do you explain the fact that someone with Cushing's disease bruises easily?*

A. Decreased skin turgor

B. A loss of neurological sensation

C. Decreased prothrombin levels

D. Protein wasting and collagen loss

17-69 *Sandra has secondary obesity. Which of the following may have caused this?*

A. An intake of more calories than are expended

B. Polycystic ovary disease

C. Her antihypertensive medications

D. Her sedentary lifestyle

17-70 *Which hormone is secreted by the adrenal cortex?*

A. Thyroid-stimulating hormone

B. Growth hormone

C. Follicle-stimulating hormone

D. Aldosterone

17-71 *Morton has type 2 diabetes. His treatment, which includes diet, exercise, and oral antidiabetic agents, is insufficient to achieve acceptable glycemic control. Your next course of action is to*

A. increase the dosage of the oral antidiabetic agents.

B. add a dosage of insulin at bedtime to the regimen.

C. discontinue the oral antidiabetic agents and start insulin therapy.

D. suggest treatment using an insulin pump.

17-72 *Sigrid, age 48, appears with a 3-month history of heat intolerance, increased sweating, palpitations, tachycardia, nervousness, irritability, fatigue, and muscle weakness. Which test would you order first?*

A. A blood chemistry panel

B. Thyroid-stimulating hormone level

C. Liver function studies

D. Electrocardiogram

17-73 *To lower the serum concentration of thyroid hormones and reestablish a eumetabolic state in the client with Graves' disease, which of the following therapies may be used?*

A. Radiation

B. Antithyroid drugs

C. Chemotherapy

D. Parathyroid surgery

17-74 *Which blood test should be obtained before initiating antithyroid drugs for Graves' disease?*

A. Serum electrolytes

B. Liver function studies

C. White blood cell count

D. Complete chemistry profile

17-75 *Marsha, age 24, is preparing for radioactive iodine therapy for her Graves' disease. Which test must she undergo first?*

A. Beta human chorionic gonadotropin

B. Basal metabolism rate

C. Lithium level

D. Serum calcium

17-76 *After establishing clinical and biochemical euthyroidism after a thyroidectomy, you should perform* *a measurement of the serum thyroid-stimulating hormone level every*

A. 3 months.

B. 6 months.

C. 1 year.

D. 2 years.

17-77   *Minnie is pregnant. She has hypothyroidism and has been on the same levothyroxine medication for years. What might you expect to do with her levothyroxine medication?*

A. Increase the dosage.

B. Maintain her established dose.

C. Decrease her dosage.

D. Increase the dose during the first trimester, then decrease it during the second and third trimesters.

17-78   *Alice, age 48, has a benign thyroid nodule. The most common treatment involves*

A. surgery.

B. administration of levothyroxine therapy.

C. watchful waiting with an annual follow-up.

D. radioactive iodine therapy.

17-79   *Henry, age 72, has a fasting blood sugar (FBS) level of 176 mg/dL. He has never been given a diagnosis of diabetes before. Your next step would be to*

A. repeat the FBS.

B. order an oral glucose tolerance test.

C. start him on an oral hypoglycemic agent.

D. order a glycohemoglobin measurement.

17-80   *Sidney has been taking a sulfonylurea for 5 years for his type 2 diabetes. He asks how long he needs to be taking the medication before he tries another medication. You tell him,*

A. "Sulfonylureas are usually effective for 7–10 years in most clients."

B. "You'll probably be on this medication for the rest of your life."

C. "After about 5 years, you will need to start on insulin therapy."

D. "After a few years, you can stop altogether and just regulate your diabetes with your diet."

17-81   *Mark has insulin-dependent type 1 diabetes and has mild hyperglycemia. What effect does physical activity (exercise) have on his blood glucose level?*

A. It may cause it to vary a little.

B. It may decrease it.

C. It may elevate it.

D. It may fluctuate greatly either way.

17-82   *Which of the following statements is true about the insulin lispro?*

A. It works faster than regular insulin because its amino acid composition has been slightly modified.

B. When taken 30 minutes before a meal, it reduces after-meal hyperglycemia.

C. Its duration of action is about 4–5 hours.

D. It is taken with the first bite of food.

17-83   *Jane has insulin-dependent diabetes mellitus and has been experiencing hyperglycemia before dinner. A possible solution to this problem is to*

A. adjust her morning dose of rapid-acting insulin.

B. increase her midafternoon snack.

C. add physical activity between lunch and dinner.

D. reduce the amount of carbohydrate at dinner.

17-84   *Jane, who has insulin-dependent diabetes mellitus, has been hypoglycemic at bedtime. You know she misunderstands your teaching when she tells you,*

A. "I could adjust my insulin dose before dinner."

B. "I could try adding a carbohydrate at dinner."

C. "I could add an afternoon snack."

D. "I could change the time of dinner."

17-85   *Mason, age 52, has diabetes and is overweight. You now find that he is hypertensive. How should you treat his hypertension?*

A. You should treat it the same as in a client without diabetes.

B. Because insulin affects most of the antihypertensive drugs, you should try diet and exercise first before any antihypertensives are ordered.

C. You should treat it very aggressively.

D. Initiate therapy when the blood pressure is 5–10 mm Hg more than the conventional therapeutic guidelines.

17-86 *Which of the following steps will not prevent or slow the progression of diabetic nephropathy?*

A. Control of blood pressure

B. Use of ACE inhibitors

C. Restriction of protein intake

D. Use of calcium channel blockers

17-87 *Older clients with diabetes are predisposed to which of the following types of ear infections?*

A. Simple otitis externa

B. Malignant otitis externa

C. Otitis media

D. Serous otitis media

17-88 *Which of the following is a characteristic of virilization in a woman?*

A. A squeaky voice

B. Decreased muscle mass

C. Clitoral enlargement

D. Excessive hair distribution

17-89 *Which of the following statements regarding osteoporosis and gender is true?*

A. Men and women are equally prone to osteoporosis.

B. Because of menopause, women are more prone to osteoporosis.

C. Men who develop osteoporosis usually have fractures of the wrist and ankle.

D. Women who have had hysterectomies are more prone to developing osteoporosis.

17-90 *Margie has hypoparathyroidism. Which of the following would you assess during your examination?*

A. Skin turgor

B. Heart tones

C. Chvostek's sign

D. Homans' sign

17-91 *Mary, age 72, has been taking insulin for several years. She just called you because she realized that yesterday she put her short-acting insulin in the long-acting insulin box and vice versa. She just took 22 units of regular insulin when she was supposed to take only 5 units. She says that she tried to do a finger-stick to test her glucose level but was unable to obtain*

any blood. She states that she feels fine. What do you tell her to do first?

A. "Keep trying to get a fingerstick and call me back with the results."

B. "Call 911 before you collapse."

C. "Drive immediately to the ER."

D. "Drink 4 oz of fruit juice."

17-92 *Pancreatic juice carries all of the following digestive enzymes except*

A. pancreatic amylase.

B. pancreatic lipase.

C. pancreatic protease.

D. pancreatic trypsin.

17-93 *The process of aging results in*

A. an increase in liver weight and mass.

B. a decreased absorption of fat-soluble vitamins.

C. an increase in enzyme activity.

D. constricted pancreatic ducts.

17-94 *After an oral cholecystogram, Sam complains of burning on urination. This is because of*

A. a mild reaction to the contrast medium.

B. biliary obstruction.

C. contraction of the gallbladder.

D. the presence of dye in the urine.

17-95 *How long after the acute illness of hepatitis A do immunoglobulin M anti–hepatitis A virus titers disappear?*

A. 1 week

B. 3–6 months

C. 1 year

D. 2 years

17-96 *If a client has hepatitis, abdominal pain in the right upper quadrant is a result of what pathophysiological basis?*

A. Reduced prothrombin synthesis by injured hepatic cells

B. Bile salt accumulation

C. Release of pyrogens

D. Stretching of Glisson's capsule

17-97 *You suspect myxedema in your client because she exhibits*

A. smooth, moist skin.

B. pitting edema.

C. abnormal deposits of mucin in the skin.

D. abdominal bloating.

17-98 *Which of the following antithyroid drugs blocks thyroid hormone production and release?*

A. Propylthiouracil

B. Methimazole (Tapazole)

C. Saturated solution of potassium iodide

D. Radioactive iodine (^{131}I)

17-99 *You suspect that Sharon has hypoparathyroidism because, in addition to her other signs and symptoms, she has*

A. elevated serum phosphate levels.

B. elevated serum calcium levels.

C. decreased neuromuscular irritability.

D. increased bone resorption, as implied by her bone density test.

17-100 *Dan, age 45, is obese and has type 2 diabetes and has been having trouble getting his glycohemoglobin under control. He's heard that Exenatide (Byetta) causes weight loss and wants to try it. What do you tell him?*

A. "Let's adjust your oral antidiabetic agents instead."

B. "That's a myth. People usually change their eating habits when taking this and that's what causes the weight loss."

C. "With type 2 diabetes, you never want to be on injectable insulin."

D. "Let's try it. You're glycohemoglobin will be lowered and you'll lose weight."

17-101 *If a thyroid gland is palpable and you listen over the thyroid gland with the bell of the stethoscope while the client is holding his/her breath, what are you are listening for?*

A. A bruit, which may indicate increased vascularity of hyperthyroidism

B. Absence of sound, which may indicate a thyroid nodule

C. An echo from surrounding vessels indicating high blood pressure

D. A "thrill" indicating increased vascularity

17-102 *Presence of Trousseau's sign is often preceded by*

A. a spasm of the facial muscle.

B. muscle cramps in the legs and feet.

C. abdominal pain.

D. headache.

17-103 *Judy has the visiting nurse prefill her insulin syringes because of her visual and dexterity difficulties. On Judy's routine visit for her blood work, she asks you about storing these prefilled syringes. How do you respond?*

A. "Keep them at room temperature with the needle angled down, just like you do with a bottle of wine."

B. "They can be kept in the refrigerator for 1 week when the visiting nurse should fill new ones."

C. "They can be stored in a vertical position in the refrigerator for 30 days with the needle pointing upward."

D. "They should be placed in the refrigerator without the needles on—those should be added just prior to administration."

17-104 *Diabetic clients with neuropathy require special foot care because most ulcers begin at the site of*

A. an ingrown toenail.

B. a previous sore.

C. a mole.

D. a callus.

17-105 *Why is there an increased parathyroid hormone secreted during pregnancy?*

A. To meet the increased stress demands on the mother

B. To meet the increased requirements for calcium and vitamin D for fetal skeletal growth

C. To help prevent neural tube defects in the fetus

D. To help promote neurological growth of the developing brain in the fetus

17-106 *Which of the following hormones is secreted by the posterior pituitary gland?*

A. Antidiuretic hormone (ADH)

B. Thyroid-stimulating hormone (TSH)

C. Adrenocorticotropic hormone (ACTH)

D. Growth hormone (GH)

Answers

17-1 Answer C

The thyroid-stimulating hormone (TSH) test measures the pituitary's response to peripheral levels of thyroid hormone. If the circulating level of T_4 is low, the pituitary will increase the production of TSH to try to stimulate the thyroid gland to produce more thyroid hormone.

17-2 Answer B

Brittle hair is a sign of hypothyroidism. A thyroid bruit; gynecomastia; and warm, smooth, moist skin are all signs of hyperthyroidism.

17-3 Answer C

A low level of thyroid-stimulating hormone (TSH) indicates hyperthyroidism. Hyperthyroidism is an excess of circulating thyroid hormones, which will suppress the level of TSH produced by the pituitary. The TSH would be increased in primary hypothyroidism. In myxedema, there would be a deficiency of thyroxine. Most thyroid nodules secrete thyroid hormone, so levels of thyroid hormones would be elevated.

17-4 Answer C

Clients using an insulin pump need to monitor their blood glucose levels at least four times a day. The client can develop diabetic ketoacidosis in as little as 4 hours if there is mechanical failure of the pump because the only insulin used in the pump is rapid acting.

17-5 Answer B

BIDS refers to bedtime insulin, daytime sulfonylurea. It is a form of therapy in which a sulfonylurea medication is taken in the morning and insulin is taken at bedtime. The bedtime insulin suppresses hepatic glucose output and controls the blood glucose levels overnight, allowing the beta cells to recuperate so that they will function more effectively in the morning. The sulfonylurea stimulates the insulin secretion of the pancreas in response to eating, thus giving an extra jolt to diabetes control. This combination therapy has been shown to reduce hyperglycemia and the dosage of insulin required.

17-6 Answer C

There is a major link between diabetes mellitus and coronary artery disease (CAD). There are many theories about the pathophysiology of diabetes mellitus and how it leads to CAD. Some of these mechanisms include the following: Hyperinsulinemia causes a large number of vascular smooth muscle cells to be formed and deposited on the walls of vessels, causing buildup and eventual blockage, reducing blood flow; hyperinsulinemia increases (not decreases) sympathetic tone and cardiac contractility by increasing plasma catecholamine, epinephrine, and norepinephrine levels; and an increase in the glucose level causes the distal nephrons of the kidneys to absorb more (not less) sodium, resulting in more fluid, expanding the intravascular volume and increasing blood pressure.

17-7 Answer B

Morris should be started on an ACE inhibitor such as captopril (Capoten) or enalapril (Vasotec). ACE inhibitors have renoprotective effects by reducing the intraglomerular pressure. They do this by inhibiting the renin-angiotensin system, which causes efferent dilation, and by improving glomerular permeability, which causes a reduction of glomerulosclerosis. ACE inhibitors have this beneficial effect on clients with diabetes who are normotensive and hypotensive. Diabetic nephropathy is the leading cause of end-stage renal disease in the United States. Monitoring for microalbuminuria is a method for identifying early nephropathy. Ordering a 24-hour urinalysis will not give you any additional information. You do want to stress tight glycemic control and possibly send Morris to a dietitian, but he needs to be started on an ACE inhibitor now because he is already exhibiting microalbuminuria.

17-8 Answer A

In an outpatient setting, primary hyperparathyroidism is the most common cause of hypercalcemia. Some of the clinical manifestations include hypertension, left ventricular hypertrophy, peptic ulcer disease, pancreatitis, fatigue, and anxiety. A dual-energy x-ray absorptiometry (DEXA) scan is required to detect skeletal involvement in mild PHPT. Bone cysts and subperiosteal resorption are no longer common findings, but bone loss is usually found in varying degrees. The client's history and physical examination are not usually helpful in diagnosing this condition. Persistent hypercalcemia and an elevated parathyroid hormone (PTH) level are necessary for a diagnosis of PHPT.

17-9   Answer C

The Diabetes Control and Complications Trial recommends intensive management of diabetes for persons who already have a diagnosis of beginning nephropathy, neuropathy, or retinopathy. Intensive management of diabetes is recommended for clients with diabetes to prevent or reduce the risk for developing retinopathy, nephropathy, or neuropathy. Having one of these conditions does not preclude therapy. Intensive therapy may slow the progression of the disease if already present. However, because the most significant adverse effect of intensive treatment is an increase in the risk of severe hypoglycemic episodes, intensive therapy is not recommended for children younger than age 13; older adults; or people with heart disease, advanced complications, or a history of frequent severe hypoglycemia.

17-10   Answer C

The only treatment option that is curative for PHPT is a parathyroidectomy. It is successful in 90%–98% of the cases. The type II calcimimetic cinacalcet treats the underlying cause of PHPT by binding to the calcium-sensing receptor on the surface of the parathyroid glands, which increases the sensitivity to extracellular calcium, which then reduces the excess secretion of PTH. It is used for the treatment of secondary hyperparathyroidism but not for PHPT. Although the first generation of bisphosphonates was found to be not effective for the treatment of the skeletal manifestations of PHPT, the newer bisphosphonates such as alendronate (Fosamax) increase the bone density a little, but they don't affect PTH secretion and thus will not reduce serum calcium. Hormone therapy is not used by itself. Low doses of estrogen have been shown to reduce calcium, prevent bone loss, and improve bone density.

17-11   Answer A

Clients with pheochromocytoma should be told to void in small amounts and to avoid a full bladder. In addition, to prevent stimulating a paroxysm in pheochromocytoma, also advise the client to avoid smoking; drugs that may influence catecholamine release, such as histamines, some anesthetics, atropine, opiates, steroids, and glucagon; and activities that might displace abdominal organs, such as bending, exercising, straining, and vigorous palpation of the abdomen. For women, pregnancy should be discouraged.

17-12   Answer C

The most common cause of chronic hypocalcemia is hypoalbuminemia. Other causes of hypocalcemia include vitamin D deficiency, alkalosis, hypoparathyroidism, malabsorption syndromes, pancreatitis, laxative abuse, peritonitis, pregnancy, renal failure, phosphate excess, burn trauma, osteomalacia, and overwhelming infections.

17-13   Answer B

When serum calcium levels return to normal, urinary calcium should be assessed. Hypercalciuria (greater than 250 mg in a 24-hour urine sample) indicates that the client's vitamin D dosage should be decreased. Once the dosages of calcium and vitamin D are regulated to achieve normal serum calcium levels, urinary calcium levels should be assessed every 3 months.

17-14   Answer C

Gynecomastia may be the first sign of testicular cancer. It is also associated with breast, adrenal, pituitary, lung, and hepatic malignancies. Hypogonadism produces low testosterone levels in men with normal estrogen levels. Alteration in breast tissue responsiveness to hormonal activity can result in gynecomastia. Gynecomastia can occur secondary to cirrhosis, chronic obstructive lung disease, malnutrition, hyperthyroidism and other endocrine imbalances, tuberculosis, and chronic renal disease.

17-15   Answer A

Medications such as cimetidine (Tagamet), digoxin (Lanoxin), spironolactone (Aldactone), phenothiazines, antituberculosis agents, as well as marijuana, heroin, and alcohol can produce gynecomastia. In addition, men receiving estrogen therapy for the treatment of prostate cancer are likely to experience gynecomastia.

17-16   Answer B

The Ferriman-Gallivey scale has been used to define and grade hirsutism. The clinician evaluates hair growth in nine androgen-sensitive hair-growth areas. No hair growth is indicated by 0, and 4 is designated for frank virile hair growth. A score of 8 is diagnostic for hirsutism.

17-17   Answer B

Polydipsia occurs in diabetes as a result of high serum glucose levels that have an osmotic effect on fluids, drawing fluid from the cells into the intravascular space and creating a dehydrated state that, in turn, triggers the thirst mechanism for compensation. With a deficiency of antidiuretic hormone, as in diabetes insipidus, copious amounts of urine are excreted by the client, stimulating the thirst mechanism to replace fluid losses. Certain drugs such as phenothiazines and anticholinergics can cause dry mouth, increasing the client's thirst to the point of drinking compulsively. Excessive ingestion of salt, glucose, and other hyperosmolar substances can disrupt fluid and electrolyte imbalance, increasing the thirst mechanism to compensate for fluid loss or gain.

17-18   Answer A

The most common cause of hyperthyroidism is an autoimmune condition known as Graves' disease. It accounts for 90% of hyperthyroid conditions in young adults. Graves' disease is a result of a diffuse toxic goiter. A toxic uninodular goiter is the second most common cause of hyperthyroidism. Other causes include toxic hyperfunctioning multinodular goiter, subacute thyroiditis, metastatic follicular thyroid carcinoma, ingestion of iodide-containing drugs and contrast media, a pituitary tumor, a human chorionic gonadotropin-secreting tumor, and a testicular embryonal carcinoma.

17-19   Answer B

Treatment for ophthalmopathy in Graves' disease often includes diuretics and ophthalmic prednisone drops; severe cases may require radiation or surgical decompression. Propranolol (Inderal) is usually given initially to control symptoms of tachycardia, palpitations, or tremors during the initiation of radioactive iodine therapy. It is not used to help control symptoms related to ophthalmopathy in Graves' disease. Radioactive iodine may worsen the ophthalmopathy in Graves' disease. Clients with ophthalmopathy require a referral to an ophthalmologist.

17-20   Answer C

Iodine deficiency is the most common worldwide cause of hypothyroidism. In the United States, where iodine ingestion is adequate, autoimmune processes are the primary cause of hypothyroidism. Hashimoto's thyroiditis, a type of primary hypothyroidism, is the most common form of autoimmune thyroid disease. Iatrogenic hypothyroidism, which occurs after treatment with radioactive iodine for hyperthyroidism or surgery for hyperthyroidism, thyroid nodules, or carcinoma, is the next most common cause of hypothyroidism.

17-21   Answer C

Although a serum glucose test is an excellent test for clients with diabetes, it reports only the serum glucose of that day. The American Diabetes Association (ADA) therefore recommends that the glycohemoglobin (Hemoglobin A_{1C}) test be performed quarterly because it reports the serum glucose concentration of the previous 3 months. The ADA also recommends an annual urine test to assess for urine protein that might indicate an early sign of kidney damage. Liver function studies should be done on an annual basis as part of a routine examination.

17-22   Answer D

Eighty percent of cases of type 2 diabetes are associated with excess body weight. Although heredity is an important consideration, a normal-weight client with two parents who have diabetes has a better chance of avoiding the disease than an overweight client with healthy parents.

17-23   Answer C

The first line of therapy for a client with type 2 diabetes is usually a sulfonylurea medication, which lowers blood sugar levels by prompting the pancreas to pump out more insulin. If the sulfonylurea fails to control the blood sugar, metformin (Glumetza, Glucophage) is added to the regimen to reduce the amount of glucose the liver releases into the blood. Once clients have failed on either metformin or other oral agents, Exenatide (Byetta), an incretin mimetic, should be initiated.

17-24   Answer C

Although paresthesias (tingling or numbness in the hands or feet) may be one of the warning signs of diabetes, the classic symptoms remain the three polys—polyuria, polydipsia, and polyphagia.

17-25   Answer D

Although the diabetic diet has "relaxed" over the years, it is still not possible to eat everything. It is acceptable to substitute two Oreo cookies for a fresh pear. In the past, sugar was forbidden to clients with diabetes. The belief was that simple carbohydrates, like candy, were quickly digested, allowing blood sugar to soar, whereas the body took more time to process complex carbohydrates such as bread. Research now shows that both types of carbohydrates—simple and complex—affect glucose levels at comparable speeds. It is still important to monitor the amount of total carbohydrates per meal because they have the greatest impact on blood sugar. Drinking alcohol may increase the risk of low blood sugar, so if your client has an occasional glass of wine, stress the fact that alcohol should not be consumed on an empty stomach.

17-26   Answer B

Jogging is not a wise choice for clients with diabetes because of the potential underlying nerve damage to their feet or eyes. Although tennis is physically taxing, it does not require a constant bouncing up and down on the feet, and even if played at night, courts are well lit. Swimming and dancing are excellent forms of exercise.

17-27   Answer C

Beta blockers should not be used to control hypertension in clients with diabetes because of their blockade of hypoglycemic responses. ACE inhibitors are the first choice for clients with diabetes who have hypertension because they slow the progression of diabetic nephropathy. Calcium channel blockers provide pressure reduction without adverse effects on lipids and glucose control. Alpha-blocking agents provide a smooth control and an improved lipid profile.

17-28   Answer C

Lantus (insulin glargine) has an onset of action in just over 1 hour and stays in your system for 24 hours. Regular insulin is the only insulin that may be administered by the IV route. Lantus may not be mixed with any other insulin.

17-29   Answer C

Jenny's fasting blood sugar (FBS) test should be repeated before you order a glucose tolerance test (GTT) to confirm a diagnosis of diabetes. Diabetes is not diagnosed with a single high glucose reading. Hyperglycemia is an adverse reaction to hydrocholorothiazide, but the first action would be to repeat the FBS. If it is high for a second reading, the diuretic should be changed. A GTT may be ordered to diagnose diabetes mellitus if the second FBS is high. Certainly insulin therapy would not be started until Jenny was given a positive diagnosis, and even then oral hypoglycemic agents would be tried first.

17-30   Answer B

Stress causes the adrenal glands to secrete more cortisol, which leads to gluconeogenesis and insulin antagonism, raising the blood sugar. It is possible then that Harriet will have an increased blood sugar level. She will not need less daily insulin or more carbohydrates and will not have an insulin reaction, such as hypoglycemia, more readily than usual. Harriet may, in fact, need to increase her insulin use.

17-31   Answer A

Pubertal gynecomastia is common and is characterized by tender discoid breast tissue enlargement of about 2–3 cm in diameter beneath the areola. The swelling usually subsides spontaneously within a year, and watchful waiting along with reassurance is recommended for that time period.

17-32   Answer C

Galactorrhea is lactation that occurs in the absence of nursing. A small amount of breast milk can be expressed from the nipple in many parous women and is not of concern. Normal breast milk may vary in color and not always be white. If there are significant amounts, or if galactorrhea occurs in nulliparous women or in conjunction with amenorrhea, headache, or visual field abnormalities, it might imply a systemic illness.

17-33   Answer B

Starting Steve on an antianxiety agent, starting him on a diuretic and/or beta blocker, or rechecking his blood pressure in 1 week will only delay the correct diagnosis. Steve's signs and symptoms are diagnostic of a pheochromocytoma, which can be detected with an assay of urinary catecholamine levels (total and fractionated), metanephrine, vanillylmandelic acid, and creatinine levels. A 24-hour urine specimen is usually obtained, but an overnight or shorter collection may also be obtained. Pheochromocytoma typically causes attacks of severe headache (85%), palpitations (65%), and profuse sweating (65%). The absence of all three of these symptoms can exclude the diagnosis of pheochromocytoma to a 99% certainty.

17-34   Answer C

Painless ulcerations are very common in clients with diabetes, and the only way to assess for them in the feet is for clients to use a mirror to examine the bottoms of their feet. Leah should not be walking barefoot because her sensations are probably decreased as a result of neuropathy, and she should try to avoid the development of calluses because preparations used to remove them are very caustic.

17-35   Answer D

The dawn phenomenon is an early-morning increase in blood glucose concentration occurring with no corresponding hypoglycemia during the night. It is secondary to the nocturnal elevations of growth hormone. The Somogyi phenomenon is a rebound effect caused by too much insulin at night, resulting in hypoglycemia during the night. This results in the secretion of certain anti-insulin hormones, including epinephrine, glucagon, glucocorticoids, and growth hormones, which results in hyperglycemia. Insulin shock is a hypoglycemic reaction. Diabetic ketoacidosis implies that there is hyperglycemia at all times during the day, not only in the early morning.

17-36   Answer C

Laryngeal nerve damage is a potential danger after a subtotal thyroidectomy. You should assess the client's speaking ability, including the ability to speak aloud, along with the quality and tone of the voice. The location of the laryngeal nerve increases the risk of damage during thyroid surgery. Hoarseness may be present because of edema or the endotracheal tube during surgery and will subside, but permanent hoarseness or loss of vocal volume is a sign of laryngeal nerve damage.

17-37   Answer C

Serum laboratory findings in the client with Cushing's syndrome usually include increased cortisol, increased sodium, decreased potassium, decreased glucose, and normal blood urea nitrogen levels.

17-38   Answer D

Addisonian crisis is a serious, life-threatening response to acute adrenal insufficiency and may be precipitated by abruptly stopping glucocorticoid medications. Other causes include major stressors, especially if the person has poorly controlled Addison's disease, and hemorrhage into the adrenal glands from either septicemia or anticoagulant therapy. The primary problems in Addisonian crisis are severe hypotension, circulatory collapse, shock, and coma. Treatment involves rapid intravenous replacement of fluids and glucocorticoids.

17-39   Answer D

Visceral neuropathies include anhidrosis (absence of sweating) on the hands and feet, increased sweating on the face or trunk, dysphagia, anorexia, heartburn, constricted pupils, nausea and vomiting, constipation, and diabetic diarrhea. Macrocirculation changes include an early onset of atherosclerosis and peripheral vascular insufficiency with claudication, ulcerations, and gangrene of the legs. Microcirculation changes include diabetic retinopathy with retinal ischemia and loss of vision and diabetic nephropathy with hypertension, albuminuria, edema, and progressive renal failure. Somatic neuropathies include changes in sensation in the feet and hands; palsy of cranial nerve III with headache, eye pain, and inability to move the eye up, down, or to the middle; pain or loss of cutaneous sensation over the chest; and motor and sensory deficits in the anterior thigh and medial calf.

17-40   Answer C

Diabetic neuropathies involve three pathological changes: a thickening of the walls of the blood vessels that supply nerves, which causes a decrease in nutrients; the formation and accumulation of sorbitol within the Schwann cells, which impairs nerve conduction; and demyelinization of the Schwann cells that surround and insulate nerves, which results in slowed nerve conduction. The locations of the lesions determine where the neuropathies occur.

17-41   Answer D

Clients with diabetes are more prone to cardiovascular disease than those without diabetes. The most likely reason for this is that the high levels of glucose and fat that occur with poor control result in atherosclerotic changes in the blood vessels. The client with diabetes may also be overweight, but that is not the primary contributing factor to the development of cardiovascular disease. Diabetes is associated with a greater incidence of high blood lipid levels, high blood pressure, and obesity, all of which are risk factors for cardiovascular disease. Diabetes affects both small and large blood vessels, which contributes to the process of atherosclerosis. In women, diabetes negates the protective effects of estrogen. The amount of protein in the diet of a client with diabetes is restricted to help prevent or delay renal complications, not cardiovascular ones. The reason why clients with diabetes, especially older adults, are more prone to cardiovascular disease than those without diabetes is the high levels of glucose and fat, which result in atherosclerotic changes in the blood vessels.

17-42   Answer B

For insulin-dependent clients with diabetes, an increase in their daily insulin dosage is usually required in the presence of an acute infection. Betty should begin by increasing her regular insulin dosage by just two units and then monitor her blood sugar level.

17-43   Answer D

Signs and symptoms of diabetic ketoacidosis include Kussmaul's breathing (very deep respiratory movements), hyperglycemia, glycosuria, polyuria, polydipsia, anorexia, and headache, as well as ketonuria and a decreased blood pH.

17-44   Answer B

Marie is experiencing the Somogyi phenomenon (nocturnal rebound hyperglycemia). If her blood glucose level at 2 a.m. to 4 a.m. is greater than 70 mg/dL, the evening dosage of neutral protamine Hagedorn insulin should be increased and changed from before dinner to before bedtime. These actions should prevent most cases of nocturnal rebound hypoglycemia, which results in morning hyperglycemia. A fasting blood sugar test will not confirm the Somogyi phenomenon. The blood sugar level needs to be checked during the night to "catch" the Somogyi phenomenon.

17-45   Answer C

ACE inhibitors are given to clients with diabetes who have persistent proteinuria. When diabetes is diagnosed, it may have been present for 10 years. Most clinicians will order an ACE inhibitor for clients with diabetes even without hypertension due to the renoprotective mechanism. Proteinuria is one of the early signs of diabetic nephropathy, with or without the presence of hypertension. Urine protein must be measured to monitor the effectiveness of the ACE inhibitor. ACE inhibitors may be effective in decreasing urinary excretion of albumin even in clients without hypertension; therefore, a urinalysis should be performed and a serum creatinine level determined at least yearly. Detection of microalbuminuria alerts one that nephropathy is developing. When the serum creatinine level reaches about 3 mg/dL, a referral to a diabetologist and nephrologist should be done. Intensive treatment can delay or improve diabetic nephropathy in its early stages. There is evidence that, with good control of hypertension, proteinuria can be reduced and the expected decline in the glomerular filtration rate can be slowed.

17-46   Answer D

During inspection of the integumentary system of clients with endocrine disorders, coarse hair may be an indicator of hypothyroidism. Fine hair is seen in clients with hyperthyroidism; hirsutism with Cushing's syndrome; hyperpigmentation with Addison's disease or Cushing's syndrome; hypopigmentation with diabetes mellitus, hyperthyroidism, or hypothyroidism; and purple striae over the abdomen and bruising with Cushing's syndrome.

17-47   Answer A

Trousseau's sign assesses for hypocalcemia. It is assessed by inflating a blood pressure cuff above the client's antecubital space to occlude the blood supply to the arm, then deflating it. Decreased calcium levels (hypocalcemia/tetany) cause the client's hand and fingers to contract in a carpal spasm. Hypocalcemia may also be assessed by checking for Chvostek's sign, which is performed by tapping fingers in front of the client's ear at the angle of the jaw. If hypocalcemia is present, the client's lateral facial muscle will contract.

17-48   Answer B

Acute pancreatitis is an inflammation of the pancreas caused by the release of activated pancreatic enzymes into the surrounding parenchyma with the subsequent destruction of tissue, blood vessels, and supporting structures. Although pancreatitis may be acute or chronic, acute symptoms include continuous abdominal pain for several days' duration that increases in the epigastric area and radiates to the back, nausea, vomiting, sweating, weakness, pallor, abdominal tenderness, distention, and a low-grade fever. Pancreatitis occurs primarily in middle-aged adults and slightly more often in women than in men. The pain is in the upper right quadrant with cholecystitis and is intermittent, usually after a fatty meal. The gastrointestinal (GI) manifestations of cirrhosis include parotid enlargement, esophageal or rectal varices, peptic ulcers, and gastritis. The clinical manifestation of Cushing's syndrome related to the GI system is a peptic ulcer, which would result in intermittent pain related to meals.

17-49 Answer C

Although it is generally accepted that self-monitoring of blood glucose (SMBG) is a necessary component of the management of type 1 diabetes, its use in type 2 diabetes is controversial. Although individuals with type 2 diabetes may be treated with diet, oral agents, insulin, or combination therapy, the frequency of SMBG depends on the particular therapeutic interventions. The minimum recommended frequency is three times a week at selected intervals. The frequency obviously depends on the client's success in achieving treatment goals.

17-50 Answer D

Baseline pulmonary function testing needs to be done initially and then at 6 months. Inhaled insulin is available in 1- and 3-mg packets. It is dosed before meals and should not be used in anyone who smokes or who has given up smoking in the previous 6 months. It is contraindicated in anyone with active lung disease. It may be used in someone who is hesitant to begin injection therapy and can be used alone. The 1-mg blister pack is the equivalent of three units of rapid-acting SC insulin and the 3-mg pack is equivalent to eight units.

17-51 Answer C

The major risk factor for development of thyroid cancer is exposure to radiation, usually from treatment to the head and neck. Until 1950, radiation treatments were given to children for an enlarged thymus, enlarged tonsils, and acne. Several million children were exposed in this manner. It may also occur in individuals who have had radiation therapy to the face or upper chest. There is also an increased incidence of thyroid cancer in areas where iodine deficiency and goiter are more common.

Cigarette smoking is a risk factor for bladder and lung cancer but not thyroid cancer.

17-52 Answer A

Cushing's syndrome results in an excessive amount of adrenocorticotropic hormone, which stimulates the secretion of glucocorticoids, mineralocorticoids, and androgenic steroids from the adrenal cortex. In the presence of excessive cortisol, fungal infections of the skin, nails, and oral mucosa, such as onychomycosis and tinea versicolor, are common and, in addition, skin wounds heal very slowly. Other symptoms include fatigue and weakness and excessive hair growth. Addison's disease, which is a deficiency in the secretion of adrenocortical hormones, usually results in an increased pigmentation of the entire skin.

17-53 Answer D

Podagra is gout of the first metatarsophalangeal joint, the joint most frequently affected in the initial attack. Podagra is experienced by 90% of clients with gout. An acute attack of gout is usually monoarticular (affecting only one joint). Subsequent attacks may progress to include several joints (polyarticular).

17-54 Answer A

The medication of choice for an initial acute attack of gout is an NSAID. Indomethacin (Indocin) is the most commonly prescribed NSAID for this use. An initial dose of 50–75 mg is given, followed by 25–50 mg every 8 hours for 5–10 days. An alternative to indomethacin is naproxen (Naprosyn). The first dose of naproxen is 750 mg, followed by 250 mg every 8 hours for 5–10 days. Colchicine is an effective medication to terminate an acute attack only if administered within 48 hours of the initial onset of symptoms. Unfortunately, the attack is usually not diagnosed within this time frame. Corticosteroids can provide dramatic systematic relief but are contraindicated in septic conditions; therefore, they should not be administered before analysis of the synovial aspirate. Allopurinol (Zyloprim) is used to decrease uric acid production. Although it is effective, it may take weeks to decrease the uric acid level and therefore is not the initial choice in an acute attack.

17-55 Answer C

Foods high in purine should be avoided by clients with gout. Broccoli is not high in purine. Foods high in purine include all meats and seafood, meat extracts and gravies, yeast and yeast extracts, beans, peas, lentils, oatmeal, spinach, asparagus, cauliflower, and mushrooms. Wine and alcohol in excessive amounts impair the kidney's ability to excrete uric acid and should be used in moderation.

17-56   Answer C

Women with type 2 diabetes need to use insulin during their pregnancy to maintain good glycemic control. It would be ideal, although unrealistic, to put all women with type 2 diabetes who are thinking of conceiving on insulin. There is a risk of having a malformed infant if conception occurs when the blood sugar is not well controlled. Insulin is used, rather than oral antidiabetic medications, to achieve good glycemic control because the effects of most of the oral antidiabetic preparations on the human embryo and fetus are not well known. Many clients do not require antidiabetic therapy for the first several weeks after delivery, and most women can return to their preconception regimen within 6–12 weeks. Sulfonylureas and ACE inhibitors may be transferred to the fetus via breast milk, so they should not be resumed until breastfeeding is discontinued.

17-57   Answer B

The American Diabetes Association position statement on aspirin therapy in diabetes recommends aspirin use as a secondary prevention strategy in men and women with diabetes who have evidence of large-vessel disease, such as a history of myocardial infarction, vascular bypass procedures, and stroke. They also recommend aspirin therapy as a primary prevention strategy in high-risk men and women with type 1 or type 2 diabetes who have a family history of coronary heart disease and for individuals who smoke, are hypertensive or obese, or who have albuminuria, cholesterol levels greater than 200 mg/dL, low-density lipoprotein cholesterol levels greater than 130 mg/dL, high-density lipoprotein cholesterol levels less than 40 mg/dL, and triglyceride levels greater than 250 mg/dL.

17-58   Answer D

Fluid intake should exceed 3000 mL daily to prevent formation of uric acid kidney stones. Clients should avoid dehydration because it may precipitate an acute attack. Because both wine and alcohol in excessive amounts impair the kidney's ability to

excrete uric acid, they should be used in moderation. Clients must be aware that binge drinking may provoke an acute attack. If the client is obese, weight loss should be encouraged because loss of excess body fat may normalize serum uric acid without pharmacological intervention. Weight loss will also decrease stress on weight-bearing joints. Caution as to severe, rapid weight loss should be given because secondary hyperuricemia may result. A very low caloric-restricted diet may precipitate an acute attack.

17-59   Answer B

The fetus with intrauterine growth retardation has very scant carbon stores in the form of glycogen and body fat and is prone to hypoglycemia even with appropriate endocrine adjustments at birth. In addition, an infant whose mother has diabetes (and had no problem with intrauterine growth retardation) has abundant glucose stores in the form of glycogen and fat and also develops hypoglycemia because of an imbalance in insulin-glucagon secretion resulting from hyperinsulinemia caused by islet cell hyperplasia. Other causes of hypoglycemia are associated with islet cell hyperplasia, inborn errors of metabolism such as glycogen storage disease and galactosemia, and as a complication of birth, asphyxia, hypoxia secondary to cardiorespiratory disease, or other stresses such as bacterial and viral sepsis.

17-60   Answer B

A client with insulin-dependent diabetes mellitus who misses a meal needs to eat about 15–30 g of complex carbohydrates to forestall hypoglycemia. If the client's appetite is poor, this may be accomplished through juice, flavored gelatin, soft drinks, or frozen juice bars.

17-61   Answer C

Calcium does not affect an oral glucose tolerance test (OGTT). The following medications may interfere with the results of an OGTT and should be discontinued for 3 days before the test: vitamin C, aspirin, oral contraceptives, corticosteroids, synthetic estrogens, phenytoin (Dilantin), thiazide diuretics, and nicotinic acid.

17-62   Answer C

Fiber is important in the dietary management of diabetes. A diet high in fiber, especially soluble fiber, helps improve carbohydrate metabolism, lowers total cholesterol level, and lowers low-density lipoprotein cholesterol. Soluble fiber is found in dried beans, oats, barley, and in some vegetables and fruits (peas, corn, zucchini, cauliflower, broccoli, prunes, pears, apples, bananas, and oranges). It should not be assumed that individuals will get enough fiber in their diet because most dietary habits are not perfect. An intake of 20–30 g of fiber per day is recommended.

17-63   Answer D

Women who have diabetes and frequently develop vaginitis should avoid douching. They should also maintain good personal hygiene, wipe from front to back after voiding, wear cotton underwear, avoid wearing tight jeans with nylon pantyhose, and void after intercourse.

17-64   Answer D

The cause of Graves' disease is an autoimmune response wherein the body produces antibodies that act against its own organs and tissues. Thyroid-stimulating immunoglobulins are found in 95% of persons with Graves' disease and are evidence of this autoimmune process. Although thyroid carcinoma and pituitary tumors can cause hyperthyroidism, they do not cause Graves' disease. Hyperplasia of the thyroid results from hyperthyroidism; it does not cause it.

17-65   Answer B

Marisa can have snacks that are sufficient in calories to maintain her normal weight. She should consume adequate amounts of carbohydrates, fats, and proteins in a well-balanced diet. The majority of the fats should be unsaturated to decrease the incidence of vascular changes. The carbohydrates should be complex rather than simple to provide a more constant blood glucose level. She can still go out with her friends and consume most of the same snacks. Pizza, hamburgers, and many other "fast foods" are on the American Diabetes Association diet.

17-66   Answer A

Proteinuria is the first symptom indicative of renal nephropathy in clients who have had diabetes for about 10 years (although some studies suggest 5 years). There is increased permeability of the capillaries, with resultant leakage of albumin into the glomerular filtrate, causing albuminuria. The

development of Kimmelstiel-Wilson nodules occurs in persons with type 1 diabetes but does not necessarily precede the proteinuria. As renal function deteriorates, both the serum creatine and the blood urea nitrogen levels increase.

17-67   Answer C

Diane's symptoms today are the result of excessive levels of circulating cortisol. Ordinarily, there is a feedback loop that controls the circulating adrenocorticotropic hormone (ACTH) and cortisol levels. In Cushing's disease, the anterior pituitary is constantly producing excessive ACTH, which increases the levels of both cortisol and adrenal androgens. Her symptoms were precipitated by the administration of pharmaceutical cortisone preparations given in large doses over a long period of time.

17-68   Answer D

When clients have been on long-term cortisol therapy, increased protein breakdown or catabolism leads to loss of adipose and lymphatic tissue. The collagen loss is a result of protein wasting, which causes individuals to bruise easily. The skin is susceptible to rupture because the loss of collagenous support around the vessels makes them vulnerable. The skin becomes thin and atrophic.

17-69   Answer B

Secondary obesity is rare; possible causes include Cushing's disease, polycystic ovary disease, hypothalamic disease, hypothyroidism, and insulinoma. Some medications associated with weight gain include glycocorticoids, tricyclic antidepressants, and phenothiazines. Essential obesity is the most prevalent type and is the result of the intake of more calories than are expended. This type of obesity results from the multiple interactions of genetic and environmental factors (cultural, metabolic, social, and psychological factors).

17-70   Answer D

Aldosterone is a mineralocorticoid hormone secreted by the adrenal cortex. Follicle-stimulating hormone, thyroid-stimulating hormone, and growth hormones are all secreted by the anterior pituitary gland.

17-71   Answer B

If treatment with diet, exercise, and oral antidiabetic agents is insufficient to achieve acceptable glycemic control in clients with type 2 diabetes, adding a dose of insulin at bedtime to the regimen may be necessary. As a first step, the addition of a bedtime injection of an intermediate-acting insulin such as neutral protamine Hagedorn (NPH) is recommended. Initially, the dosage is 10–15 units at bedtime; then the dose is adjusted to reduce overnight hepatic glucose production and achieve a normal or near-normal fasting blood glucose concentration. If this regimen does not achieve the desired effect, the oral antidiabetic agents should be discontinued and insulin therapy (two or more times a day) should be started. Finally, more intensified insulin regimens may be required in some clients, using multiple daily injections or insulin pump therapy.

17-72   Answer B

For a client with the symptoms experienced by Sigrid, a thyroid-stimulating hormone (TSH) level measurement should be ordered first because the symptoms suggest hyperthyroidism. The TSH level is the single best screening test for hyperthyroidism. Other laboratory and isotope tests for hyperthyroidism include a free T_4 or T_4 level, T_3 resin uptake, and thyroid autoantibodies including TSH receptor antibody (TSH or TRab). Tests not routinely performed but that may be helpful in selected cases such as hyperthyroidism during pregnancy include radioactive iodine uptake and a thyroid scan (with iodine-123 [^{123}I] or technetium-99m), which help to determine the etiology of the hyperthyroidism and assess the functional status of any palpable thyroid irregularities or nodules associated with the toxic goiter. Liver function studies and a chemistry panel will probably not show any abnormalities. An electrocardiogram may be ordered because of the palpitations, but once the thyroid is stabilized, the cardiac rhythm usually returns to normal.

17-73   Answer B

The treatment of Graves' disease (hyperthyroidism) is directed toward lowering the serum concentrations of thyroid hormones to reestablish a eumetabolic state. Therapies that may be used include antithyroid drugs (ATDs), radioactive iodine (^{131}I), and thyroid surgery. Chemotherapy is not used. For clients with hyperthyroidism and a low radioactive iodine uptake, none of these therapies is indicated because low-uptake hyperthyroidism usually implies thyroiditis, which generally resolves spontaneously. Therapy with beta-blocking agents is usually sufficient to control the symptoms of hyperthyroidism in these individuals. In addition, lithium carbonate and stable iodine have been used to block release of thyroid hormone from the thyroid gland in clients who are intolerant to ATDs.

17-74   Answer C

Clients should be cautioned about the adverse effects of antithyroid drugs (ATDs) before the initiation of therapy. Some providers obtain a white blood cell (WBC) count before initiating ATDs because mild leukopenia is common in Graves' disease. A baseline WBC count may be useful for comparison if any problems arise. Serum electrolyte measurements and liver function studies will probably not be affected by ATD therapy.

17-75   Answer A

Radioactive iodine therapy is the most commonly used treatment in the United States for Graves' disease (hyperthyroidism); however, it is contraindicated during pregnancy. Therefore, for women, a pregnancy test (beta human chorionic gonadotropin) needs to be performed before initiating therapy. Women of childbearing age should also be told to delay conception for a few months after radioactive iodine therapy. It is also contraindicated in women who are breastfeeding. Older adults or clients at risk for developing cardiac complications may be pretreated with antithyroid drugs (ATDs) before therapy to deplete the thyroid gland of stored hormone, thereby minimizing the risk of exacerbation of hyperthyroidism because of radioactive iodine (^{131}I)–induced thyroiditis. Marsha's basal metabolism rate will be affected by her Graves' disease but has no bearing on her preparation for radioactive iodine therapy. Lithium levels are usually not performed before radioactive iodine therapy. They may be done if lithium is being used to block the release of thyroid hormone from the thyroid gland in clients who are intolerant of ATDs. Although parathyroid hormone secretion is dependent on the serum calcium level, it is usually not necessary to obtain a serum calcium level measurement before radioactive iodine therapy.

17-76   Answer C

After establishing clinical and biochemical euthy-roidism after a thyroidectomy, you should perform a serum thyroid-stimulating hormone (TSH) level every year. If it is necessary to adjust a client's dosage of levothyroxine, a repeat TSH level measurement should be done in 2–3 months to assess the therapeutic response. Once clinical and biochemical euthyroidism is reestablished, you may return to obtaining an annual serum TSH level.

17-77   Answer A

During pregnancy, many clients with hypothyroidism require an increase in levothyroxine, which would require an increase in the dosage of levothyroxine medication. This need would be detected by performing a thyroid-stimulating hormone (TSH) level test. The woman's TSH level should be checked every trimester to make sure the TSH level is normal. Adjustments to the medication dosage should be made as indicated. Usually, the levothyroxine medication dosage is returned to the prepregnancy dosage immediately after delivery. A serum TSH level reading should be obtained at the 6-week postpartum visit.

17-78   Answer C

Thyroid specialists agree that most benign thyroid nodules require no management beyond watchful waiting and an annual follow-up to evaluate their size. In rare cases, surgery may be indicated if a nodule enlarges to the point of interfering with breathing. Surgery may also be a cosmetic choice. There are conflicting studies regarding the use of levothyroxine to shrink thyroid nodules; because of this, the practice remains unclear. The choice of treatment for malignant thyroid nodules usually calls for subtotal or total thyroidectomy followed by radioactive iodine therapy to destroy residual thyroid tissue.

17-79   Answer A

If a client has a fasting blood sugar (FBS) level greater than 126 mg/dL, experts now prefer that the FBS test be repeated 8 hours after caloric intake. An oral glucose tolerance test, which is inconvenient and distasteful, is usually used for pregnant clients and those participating in research. Medication should not be started until the diagnosis of diabetes has been confirmed by two consecutive FBS tests. Measurement of glycohemoglobin or other glycosylated proteins is not recommended for diagnosing diabetes. It is, however, the gold standard measure of long-term glycemic control in persons with diagnosed diabetes.

17-80   Answer A

For sulfonylurea medications to be effective, reasonable pancreatic insulin reserve is necessary. This reserve tends to dwindle over time; therefore, sulfonylureas tend to be effective for only 7–10 years in most clients. After they lose their effectiveness as a sole agent, another antidiabetic agent may be added to the regimen, insulin may be started, or both. It is unlikely that after being on an oral hypoglycemic agent for 7–10 years, the client will no longer require it and that diet alone would be effective.

17-81   Answer B

Clients with insulin-dependent diabetes mellitus (IDDM) type 1 who have mild hyperglycemia may experience a drop in their blood glucose level during physical activity, whereas those with marked hyperglycemia may experience a rise in their blood glucose level. Clients with IDDM should check their blood glucose level before exercising and refrain from exercising if their blood glucose levels are too high (greater than 300 mg). For individuals without diabetes, the blood glucose level generally varies little during physical activity unless the activity is intense and of very long duration, such as marathon running.

17-82   Answer A

Insulin lispro is a rapid-acting human insulin whose amino acid composition has been slightly modified to make it work faster. It is administered 5–10 minutes before meals and reduces after-meal hyperglycemia to a greater extent than does regular insulin. Its duration of action is about 3 hours, rather than the 5–6 hours of regular insulin. Because of this, lispro reduces the risk of hypoglycemia between meals and during the night.

17-83   Answer C

If Jane has insulin-dependent diabetes mellitus and has been experiencing hyperglycemia before dinner, a possible solution to this problem is to add physical activity between lunch and dinner. In addition, she may try the following strategies:

adjust her afternoon dose of rapid-acting insulin, reduce her carbohydrate consumption at lunch, reduce or omit her midafternoon snack, or change the time of her lunch or midafternoon snack. Adjusting her morning dose of rapid-acting insulin may be necessary if she is hyperglycemic before lunch. Reducing the amount of carbohydrate at dinner may be necessary if she is hyperglycemic at bedtime.

17-84   Answer C

Jane, who has insulin-dependent diabetes mellitus, has been hypoglycemic at bedtime. To correct this, she could try all of the strategies listed as options, except adding an afternoon snack. This would be a strategy to try if the client were hypoglycemic before dinner. Strategies to try to correct hypoglycemia at bedtime include adjusting her insulin dose before dinner, adding carbohydrates at dinner, changing the time of dinner or evening snack, or adding an evening snack.

17-85   Answer C

Because hypertension is implicated in accelerating the microangiopathy of diabetes (especially retinopathy and nephropathy), therapy for hypertension in a client with diabetes should be more aggressive and initiated at a blood pressure 5–10 mm Hg less than the conventional therapeutic guidelines indicate (either systolic or diastolic pressure consistently over 140/90 mm Hg).

17-86   Answer D

Calcium channel blockers do not slow the progression of diabetic nephropathy in clients with diabetes. The steps that can be taken to avoid or slow the progression of diabetic nephropathy include maintaining excellent blood pressure control, using ACE inhibitors, restricting protein, and maintaining excellent glucose control.

17-87   Answer B

Older clients with diabetes are predisposed to malignant otitis externa, caused by *Pseudomonas aeruginosa*. It is an invasive and necrotizing infection with a high mortality, mainly because of meningitis. The client complains of pain in the ear with or without a purulent drainage, swelling of the parotid gland, trismus (tonic contraction of the muscles of mastication), and paralysis of the 6th through 12th cranial nerves.

17-88   Answer C

Virilization involves an increased androgen response, including increased muscle mass, clitoral enlargement, lowered voice, and behavioral changes. Hirsutism is excessive hair distribution.

17-89   Answer A

Men and women are equally prone to osteoporosis, but it usually occurs later in life in men. Men develop the classic fractures of osteoporosis: Colles', vertebral, and hip. In women, the loss of sex steroids at menopause or after a hysterectomy leads to an increase in bone turnover through activation of bone remodeling. This results in an overall bone loss and loss of cancellous (trabecular) bone. In addition, with loss of estrogen, the amount of bone resorbed is greater than that replaced, leading to a continuing decline in overall bone mass and worsening microarchitecture. Hormone replacement for older men is not an option as it is in women because of the detrimental effects of testosterone on blood pressure and serum lipids. Prevention of osteoporosis in men is limited to maintenance of exercise, calcium supplementation, and cessation of smoking.

17-90   Answer C

Chvostek's sign is seen in tetany and is a spasm of the facial muscles after a tap on one side of the face over the facial nerve. To diagnose hypoparathyroidism, the following are usually present: a positive Chvostek's sign and positive Trousseau's sign, tetany, carpopedal spasms, tingling of the lips and hands, muscular and abdominal cramps, low serum calcium level, high serum phosphate level, and reduced urine calcium excretion.

17-91   Answer D

The first action a client should take for treating hypoglycemia (which is assumed because Mary took more than four times the usual dose of her short-acting insulin) is to ingest 10–15 g of a rapidly absorbable carbohydrate, such as three to five pieces of hard candy, two to three packets of sugar, or 4 oz of fruit juice, to abort the episode. This should be repeated in 15 minutes, as needed. Mary should continue to try to obtain her blood glucose level and should certainly not drive. You should ask Mary to call you back in about 30 minutes to 1 hour after ingesting the carbohydrate and after checking her glucose level (or sooner if she feels any different).

17-92   Answer C

Pancreatic protease is not carried in pancreatic juice. Pancreatic juice carries pancreatic amylase, pancreatic lipase, and pancreatic trypsin. Proteolytic enzymes are activated by trypsin, which is activated in the intestine. Pancreatic amylase splits carbohydrates into dextrins and maltose. Pancreatic lipase hydrolyzes fat to yield glycerol and fatty acids. Pancreatic trypsin is one of a group of enzymes, including chymotrypsin and carboxypolypeptidase, that split proteins.

17-93   Answer B

The process of aging results in a decreased absorption of fat-soluble vitamins. There is a decrease in the number and size of hepatic cells, leading to a decrease in liver weight and mass. There is also a decrease in enzyme activity, which diminishes the liver's ability to detoxify drugs. This increases the risk of toxic levels of many medications in older adults. There is calcification of the pancreatic vessels and the ducts distend and dilate. These changes lead to a decrease in the production of lipase.

17-94   Answer D

After an oral cholecystogram, some persons experience burning on urination because of the presence of dye in the urine. This is helped by forcing fluids. An oral cholecystogram is done to assess for biliary obstruction. Contraction of the gallbladder may be desirable during a cholecystogram to obtain a better reading and may be accomplished by having the client consume a high-fat meal during the procedure. A reaction to the contrast medium would produce symptoms such as urticaria, nausea, vomiting, or dyspnea.

17-95   Answer B

Immunoglobulin M (IgM) anti–hepatitis A virus (HAV) titers peak during the first week of the infection with acute hepatitis A and usually disappear within 3–6 months. Detection of IgM anti-HAV is a valid test for demonstrating acute hepatitis A. IgG anti-HAV titers peak after 1 month of the disease but may stay elevated for years; therefore, they are an indicator of past infection.

17-96   Answer D

For the client with hepatitis, abdominal pain in the right upper quadrant is caused by stretching of Glisson's capsule surrounding the liver, which occurs because of inflammation; bleeding tendencies are a result of reduced prothrombin synthesis by injured hepatic cells; pruritus is caused by bile salt accumulation in the skin; and fever is the result of the release of pyrogens in the inflammatory process.

17-97   Answer C

Myxedema is characterized by abnormal deposits of mucin in the skin and other tissues; a dry, waxy type of swelling in the skin; and nonpitting edema in the pretibial and facial areas. Myxedema is most common in hypothyroid women in their 60s. Untreated myxedema has been associated with severe atherosclerosis and has been attributed to the increase in serum cholesterol concentrations, particularly of low-density lipoprotein. Thyroid hormone replacement counters these changes.

17-98   Answer C

Saturated solution of potassium iodide is an antithyroid drug that blocks the production and release of thyroid hormone. It is used to treat hyperthyroidism before thyroidectomy. Propylthiouracil and methimazole (Tapazole) treat hyperthyroidism by inhibiting thyroid hormone synthesis. Radioactive iodine (^{131}I) treats hyperthyroidism and may be used to treat thyroid cancer by destroying thyroid tissue.

17-99   Answer A

Signs of hypoparathyroidism include elevated serum phosphate levels; decreased serum calcium levels; increased neuromuscular activity, which may progress to tetany; decreased bone resorption; hypocalciuria; and hypophosphaturia.

17-100   Answer D

Unlike many oral antidiabetic agents, Byetta causes weight loss. The active ingredient is a protein that encourages digestion and the production of insulin.

17-101   Answer A

If the thyroid gland is palpable, the next step is to have the client hold his or her breath and listen over the gland with the bell of the stethoscope for bruits. A bruit may indicate an increased vascularity of hyperthyroidism. Although there may not be any sound, that doesn't mean that there is not a thyroid nodule. A thrill is feeling turbulent blood flow, whereas a bruit is listening to it.

17-102   Answer B

Trousseau's sign (carpal spasm) is one of two neuromuscular signs indicative of hypocalcemia. It is often preceded by muscle cramps in the legs and feet. Carpal spasm consists of a flexed elbow and wrist, adducted thumb over the palm, flexed metacarpophalangeal joints, adduction of hyperextended fingers, and extended interphalangeal joints. The response is elicited by inflation of a blood pressure cuff to 20 mm Hg above the level of the systolic blood pressure. Inflation is maintained for 3 minutes to elicit the response, which is secondary to ulnar and median nerve ischemia. In severe hypocalcemia, spontaneous spasms may occur in the lower extremities. Chvostek's sign is the second neuromuscular sign associated with hypocalcemia. It is an abnormal unilateral spasm of the facial muscle when the facial nerve is tapped below the zygomatic arch anterior to the earlobe.

17-103   Answer C

Clients with visual or dexterity difficulties may benefit from prefilling syringes. Prefilled insulin syringes may be stored in a vertical position in the refrigerator for up to 30 days with the needle pointing upward. Alternatives to syringes include jet injectors and penlike devices. Jet injectors are useful for clients who have needle phobias, but they are expensive. Penlike devices hold insulin cartridges and are useful if the client is visually or neurologically impaired, and they help to increase the accuracy of insulin administration. Another alternative is the insulin pump.

17-104   Answer D

Clients with neuropathy require professional nail and callus care because most ulcers begin at the site of a callus.

17-105   Answer B

Increased parathyroid hormone peaks between 15 and 35 weeks' gestation to meet increased requirements for calcium and vitamin D for fetal skeletal growth. Folic acid is a member of the vitamin B complex and is necessary to reduce the risk of neural tube defects.

17-106   Answer A

Posterior pituitary hormones include antidiuretic hormone (ADH) with the kidney as the target organ and oxytocin with the uterus and breasts as the target organs. Anterior pituitary hormones include growth hormone (GH) with bones and organs as the target organ; adrenocorticotropic hormone (ACTH) affecting the adrenal cortex; thyroid-stimulating hormone (TSH) affecting the thyroid; follicle-stimulating hormone (FSH) affecting the testes and ovaries; luteinizing hormone (LH) affecting the ovaries; and prolactin affecting the breasts.

Bibliography

Barclay, L: Starting therapy with high dose levothyroxine is safe in asymptomatic cardiac clients. *Medscape Medical News*, June 2003. www.medscape.com/viewarticle/457629, accessed 10/3/08.

Bengel, FM, et al: Cardiac oxidative metabolism, function and metabolic performance in mild hyperthyroidism: A noninvasive study using positron emission tomography and magnetic resonance imaging. *Thyroid*, July 2003.

DeNoia, V: Bisphosphonates for osteoporosis: A closer look at efficacy and safety. *Arthritis Practitioner* 3(4):20–23. July/August 2007.

Dillon, PM. Nursing Health Assessment—A Critical Thinking, Case Studies Approach, ed 2. FA Davis, Philadelphia, 2007.

Dunphy LM: Management Guidelines for Nurse Practitioners Working With Adults, ed 2. FA Davis, Philadelphia, 2004.

Dunphy, LM, et al: Primary Care: The Art and Science of Advanced Practice Nursing, ed 2. FA Davis, Philadelphia, 2007.

Holman, R, et al: The role of protein kinase C in diabetic microvascular damage. *Family Medicine*, February 2003.

Jones, R: Primary hyperparathyroidism. *Clinician Reviews* 17(7):27–33, July 2007.

Lawrence, J, and Robinson, A: Screening for diabetes in general practice. *Preventive Cardiology*, May 2003.

McKay JM: Diabetes mellitus and the elderly: A review of the 2003 California Health Care Foundation/American Geriatrics Society guidelines. *Family Medicine*, 2003.

Meigs, J, et al: The natural history of progression from normal glucose tolerance to type 2 diabetes in the Baltimore longitudinal study of aging. *Diabetes*, July 2003.

Mitzner, L: A quick guide to the newest diabetes drugs. *The Clinical Advisor* 10(5):34–42, May 2007.

Wynne, AL, Woo, TM, and Olyaei, AJ: *Pharmacotherapeutics for Nurse Practitioner Prescribers*, ed 2. FA Davis, Philadelphia, 2007.

How well did you do?

85% and above, congratulations! This score shows application of test-taking principles and adequate content knowledge.

75%–85%, keep working! Review test-taking principles and try again.

65%–75%, hang in there! Spend some time reviewing concepts and test-taking principles and try the test again.

Chapter 18: *Hematological and Immune Problems*

LYNNE M. DUNPHY
JILL E. WINLAND-BROWN

Questions

18-1 *Tina, age 2, had a complete blood count (CBC) drawn at her last visit. It indicates that she has a microcytic hypochromic anemia. What should you do now at this visit?*

A. Obtain a lead level.

B. Instruct Tina's parents to increase the amount of milk in her diet.

C. Start Tina on ferrous sulfate (Feosol) and check the CBC in 6 weeks.

D. Recheck the CBC on this visit.

18-2 *A client with HIV infection has a CD4 count of 305 and an HIV RNA level of 13,549. The client is asymptomatic. What is your course of action?*

A. Negotiate with your client a time to start therapy.

B. Recheck the laboratory results in 1 month. If the counts remain like this, start treatment.

C. Start therapy now because the client's CD4 count is less than 500 and the HIV RNA level is greater than 10,000.

D. Wait to start therapy until the client becomes asymptomatic.

18-3 *Mindy, age 6, recently was discharged from the hospital after a sickle cell crisis. You are teaching her parents to be alert to the manifestations of splenic sequestration and tell them to be alert to*

A. vomiting and diarrhea.

B. decreased mental acuity.

C. abdominal pain, pallor, and tachycardia.

D. abdominal pain and vomiting.

18-4 *The Centers for Disease Control and Prevention's definition of AIDS includes the presence of which of the following disorders, with or without laboratory evidence of HIV infection?*

A. Pneumonia in clients younger than age 60

B. Dementia in clients younger than age 60

C. Kaposi's sarcoma in clients younger than age 60

D. Primary brain lymphoma in clients older than age 60

18-5 *Pernicious anemia is a result of*

A. not enough folic acid.

B. not enough intrinsic factor.

C. not enough vitamin D.

D. not enough iron.

18-6 *A loss of DNA control over differentiation that occurs in response to adverse conditions is referred to as*

A. hyperplasia.

B. metaplasia.

C. anaplasia.

D. dysplasia.

18-7 *Which of the following cancers is associated with Epstein-Barr virus?*

A. Burkitt's lymphoma

B. Kaposi's sarcoma

C. Lymphoma

D. Adult T-cell leukemia

18-8 *Prostate cancer is associated with which of the following viruses?*

A. Herpes simplex virus types 1 and 2

B. Human herpesvirus 6

C. Human cytomegalovirus

D. Human T-lymphotropic viruses

18-9 *Which of the following is a genotoxic carcinogen?*

A. Vinyl chloride polymers

B. Chemotherapy drugs

C. Asbestos

D. Wood and leather dust

18-10   Tobacco has been linked to which of the following types of cancer?

A. Colon cancer

B. Bladder cancer

C. Prostate cancer

D. Cervical cancer

18-11   Sam is being worked up for pancreatic cancer. He states that the doctor wants to put a "scope" in and inject dye into his ducts. He wants to know more about this. What procedure is he referring to?

A. Percutaneous transhepatic cholangiography

B. An endoscopic retrograde cholangiopancreatography

C. An angiography

D. An upper gastrointestinal (GI) series

18-12   Jan is having biological therapy for her pancreatic cancer. What kind of treatment is this?

A. Surgery

B. Radiation therapy

C. Immunotherapy

D. Chemotherapy

18-13   Which of the following increases the risk of pancreatic cancer?

A. A high-carbohydrate diet

B. Cigarette smoking, diabetes, and a high-fat diet

C. Diabetes and lack of activity

D. Yo-yo dieting

18-14   One major approach to cancer prevention is

A. colonoscopy.

B. new drug trials.

C. Pap smears for women of all ages.

D. host modification.

18-15   Which ethnic group has the highest overall cancer incidence rate?

A. Native Americans

B. Asian and Pacific Islanders

C. Hispanics

D. African Americans

18-16   Joan had a modified mastectomy with radiation therapy 10 years ago. She asks when she can have her blood pressure or needle sticks taken in the affected arm. How do you respond?

A. "If it's been 10 years and you've had no problems, you can discontinue those precautions."

B. "Because you didn't have a radical mastectomy, you can do those things now."

C. "You must observe these precautions forever."

D. "As long as you do limb exercises and have established collateral drainage, you can discontinue these precautions."

18-17   Which of the following is not an effective strategy to prevent the nausea and vomiting associated with the effects of radiation and chemotherapy?

A. Decreasing the amount of liquids

B. Eating a soft, bland diet low in fat and sugar

C. Relaxation

D. Distraction

18-18   Multiple myeloma is a plasma cell malignancy in which the bone marrow is replaced, and there is bone destruction and paraprotein formation. Myeloma is a disease of older adults overall (median age at presentation, 65 years). Common presenting symptoms include

A. nausea and vomiting and chronic cough.

B. fatigue and splenomegaly.

C. lower back pain and hypercalcemia.

D. nausea and vomiting and fatigue.

18-19   What is the earliest visual sign of oral and pharyngeal squamous cell carcinomas?

A. Leukoplakia

B. Mucosal erythroplasia

C. Loss of sensation in the tongue

D. Difficulty chewing or swallowing

18-20   Fecal occult blood testing (FOBT) is most effective in identifying

A. cancers in the right colon.

B. polyps.

C. cancers in the sigmoid colon.

D. cancers in the transverse colon.

18-21   *Sickle cell anemia affects African Americans. Approximately 1 in 400 African Americans in the United States has sickle cell disease (SCD). Advances in treatment have been made, but life expectancy is still limited. The mean survival time for men with the disease is approximately*

A. 24 years.

B. 34 years.

C. 42 years.

D. 52 years.

18-22   *Clients with AIDS typically experience the neurological symptomatic triad consisting of*

A. cognitive, motor, and behavioral changes.

B. seizures, paresthesias, and dysesthesias.

C. Kaposi's sarcoma, cryptococcal meningitis, and depression.

D. seizures, depression, and paresthesias.

18-23   *Barbie, age 27, had her spleen removed after an automobile accident. You are seeing her in the office for the first time since her discharge from the hospital. She asks you how her surgery will affect her in the future. How do you respond?*

A. "Your red blood cell production will be slowed."

B. "Your lymphatic system may have difficulty transporting lymph fluid to the blood vessels."

C. "You'll have difficulty storing the nutritional agents needed to make red blood cells."

D. "You may have difficulty salvaging iron from old red blood cells for reuse."

18-24   *Sara comes today with numerous petechiae on her arms. You know that she is not taking warfarin (Coumadin). What other drugs do you ask her about?*

A. Aspirin or aspirin compounds

B. Antihypertensive agents

C. Oral contraceptives

D. Anticonvulsants

18-25   *Screening infants for anemia should occur at what age?*

A. 6 months

B. No screening is recommended.

C. 9 months

D. 12 months

18-26   *Despite successful primary prophylaxis, which infection remains a common AIDS-defining diagnosis?*

A. *Pneumocystis jiroveci* pneumonia (PCP)

B. Cryptococcosis

C. Cryptosporidiosis

D. Candidiasis

18-27   *Which of the following indicates that Jim, a 32-year-old client with AIDS, has oropharyngeal candidiasis?*

A. Small vesicles

B. Fissured, white, thickened patches

C. Removable white plaques

D. Flat-topped papules with thin, bluish-white spiderweb lines

18-28   *Stu, age 49, has slightly reduced hemoglobin and hematocrit readings. What is your next action after you ask him about his diet?*

A. Repeat the laboratory tests.

B. Perform a fecal occult blood test.

C. Start him on an iron preparation.

D. Start him on folic acid.

18-29   *Sue has sickle cell anemia. In regulating her and monitoring her hemoglobin and hematocrit levels, you want to maintain them at*

A. slightly below normal.

B. strictly at normal.

C. slightly above normal.

D. around normal with only minor fluctuations.

18-30   *A metastatic tumor from below the diaphragm is suspected when you palpate which of the following nodes in the left supraclavicular space?*

A. Wringer's node

B. Sims' node

C. Wiskott-Aldrich node

D. Virchow's node

18-31 *An increase of which immunoglobulin (Ig) signifies atopic disorders such as allergic rhinitis, allergic asthma, atopic dermatitis, and parasitic infestation?*

A. IgG

B. IgM

C. IgA

D. IgE

18-32 *Which hypersensitivity reaction results in a skin test that is erythematous with edema within 3–8 hours?*

A. Anaphylactic reaction

B. Cytotoxic reaction

C. Immune complex–mediated reaction

D. Delayed hypersensitivity reaction

18-33 *You are examining Joseph, age 9 months, and note a palpable right supraclavicular node. You know that this finding is suspicious for*

A. candidiasis.

B. cryptococcosis.

C. lymphoma of the mediastinum.

D. abdominal malignancy.

18-34 *Samuel, age 5, is receiving radiation therapy for his acute lymphocytic leukemia. He is at increased risk of developing which type of cancer as a secondary malignancy when he becomes an adult?*

A. Chronic lymphocytic leukemia

B. Brain tumor

C. Liver cancer

D. Esophageal cancer

18-35 *Robin has HIV infection and is having a problem with massive diarrhea. You suspect the cause is*

A. cryptococcosis.

B. toxoplasmosis.

C. cryptosporidiosis.

D. cytomegalovirus.

18-36 *What is the meaning of the term "shift to the left" or "left shift"?*

A. This indicates a rise in basophils.

B. This indicates a rise in monocytes.

C. This indicates a rise in neutrophils.

D. This indicates a rise in lymphocytes.

18-37 *Jill has just been given a diagnosis of HIV infection and has a normal initial Pap test. When do the Centers for Disease Control and Prevention (CDC) guidelines state that she should have a repeat Pap test?*

A. In 3 months

B. In 6 months

C. In 1 year

D. She should have a colposcopy every year rather than a Pap test.

18-38 *Maurice is an intravenous drug abuser with chronic hepatitis B (HBV). The development of which type of hepatitis poses the greatest risk to a client with HBV?*

A. Hepatitis A

B. Hepatitis C

C. Hepatitis D

D. Hepatitis E

18-39 *Sally has HIV infection and asks which method of birth control, other than abstinence, would be best for her. You suggest*

A. latex condoms.

B. the spermicide nonoxynol-9.

C. an intrauterine device (IUD).

D. an oral contraceptive.

18-40 *Prophylaxis for the first episode of Pneumocystis jiroveci pneumonia in an adult or adolescent client infected with HIV is*

A. isoniazid (Nydrazid) 300 mg PO and pyridoxine (vitamin B_6 [Beesix]) 50 mg PO qd for 12 days.

B. clarithromycin (Biaxin) 500 mg PO bid for 2 weeks.

C. rifampin (Rimactane) 600 mg PO qd for 12 months.

D. trimethoprim-sulfamethoxazole (TMP-SMZ) (Bactrim) DS 1 tablet PO qd for 10 days.

18-41 *Which of the following is an X-linked recessive disorder commonly seen in African American men?*

A. Sickle cell anemia

B. Glucose-6-phosphate dehydrogenase deficiency

C. Pyruvate kinase deficiency

D. Bernard-Soulier syndrome

18-42 *When Judy tells you that she has hemophilia, you know that*

A. both of her parents also have the disease.

B. her maternal grandfather probably had the disease and it skipped a generation.

C. her father had the disease and her mother was a carrier.

D. her mother had the disease.

18-43 *Frank, a 66-year-old white male who is on diuretic therapy, presents with an elevated hematocrit. He also has splenomegaly on examination, as well as subjective complaints of blurred vision, fatigue, headache, and tinnitus. You suspect*

A. multiple myeloma.

B. Waldenström's macroglobulinemia.

C. dehydration related to use of diuretics.

D. polycythemia vera.

18-44 *Which is the most abundant immunoglobulin (Ig) found in the blood, lymph, and intestines?*

A. IgG

B. IgA

C. IgM

D. IgD

18-45 *Which of the following white blood cell types is elevated in parasitic infections, hypersensitivity reactions, and autoimmune disorders?*

A. Neutrophils

B. Eosinophils

C. Basophils

D. Monocytes

18-46 *Lorie, age 29, appears with the following signs: pale conjunctiva and nailbeds, tachycardia, heart murmur, cheilosis, stomatitis, splenomegaly, koilonychia, and glossitis. What do you suspect?*

A. Vitamin B_{12} deficiency

B. Folate deficiency

C. Iron-deficiency anemia

D. Chronic fatigue syndrome

18-47 *Antibodies (inhibitors) directed against factor VIII can arise spontaneously in a number of situations. These include*

A. clients who have mitral regurgitation.

B. as sequelae to a strep infection.

C. clients on antibiotics.

D. women who are several weeks postpartum after a normal labor and delivery.

18-48 *Skip, age 4, is brought in to the office by his mother. His symptoms are pallor, fatigue, bleeding, fever, bone pain, adenopathy, arthralgias, and hepatosplenomegaly. You refer him to a specialist. Which of the following tests do you expect the specialist to perform to confirm a diagnosis?*

A. An enzyme-linked immunosorbent assay

B. A monospot test

C. A prothrombin time, partial thromboplastin time, bleeding time, complete blood count, and peripheral smear

D. A bone marrow smear

18-49 *When a neonate is initially protected against measles, mumps, and rubella because the mother is immune, this is an example of which type of immunity?*

A. Natural active

B. Artificial active

C. Natural passive

D. Artificial passive

18-50 *Systemic lupus erythematosus is diagnosed on the basis of*

A. positive antinuclear antibody (ANA), malar rash, and photosensitivity.

B. positive ANA, weight loss, and night sweats.

C. negative ANA, photosensitivity, and renal disease.

D. leukopenia, negative ANA, and photosensitivity.

18-51 *The T in the TNM staging system refers to*

A. tolerance.

B. primary tumor.

C. tumor marker.

D. turgor.

18-52   *Bladder cancer can be detected early by*

A. an annual urine culture.

B. a bladder tumor marker blood test.

C. an annual cystoscopy.

D. none of the above; there is no early detection.

18-53   *Which bone tumor arises from cartilage and is usually located in the pelvis, femur, proximal humerus, or ribs?*

A. Osteosarcoma

B. Chondrosarcoma

C. Ewing's sarcoma

D. Fibrosarcoma

18-54   *Which tumor marker may detect a tumor of the ovary or testis?*

A. Alpha fetoprotein

B. Carcinoembryonic antigen

C. Human chorionic gonadotropin

D. Cancer antigen 125

18-55   *Select a statement that is true about the erythrocyte sedimentation rate (ESR).*

A. It is a very specific indicator of inflammation.

B. A rise in the ESR is a normal part of aging.

C. It is useful in detecting pancreatic cancer.

D. It is diagnostic for rheumatoid arthritis.

18-56   *Julie's brother has chronic lymphatic leukemia. She overheard that he was in stage IV and asks what this means. According to the Rai classification system, stage IV is a stage*

A. at which the lymphocytes are greater than 10,000 mm³.

B. with an absolute lymphocytosis, in which the client may live 7–10 years or more.

C. of thrombocytopenia, in which the life expectancy may be only 2 years.

D. of anemia.

18-57   *Before initiating cancer therapy, the first crucial step is to*

A. stage the disease.

B. define the goals of therapy.

C. confirm the diagnosis using tissue biopsy.

D. choose a treatment plan from the many therapeutic options.

18-58   *Which cancer can be cured with chemotherapy alone?*

A. Breast cancer

B. Malignant melanoma

C. Bladder cancer

D. Testicular cancer

18-59   *You have a new client, Robert, age 67, who presents with a generalized lymphadenopathy. You know that this is indicative of*

A. disseminated malignancy, particularly of the hematological system.

B. cancer of the liver.

C. Sjögren's syndrome.

D. pancreatic cancer.

18-60   *Some pharmacological adjuncts to analgesics in clients with uncontrolled cancer pain include*

A. anticonvulsants and tricyclic antidepressants.

B. anticonvulsants, tricyclic antidepressants, and corticosteroids.

C. selective serotonin receptor inhibitors.

D. benzodiazepines.

18-61   *Mandy's 16-year-old daughter has hepatitis A. Which of the following statements made by Mandy indicates that she understands the teaching you've just completed?*

A. "I guess she needs to be hospitalized until she's recovered."

B. "We'll keep her at home with strict isolation precautions."

C. "We'll stop at the store and buy plastic eating utensils."

D. "We'll stop at the drugstore and pick up prescription medications immediately."

18-62   *Julia asks how smoking increases the risk for folic acid deficiency. You respond that smoking*

A. causes small-vessel disease and constricts all vessels that transport essential nutrients.

B. decreases vitamin C absorption.

C. affects the liver's ability to store folic acid.

D. causes nausea, thereby inhibiting the appetite and ingestion of foods rich in folic acid.

18-63 Which of the following is not an inherited condition that causes hemolytic anemia?

A. Hereditary spherocytosis

B. Pernicious anemia

C. Glucose-6-phosphate dehydrogenase deficiency

D. Sickle cell anemia

18-64 Caroline, an older adult, is homeless and has iron-deficiency anemia. She smokes and drinks when she can and has an ulcer. Which of the following is not one of the risk factors of iron-deficiency anemia?

A. Smoking

B. Poverty

C. Ulcer disease

D. Age older than 60

18-65 Sickle cell anemia is an autosomal recessive disorder caused by the hemoglobin S gene. An abnormal hemoglobin leads to chronic hemolytic anemia with numerous clinical manifestations and becomes a chronic multisystem disease, with death from organ failure, usually between ages 40 and 50. The hemoglobin S gene is carried by

A. approximately 4% of the U.S. population.

B. approximately 8% of American blacks.

C. approximately 4% of Latinos.

D. approximately 12% of Native Americans.

18-66 Which is the best serum test to perform to spot an iron-deficiency anemia early before it progresses to full-blown anemia?

A. Hemoglobin

B. Hematocrit

C. Ferritin

D. Reticulocytes

18-67 Which of the following laboratory studies is used to determine if a client has had hepatitis?

A. Serum protein

B. Protein electrophoresis

C. Antibody testing

D. Globulin levels

18-68 Under which of the following circumstances is the reticulocyte count elevated?

A. Aplastic anemia

B. Iron-deficiency anemias

C. Poisonings

D. Acute blood loss

18-69 The primary reason for newborn screening for sickle cell disease is to

A. present the parents with the option for genetic screening in the future.

B. test siblings if it is proved that the newborn has sickle cell disease.

C. allow for the prevention of septicemia with prophylactic medication.

D. prevent a sickle cell crisis.

18-70 Samantha is being given platelets because of acute leukemia. One "pack" of platelets should raise her count by how much?

A. 2000–4000 mm³

B. 5000–8000 mm³

C. 9000–12,000 mm³

D. About 15,000 mm³

18-71 When the donor and recipient of a transplant are identical twins, this is referred to as a(n)

A. isograft.

B. autograft.

C. allograft.

D. xenograft.

18-72 Your client, Mr. Jones, has Sjögren's syndrome. Which treatment do you suggest?

A. Artificial tears and chewing sugarless gum

B. Frequent rinsing out of the mouth with mouthwash

C. Drinking at least one glass of milk per day

D. Removing wax from the ears at regular intervals

18-73   *The first choice of therapy for a client who is positive for HIV and has oral candidiasis is*

A. fluconazole (Diflucan) 100 mg PO qd.

B. ketoconazole (Nizoral) 200 mg PO qd.

C. clotrimazole troches (10 mg) five times daily or nystatin (Mycostatin) suspension 500,000–1,000,000 units three to five times daily.

D. griseofulvin (Grisactin) 500 mg bid.

18-74   *A client with HIV infection has a fever of unknown origin (FUO). Which of the following is a possible cause of an FUO in a client with HIV?*

A. Drug fever

B. Upper respiratory infection

C. Nothing specific; this is a systemic disease manifestation

D. Urinary tract infection

18-75   *The three most common signs and symptoms of primary HIV infection are*

A. weight loss, pharyngitis, and fatigue.

B. fever, fatigue, and pharyngitis.

C. night sweats, rash, and headache.

D. myalgias, fatigue, and fever.

18-76   *Mrs. Jameson complains of unilateral blurry vision and partial blindness in the left eye. On physical examination, you find decreased peripheral vision on her left side. Funduscopic examination reveals cotton-wool spots. Your most likely diagnosis is*

A. cryptococcosis.

B. toxoplasmosis.

C. cytomegalovirus infection.

D. herpes simplex virus infection.

18-77   *The "gold standard" for definitive diagnosis of sickle cell anemia is*

A. a reticulocyte count.

B. the sickle cell test.

C. a hemoglobin electrophoresis.

D. a peripheral blood smear.

18-78   *Jimmy is a 6-month-old with newly diagnosed sickle cell disease. His mother brings him to the clinic for*

a well-baby visit. Which of the following should you do on this visit?

A. Tell the parents that Jimmy will not be immunized because of his diagnosis.

B. Tell the parents that Jimmy should not go to day care.

C. Immunize Jimmy with diphtheria, tetanus, and pertussis; *Haemophilus influenzae* type b (HIB); hepatitis B (HBV); and poliomyelitis vaccines.

D. Immunize Jimmy with measles, mumps, and rubella; HIB; and HBV vaccines only.

18-79   *Health maintenance in adults with sickle cell anemia includes which of the following?*

A. Early sterilization should be performed to prevent transmission of the disease.

B. Administer hepatitis A vaccine.

C. Avoid use of oral contraceptives because of increased risk of clotting.

D. Give folic acid 1 mg PO daily.

18-80   *Which of the following situations might precipitate a sickle cell crisis in an infant?*

A. Taking the infant to visit a relative

B. Hepatitis B immunization

C. Taking the infant to a home Miami Dolphins football game

D. Having the infant sleep on its back

18-81   *Pernicious anemia is a result of*

A. not enough folic acid.

B. not enough intrinsic factor.

C. not enough vitamin D.

D. not enough iron.

18-82   *The test in which a small, radioactive tracer dose of cyanocobalamin is given by mouth and then a 24-hour urine sample is collected and assayed for radioactivity is the*

A. Coombs' test.

B. oligonucleotide probe test.

C. spherocytic test.

D. Schilling test.

18-83   *Sandra, age 19, is pregnant. She is complaining of breathlessness, tiredness, and weakness and is pale.*

After diagnosing anemia, you order medication and tell her to take it

A. only with meals because it can be irritating to the stomach.

B. in the morning if she experiences morning sickness.

C. 1 hour before eating or between meals.

D. at bedtime.

18-84 *What is the mechanism of action of steroid hormones in cancer chemotherapy?*

A. They interfere with DNA or RNA synthesis.

B. They interfere with DNA replication by attacking DNA synthesis throughout the cell cycle.

C. They inhibit protein synthesis.

D. They alter the host environment for cell growth.

18-85 *Allie, age 5, is being treated with radiation for cancer. Her mother asks about the effect radiation will have on Allie's future growth. Although she knows that a specialist will be handling Allie's care, her mother asks for your opinion. How do you respond?*

A. "Let's worry about the cancer first, then see how her growth is affected."

B. "Chemotherapy may affect her future growth, but not radiation."

C. "She will probably have growth hormone problems, in which case she can then begin growth hormone therapy."

D. "That's the least of your worries now; everything will turn out OK."

18-86 *A platelet count less than 150,000/mm³ may indicate*

A. possible hemorrhage.

B. hypersplenism.

C. polycythemia vera.

D. malignancy.

18-87 *Macrocytic normochromic anemias are caused by*

A. acute blood loss.

B. an infection or tumor.

C. a nutritional deficiency of iron.

D. a deficiency of folic acid.

18-88 *Thalassemia is caused by*

A. blood loss.

B. impaired production of all blood-forming elements.

C. increased destruction of red blood cells.

D. autoimmune antibodies.

18-89 *Which type of leukemia produces symptoms with an insidious onset including weakness, fatigue, massive lymphadenopathy, pruritic vesicular skin lesions, anemia, and thrombocytopenia?*

A. Acute lymphocytic leukemia

B. Acute myelogenous leukemia

C. Chronic lymphocytic leukemia

D. Chronic myelogenous leukemia

18-90 *Physiological changes in the immune system of older adults include*

A. an increase in immunoglobulin A and G antibodies.

B. a high rate of T-lymphocyte proliferation.

C. an increase in the number of cytotoxic T cells.

D. an increase in CD8, which affects regulation of the immune system.

18-91 *Shelley has esophageal cancer and asks you if alcohol played a part in its development. How do you respond?*

A. "Your cancer was caused by your cigarette smoking, nothing else."

B. "Alcohol is also a carcinogen."

C. "Alcohol directly alters the DNA and causes mutations."

D. "Alcohol modifies the metabolism of carcinogens in the esophagus and increases their effectiveness."

18-92 *Maria asks if being overweight predisposes her to cancer. How do you respond?*

A. "No, you have the same risk as a normal-weight individual."

B. "You have less of a risk of cancer than normal-weight individuals because you have protein stores to combat mutant cells."

C. "Yes, you have an increased risk for hormone-dependent cancers because of your obesity."

D. "Yes, you have an increased risk because you have many more cells in all the organs of your body."

18-93 *Kathy, age 64, is a sun worshipper. She tells you that because she did not get skin cancer in her youth, she certainly will not get it now. How do you respond?*

A. "You're probably right; if you haven't had it by now, you're probably safe."

B. "As you age, you have decreased pigment in your skin, which puts you at more risk."

C. "Your skin elasticity is decreased, so you have more of a chance of contracting skin cancer as you age."

D. "Skin cancer is not dependent on age; anyone can get it."

18-94 *Which of the following is a benign neoplasm?*

A. Leiomyoma

B. Osteosarcoma

C. Glioma

D. Seminoma

18-95 *Marsha states that a relative is having a carcinoembryonic antigen (CEA) test done to detect some type of cancer. She wants to know what kind. You tell her a CEA is performed to detect*

A. adenocarcinoma of the prostate.

B. medullary cancer of the thyroid.

C. adenocarcinomas of the colon, lung, breast, ovary, stomach, and pancreas.

D. multiple myeloma.

18-96 *The placement of a high dose of radioactive material directly into a malignant tumor and giving a lower dose to the normal tissues is referred to as*

A. radiotherapy.

B. teletherapy.

C. brachytherapy.

D. ionization therapy.

18-97 *In teaching your client about the American Cancer Society's CAUTION model, which identifies signs of many cancers, you teach her that the N stands for*

A. night sweats.

B. nagging cough.

C. nausea and vomiting.

D. noxious odor.

18-98 *Nancy recently had a mastectomy and refuses to look at the site. Her husband does all the dressing changes. When she comes into the office for a postoperative checkup, what would you say to her?*

A. "You'll look at it when you're ready."

B. "You must look at it today."

C. "Everything's going to be OK. It looks fine."

D. "You have to accept this eventually; just glance at it today."

18-99 *You suspect that your new client Doug has hepatitis C, although he is asymptomatic at this point in time. Your suspicion is based on his medical history, which includes which of the following factors that has been identified as a red flag for this disease?*

A. Lactose intolerance

B. Frequent sore throats and upper respiratory infections

C. A history of mononucleosis at age 17

D. Unsafe sexual behaviors

18-100 *What is the most significant reason why alcohol use is discouraged in persons with HIV infection or AIDS?*

A. Alcohol interferes with the pharmacokinetics of most AIDS drugs.

B. Filling up on the empty calories of alcohol replaces the desire for food.

C. Alcohol decreases the ability of persons to adhere to a prescribed medical regimen.

D. If clients become addicted to alcohol, when AIDS advances, they will become addicted to painkillers.

18-101 *How often should you order a complete blood count for your client?*

A. Routinely

B. Before dental work

C. In the case of infection

D. If she is pregnant

18-102 *Your client, Shirley, has an elevated mean cell volume (MCV). What should you be considering in terms of diagnosis?*

A. Iron-deficiency anemia

B. Hemolytic anemias

C. Lead poisoning

D. Liver disease

18-103 *Sherri's blood work returns with a decreased mean cell volume (MCV) and a decreased mean cellular hemoglobin concentration (MCHC). What should you do next?*

A. Order a serum iron and total iron binding capacity (TIBC).

B. Order a serum ferritin.

C. Order a serum folate level.

D. Order a serum iron, TIBC, and serum ferritin level.

18-104 *Your 18-year-old client, Mandy, has infectious mononucleosis. What might you expect her blood work to reflect?*

A. Thrombocytopenia and elevated transaminase

B. Elevated white blood cells (WBCs)

C. Decreased WBCs

D. Decreased serum globulins

18-105 *Your client, Jackson, has decreased lymphocytes. You suspect*

A. bacterial infection.

B. viral infection.

C. immunodeficiency.

D. parasitic infections.

18-106 *Your client, Ms. Jones, has an elevated platelet count. You suspect*

A. systemic lupus erythematosus.

B. infectious mononucleosis.

C. disseminated intravascular coagulation (DIC).

D. splenectomy.

18-107 *Pregnant women may be prone to thrombophilias, which may be inherited or acquired. Which of the following is an example of a factor that predisposes pregnant women to acquired thrombophilic states in pregnancy?*

A. Factor V Leiden

B. Homocystine

C. Immobilization and malignancy

D. Protein S and protein C

Answers

18-1   Answer A

The provider should always check a lead level before starting iron supplementation in children because an elevated lead level will cause anemia despite a normal iron level. Supplementation can cause iron overload. Regular milk (cow's milk) is often the cause of anemia in children; thus, a thorough diet history must be obtained. Children younger than age 1 year are usually on iron-fortified infant formulas, and when they switch to cow's milk, they do not receive sufficient iron.

18-2   Answer C

Regardless of whether the client is symptomatic or not, the Centers for Disease Control and Prevention standards call for therapy to be started when a client with HIV infection has a CD4 count less than 500 and a HIV RNA level greater than 10,000.

18-3   Answer C

Abdominal pain, pallor, and tachycardia are all manifestations of splenic sequestration. Early recognition of splenic sequestration can be a lifesaving skill. Parents can be taught to recognize signs of increasing anemia and enlarging spleen. Part of the educational plan for the parent is teaching them how to recognize increasing abdominal girth or abdominal pain, as well as how to palpate the spleen. Vomiting and diarrhea do not necessarily accompany this complication, nor does a decrease in mental acuity.

18-4   Answer C

Kaposi's sarcoma in a client younger than age 60 is considered conclusive evidence of AIDS under the Centers for Disease Control and Prevention's definition. Other disorders, with or without laboratory evidence of HIV infections that also define AIDS, include *Pneumocystis jiroveci* pneumonia; candidiasis of the esophagus, trachea, bronchi, or lungs; extrapulmonary cryptococcosis; cryptosporidiosis with persistent diarrhea; cytomegalovirus infection; herpes simplex virus infection with persistent skin lesions; *Mycobacterium avium* infection; progressive multifocal leukoencephalopathy; toxoplasmosis of the brain; and primary lymphoma of the brain in a client younger than age 60.

18-5   Answer B

Pernicious anemia is a result of the parietal cells of the stomach lining failing to secrete enough intrinsic factor to ensure intestinal absorption of vitamin B_{12}. A deficiency of folic acid in a pregnant woman can contribute to the development of neural tube defects in the fetus. It can also lead to a slowly progressive type of anemia known as megaloblastic anemia in which the red blood cells are larger than normal and deformed and have a diminished rate of production and a diminished life span. A deficiency in vitamin D interferes with use of calcium and phosphorus in bone and tooth formation and can lead to osteomalacia in adults and rickets in children. A deficiency in iron results in iron-deficiency anemia with insufficient hemoglobin; symptoms include pallor of the skin and nailbeds, fatigue, and weakness.

18-6 Answer D

A loss of DNA control over differentiation occurring in response to adverse conditions is referred to as dysplasia. Dysplastic cells show an abnormal degree of variation in size, shape, and appearance and a disturbance in the usual arrangement. An example of dysplasia is a change in the cervix in response to the human papillomavirus. Hyperplasia is an increase in the number or density of normal cells. Hyperplasia occurs in response to stress, increased metabolic demands, or elevated levels of hormones. An example of hyperplasia is the change in uterine cells in response to rising levels of estrogen during pregnancy. Metaplasia is a change in the normal pattern of differentiation such that dividing cells differentiate into cell types not normally found in that location in the body. An example of metaplasia is the replacement of normal columnar ciliated cells in the bronchial epithelium by stratified squamous cells in response to inhaled pollutants, primarily cigarette smoke. Anaplasia is the regression of a cell to an immature or undifferentiated cell type. Anaplastic cell division is no longer under DNA control. It usually occurs when a damaging or transforming event takes place inside the dividing, but still undifferentiated, cell. An example of anaplasia may be a response to an overwhelmingly destructive condition inside the cell or in the surrounding tissue.

18-7   Answer A

Burkitt's lymphoma is associated with Epstein-Barr virus. Kaposi's sarcoma is associated with human cytomegalovirus, a lymphoma is associated with the human herpesvirus 6, and adult T-cell leukemia is associated with human T-lymphotropic viruses.

18-8   Answer C

Prostate cancer is associated with the human cytomegalovirus. Carcinoma of the lip, cervical carcinoma, and Kaposi's sarcoma are all associated with herpes simplex virus types 1 and 2; lymphoma is associated with human herpesvirus 6; and adult T-cell leukemia and lymphoma, T-cell variant of hairy cell leukemia, and Kaposi's sarcoma are associated with human T-lymphotropic viruses.

18-9   Answer B

Chemotherapy drugs are genotoxic carcinogens. Carcinogens can be classified in two groups: genotoxic and promotional carcinogens. Genotoxic carcinogens directly alter DNA and cause mutations. Other examples of genotoxic carcinogens include polycyclic hydrocarbons (smoke, soot, tobacco), arsenic, and methylaminobenzene. Promotional carcinogens cause other adverse biological effects, such as hormonal imbalances, altered immunity, or chronic tissue damage. Examples include vinyl chloride polymers, asbestos, and wood and leather dust.

18-10   Answer B

Tobacco use has been linked to an increased risk for bladder, pancreatic, laryngeal, esophageal, oropharyngeal, and some types of gastric cancer. Persons who smoke pipes and cigars are especially susceptible to oropharyngeal and laryngeal cancers. Those who chew tobacco are especially susceptible to oral and esophageal cancers. Colon cancer, cervical cancer, and prostate cancer have not been linked to tobacco use.

18-11   Answer B

An endoscopic retrograde cholangiopancreatography uses an endoscope, which is inserted via the mouth and passed by the stomach and into the small intestine, where dye is injected into the pancreatic ducts and x-rays are taken to determine if any obstruction is apparent. A percutaneous transhepatic cholangiography is a procedure in which a thin needle is put into the liver through the skin on the right side of the abdomen. Dye is injected into the bile ducts to visualize any blockages. An angiography is a procedure in which x-rays are taken of the blood vessels after dye is injected. An upper gastrointestinal series is a series of x-rays of the upper digestive system taken after barium is ingested. It shows the outline of the digestive organs. All four of these procedures are used to produce pictures of the pancreas and nearby organs to assist in the diagnosis of pancreatic cancer.

18-12   Answer C

Immunotherapy is also called biological therapy. It is a form of treatment that uses the body's natural ability (immune system) to fight disease or to protect the body from adverse effects of treatment. Radiation therapy uses high-energy rays to damage cancer cells and prevent them from growing and dividing. Chemotherapy uses drugs to kill cancer cells.

18-13   Answer B

Smoking, diabetes, and a high-fat diet are risk factors for pancreatic cancer. Persons who smoke develop pancreatic cancer two to three times more often than nonsmokers. Diabetes is also a risk factor. Twice as many people with diabetes develop pancreatic cancer compared with people without diabetes. The risk of pancreatic cancer is also higher among people whose diet is high in fat and low in fruits and vegetables. Occupational exposure to petroleum and other chemicals also increases the risk of pancreatic cancer. Although a high-carbohydrate diet and lack of activity may predispose one to obesity, which may lead to diabetes, this has not been documented as a risk factor for pancreatic cancer. Yo-yo dieting is not a documented risk factor.

18-14   Answer D

Although drug trials and research and development with new drug products are important ways to work toward eradicating a disease, they do nothing for prevention. The three major approaches to cancer prevention are education, regulation, and host modification. Education reduces the cancer-causing behaviors of individuals, such as smoking. Regulations and guidelines help by prohibiting introduction of carcinogens and include methods such as encouraging nonsmoking areas, not selling cigarettes to minors, and workplace environmental guidelines. Host modification refers to increasing knowledge about cancer genetics. Health-care providers are instrumental in educating the public and sharing decisions that may be made concerning the

appropriate use of genetic testing. Colonoscopy is a screening measure aimed at detecting disease, not preventing it. The same is true of Pap smear.

18-15   Answer D

African Americans have the highest overall cancer incidence rate and the highest overall cancer mortality rate. Native Americans have the lowest overall cancer incidence and mortality rate of all of the populations in the United States. Asian and Pacific Islanders have a high rate of nasopharyngeal cancer. There is a high rate of gallbladder cancer among New Mexico Hispanics of Native American ancestry; liver cancer is more prevalent among Mexican Americans; and cervical cancer is more prevalent among women from Central and South America.

18-16   Answer C

Lymphedema may occur many years after a mastectomy (whether radical or modified) or radiation therapy on the affected side. Procedures such as venipuncture and blood pressure measurements should never be done on the affected arm because there is a greater risk for infection and compromised wound healing in that limb. About 15%–20% of women develop lymphedema after treatment for breast cancer by surgery or radiation, some not until many years later. Several interventions have been tried with lymphadenopathy, ranging from nothing to aggressive surgical procedures, and have met with limited success. Most interventions include elevation, exercises, and pneumatic compression devices.

18-17   Answer A

It is important to maintain an adequate fluid intake to prevent dehydration, which may result in vomiting; therefore, decreasing the amount of liquids in the client's diet is not an effective strategy to prevent the nausea and vomiting associated with the effects of radiation and chemotherapy. Causes of nausea and vomiting include the effects of radiation and chemotherapy, obstruction of the gastrointestinal tract by tumor growth and metastasis, other metabolic abnormalities, and stress. Nausea and vomiting should be expected and anticipatory antiemetic therapy initiated before treatment and continued around the clock after starting the cancer treatment according to the anticipated length of symptoms. It can then be used on an as-needed basis. A soft, bland diet low in fat and sugar, as well as relaxation, distraction, and guided imagery, help to reduce the adverse effects of nausea and vomiting.

18-18 Answer C

Bone pain is a common presenting symptom, most frequently manifested as low back pain or pain in the rib, and may present as a pathological fracture, especially in the femoral neck. Hypercalcemia is often present related to the leakage of calcium occurring from bone destruction. These clients are also prone to infections and fatigue. Examination may reveal pallor, bone tenderness, and soft tissue masses. Splenomegaly is absent unless amyloidosis is present. There is seldom a chronic cough. Nausea may be present related to hyperviscosity syndrome but typically not vomiting.

18-19 Answer B

Mucosal erythroplasia (red inflammatory lesions) is the earliest visual sign of oral and pharyngeal squamous cell carcinomas. Leukoplakia (thickened whitish patches on the tongue or mucous membranes) is the most common premalignant lesion, but only about 30% of people with these lesions are later found to have malignancy. Other symptoms, which typically appear after mucosal erythroplasia, include pain in the face, jaw, or ear; bleeding; stuffy nose; sore throat; loss of sensation in the tongue; difficulty chewing or swallowing; or a feeling of a mass in the mouth or throat.

18-20 Answer C

Fecal occult blood testing (FOBT) is accurate in identifying 25%–40% of colorectal cancers, specifically those in the sigmoid colon. It is less effective for identifying cancers of the right colon or transverse colon. It is not effective for identifying polyps. Persons older than age 40 should have an annual stool examination performed because this can help decrease colorectal cancer mortality rates by 33%–57%. FOBT has a false-negative and a false-positive possibility. Certain medications such as aspirin and other NSAIDs, eating red meat or raw vegetables, or bleeding hemorrhoids may cause a false-positive reading. These medications and foods should be avoided for 3 days before the administration of the test. False-negative results may occur because of polyps or the fact that some cancers do not bleed or may bleed only occasionally.

18-21 Answer C

The mean survival time for people with sickle cell disease in the United States is 42 years for men and 48 for women.

18-22 Answer A

Certainly all of the possible answer options listed may occur in clients with AIDS. However, the key word in the stem of the question is *neurological*. The neurological symptomatic triad that clients with AIDS typically experience consists of cognitive, motor, and behavioral changes. These changes are present to a greater or lesser degree in all clients with AIDS. Kaposi's sarcoma is not neurological; it is a multifocal neoplasm with vascular tumors in the skin and other organs.

18-23 Answer D

The spleen is not essential for life. When it is removed, the liver and bone marrow assume the spleen's functions. Although the bone marrow will produce and store hematopoietic stem cells, from which all cellular components of the blood are derived, it will not remove iron from old red blood cells for reuse.

18-24 Answer A

If your client has numerous petechiae, ask about the use of aspirin or aspirin compounds. Aspirin is a very effective antiplatelet agent. The recommended dosage for clients with chronic stable angina and certain other conditions is 325 mg (one tablet) per day. Many clients assume that if one tablet a day is good, two are better. Depending on the individual clotting time, even 325 mg per day may result in bleeding into the tissues. Antihypertensive agents, oral contraceptives, and anticonvulsants by themselves do not affect platelet activity.

18-25 Answer C

All infants should be screened for anemia using either hemoglobin or hematocrit testing at approximately 9 months of age. The cutoff points for a diagnosis of anemia at this age are a hemoglobin below 11 g/dL or a hematocrit below 33.0%. Cutoff points should be adjusted upward for children who live at high altitudes. You should consider repeat screening at age 3–4 years. Cutoff points for children this age are a hemoglobin of 11.2 g/dL or a hematocrit of 34.0%.

18-26   Answer A

Before the appearance of AIDS, *Pneumocystis jiroveci* pneumonia (PCP) was a rare disease that immunosuppressed persons and clients with leukemia sometimes developed. Today, PCP is usually the defining characteristic in clients with AIDS in both the United States and Europe. Cryptococcosis is a life-threatening systemic fungal infection that usually targets the central nervous system and the lungs, although it may attack anywhere. Cryptosporidiosis is a protozoal infection responsible for diarrhea in clients with AIDS. Candidiasis is the most common fungal infection, affecting 90% of all clients with AIDS, although it is common in the general population as well.

18-27   Answer C

Oral candidiasis (thrush) appears as white plaques that can be scraped off (removed), revealing an erythematous mucosal surface. Because of this, it is often referred to as a pseudomembranous lesion. Herpes simplex is an acute viral disease that causes small vesicles on the lip borders (cold sores). Leukoplakia is a disease of the mucous membranes of the cheeks, gums, or tongue with white, thickened, fissured patches that may become malignant. Flat-topped papules with thin, bluish-white spiderweb lines are lesions of lichen planus, an inflammatory pruritic benign disease of the skin and mucous membranes.

18-28   Answer B

Tests for fecal occult blood in the stools should be done on all clients suspected of having iron-deficiency anemia. In the early stages of iron-deficiency anemia, both the hemoglobin and hematocrit measures are normal to slightly reduced. It is necessary to determine whether the iron deficiency is related solely to inadequate dietary intake, decreased absorption, or chronic blood loss.

18-29   Answer A

Clients with sickle cell anemia should have their hemoglobin and hematocrit levels maintained at a level slightly below normal because this protects from some of the vaso-occlusive infarctive complications related to the viscosity characteristic of sickle cell anemia. When there is a painful sickle cell crisis, the client should be placed at rest, hydrated, given oral analgesics, and have the blood alkalinized mildly with an intravenous bicarbonate

solution. Oxygen should be given to keep the hemoglobin well oxygenated, and the amount of deoxyhemoglobin must be kept low.

18-30   Answer D

A metastatic tumor from below the diaphragm is suspected when you palpate Virchow's node in the left supraclavicular space. Virchow's node is an enlarged left supraclavicular node usually infiltrated with a metastatic tumor from below the diaphragm, especially of gastrointestinal origin. The other nodes listed do not exist. A wringer-type injury is seen in children who put their hands between the rollers of older washing machines still in use. Sims' position is a side-lying position, and Wiskott-Aldrich syndrome is a childhood immunodeficiency disease.

18-31   Answer D

An increase in immunoglobulin (Ig) E signifies atopic disorders such as allergic rhinitis, allergic asthma, atopic dermatitis, and parasitic infestation. An increase of IgG may signify bacterial infections, hepatitis A, glomerulonephritis, rheumatoid arthritis, systemic lupus erythematosus (SLE), and AIDS. An increase in IgM would occur with hepatitis A and B infections, chronic infections, SLE, rheumatoid arthritis, Sjögren's syndrome, and AIDS. An increase in IgA would occur with SLE, rheumatoid arthritis, glomerulonephritis, and chronic liver disease.

18-32   Answer C

An immune complex–mediated hypersensitivity reaction results in a skin test that produces erythema and edema within 3–8 hours. It may result from serum sickness, systemic lupus erythematosus, or rheumatoid arthritis. An anaphylactic reaction may occur with allergic rhinitis or asthma. The mediator of injury is histamine and the skin test appears as a wheal and flare. A cytotoxic reaction, such as a transfusion reaction, does not produce any reaction from a skin test. A delayed hypersensitivity (cell-mediated) reaction, such as contact dermatitis or after a tuberculosis test, produces erythema and edema within 24–48 hours.

18-33   Answer C

Palpable supraclavicular lymph nodes are not normal in infants, children, or adults. A right-sided palpable node is more commonly associated with lymphoma of the mediastinum, whereas a palpable left-sided node is more commonly associated with an abdominal malignancy. Different lymph nodes will be palpable in the presence of infectious processes such as candidiasis and cryptococcosis.

18-34 Answer B

Children receiving radiation therapy for acute lymphocytic leukemia are at an increased risk for developing a brain tumor as a secondary malignancy. This has been seen more often in children who were treated with radiation at age 5 or younger. In general, about 3%–12% of children treated for cancer will develop a new cancer within 20 years of being treated for the primary cancer.

18-35 Answer C

When clients with HIV infection have massive diarrhea, a protozoa of the *Cryptosporidium* genus is the most likely cause. The organism affects primarily the small intestine and produces massive diarrhea accompanied by nausea and fatigue. The diarrhea may exceed 4 L/day and can easily lead to dehydration and electrolyte imbalance if not treated promptly. Cryptococcosis is a fungal infection that usually appears as meningitis. Toxoplasmosis is a protozoal infection that causes encephalitis in persons with AIDS. Cytomegalovirus is a significant opportunistic infection of the herpesvirus family that can be acquired during the perinatal period, in the preschool years, or during the sexually active years.

18-36 Answer C

The term "shift to the left" or "left shift" indicates an elevated white blood count (WBC) count and a relative increase in segmented and band neutrophils. Usually seen in acute bacterial infections, it indicates clinically that the body is responding to an acute need before the neutrophils can fully mature in the bone marrow. The term originated from the Shilling hemogram, which charted the maturation of the granulocytes from the least mature (blasts) on the left to most mature (segmented neutrophils) on the right. To represent the border between the bone marrow and the circulating blood, a line was drawn between the band neutrophils and the segmented ones. When the body releases immature cells into the circulating blood, there is an increase in the cells in the circulating blood from the left of the line ("left shift"). Early hand devices for counting blood cells in a differential had the keys lined up in such a way that the technicians had to move their hand to the left to hit the keys for the more immature granulocytes.

18-37 Answer B

The Centers for Disease Control and Prevention guidelines state that if a woman infected with HIV has a normal initial Pap test, then a second evaluation should be done in 6 months to reduce the likelihood of a false-negative initial test. If the initial two Pap smears are both negative, annual Pap smears are then adequate. If severe inflammation with reactive squamous cellular change is found, another Pap smear should be done within 3 months.

18-38 Answer C

Hepatitis D (delta) virus (HDV) poses the greatest risk to a client with chronic hepatitis B (chronic HBV). Chronic HBV carriers who acquire HDV infection have a much higher incidence of cirrhosis, approaching 70%–80% compared with a 15%–30% chance of liver cirrhosis with chronic HBV alone. Modes of transmission for HDV are similar to those of HBV.

18-39 Answer A

The latex condom, when used consistently and correctly, is the preferred contraceptive method for the client infected with HIV because it provides the most effective barrier between partners. The spermicide nonoxynol-9 has not been shown to prevent viral transmission in humans, especially when used alone. Because intrauterine devices increase menstrual blood flow, they expose a woman's partner to a greater viral load. Although the effect of oral contraceptive pills on HIV transmission is not known, the estrogen and progestin can promote HIV disease progression through opportunistic infections, as well as cervical neoplasia by their immunomodulating effects.

18-40 Answer D

Prophylaxis for the first episode of *Pneumocystis jiroveci* pneumonia in an adult or adolescent client infected with HIV is trimethoprim-sulfamethoxazole (TMP-SMZ) (Bactrim) DS 1 tablet PO qd for 10 days. Clarithromycin (Biaxin) is the first choice for *Mycobacterium avium* complex infection; rifampin (Rimactane) is the first choice for combating isoniazid-resistant organisms; and isoniazid

(Nydrazid) and pyridoxine (Beesix) are the first choices for combating *Mycobacterium tuberculosis* organisms.

18-41   Answer B

Glucose-6-phosphate dehydrogenase deficiency (G6PD) is an X-linked recessive disorder commonly seen in African American men. It is an enzyme defect that causes episodic hemolytic anemia because of the decreased ability of red blood cells to deal with oxidative stresses. The other disorders listed are not X-linked. Sickle cell anemia is an autosomal recessive disorder in which an abnormal hemoglobin leads to chronic hemolytic anemia with a variety of severe clinical consequences. Pyruvate kinase deficiency is a rare autosomal recessive disorder that causes chronic hemolytic anemia, usually with the onset in childhood. Bernard-Soulier syndrome is a rare autosomal recessive intrinsic platelet disorder causing bleeding.

18-42   Answer C

Hemophilia is a classic example of an X-linked recessive disease and, as a rule, only males are affected. In rare instances, female carriers are clinically affected if their normal X chromosomes are disproportionately inactivated. Women such as Judy may also become affected if they are the offspring of a father with hemophilia and a mother who is a carrier.

18-43   Answer D

An elevated hematocrit due to contracted plasma volume, rather than increased red blood cell mass, may be due to diuretic use or may occur without obvious cause. However, the associated signs and symptoms of splenomegaly, blurred vision, fatigue, headache, and tinnitus lead you to suspect polycythemia vera. An elevated hematocrit due to contracted plasma volume is often referred to as "spurious polycythemia," and a number of conditions such as hypoxia and high altitude exposure can cause a secondary polycythemia, but splenomegaly is absent in these cases. Primary polycythemia vera is an acquired myeloproliferative disorder that causes an overproduction of all three hemapoietic cell lines. In multiple myeloma, there is a malignancy of the plasma cells, not typically characterized with an elevated hematocrit. Waldenström's macroglobulinemia is a malignant disorder of B cells that appear to be a hybrid of lymphocytes and plasma cells; these cells characteristically secrete an IgM paraprotein, and the disorder does not manifest itself with an elevated hematocrit.

18-44   Answer A

Also known as gamma globulin, immunoglobulin (Ig) G (IgG) is the most abundant Ig (75%) found in the blood, lymph, and intestines. IgG is active against bacteria, bacterial toxins, and viruses. IgA (10%–15%) is found in the blood, lymph, saliva, tears, as well as bronchial, gastrointestinal (GI), prostatic, and vaginal secretions. IgA provides local protection on exposed mucous membrane surfaces and potent antiviral activity by preventing binding of the virus to cells of the respiratory and GI tracts. IgM (5%–10%) is found in the blood and lymph and has high concentrations early in infection, decreasing within about a week. IgD (less than 1%) is found in the blood, lymph, and surfaces of B cells.

18-45   Answer B

Eosinophils are elevated in parasitic infections, hypersensitivity reactions, and autoimmune disorders. Neutrophils are increased in acute infections, the stress response, myelocytic leukemia, and inflammatory or metabolic disorders. Basophils are increased in hypersensitivity responses, chronic myelogenous leukemia, chickenpox or smallpox, after a splenectomy, and in hypothyroidism. Monocytes are increased in chronic inflammatory disorders, tuberculosis, viral infections, leukemia, Hodgkin's disease, and multiple myeloma.

18-46   Answer C

Lorie has the classic signs of iron-deficiency anemia: pale conjunctiva and nailbeds, tachycardia, heart murmur, cheilosis (reddened lips with fissures at the angles), stomatitis, splenomegaly, koilonychia (thin and concave fingernails with raised edges), glossitis, esophageal webs (Plummer-Vinson syndrome), melena, and menorrhagia. Signs of vitamin B_{12} deficiency include weakness of the extremities, ataxia, pallor, loss of vibratory and position sense, memory loss, changes in mood, and hallucinations. Signs of a folate deficiency include weakness, pallor, and glossitis, with congestive heart failure occurring if the anemia is severe. A person with chronic fatigue syndrome might have a fever, a sore throat, muscle discomfort and myalgia, and generalized headaches.

18-47   Answer D

Acquired inhibitors of coagulation are found in women who are several weeks postpartum after a normal labor and delivery, in clients with collagen vascular disease such as systemic lupus erythematosus, in older clients, and in clients with known inherited coagulation disorders, particularly factor VIII deficiency. There is no evidence that this is associated with mitral regurgitation, antibiotic usage, or as a sequela to a streptococcal infection.

18-48   Answer D

Skip has the characteristic symptoms of acute lymphoblastic leukemia. Diagnosis is made by the characteristic appearance found on a bone marrow smear. The enzyme-linked immunosorbent assay is the best test for rotavirus infection because it detects viral antigens. The monospot test is a latex agglutination test that measures production of heterophile antibodies during acute and recent episodes of Epstein-Barr virus infection. Its use is limited because of false-negative readings of 10%–20%. A prothrombin time, partial thromboplastin time, bleeding time, complete blood count, and peripheral smear are included in an initial workup of bleeding disorders.

18-49   Answer C

When a neonate is initially protected against measles, mumps, and rubella (MMR) because the mother is immune, this is an example of natural passive immunity. This type of immunity is acquired by the transfer of maternal antibodies to the fetus or neonate via the placenta or breast milk. Chickenpox and hepatitis A are examples of natural active immunity, which is acquired by infection with an antigen, resulting in the production of antibodies. MMR, polio, diphtheria, pertussis, tetanus, and hepatitis B vaccines are examples of artificial active immunity, which is acquired by immunization with an antigen, such as attenuated live virus vaccine. A gamma globulin injection following hepatitis A exposure is an example of artificial passive immunity, which is acquired by administration of antibodies or antitoxins in the immune globulin.

18-50   Answer A

Systemic lupus erythematosus (SLE) is a multisystem autoimmune disease of unknown etiology. According to the American College of Rheumatology, 4 of 11 criteria must be present at some point through the course of the disease. These include positive antinuclear antibody; malar rash; photosensitivity; renal disease; neurological disorders, especially seizures and psychosis; oral or nasal ulcers; nonerosive arthritis with inflammation; pleuritis or pericarditis; hematological disorder, specifically hemolytic anemia with reticulocytosis, leukopenia (WBC <4000 on two occasions), lymphopenia (<1500 on two occasions), or thrombocytopenia (<100,000 on two occasions); and immunological disorder, specifically anti-DNA antibody, anti-Sm antibody, and antiphospholipid antibody, including false-positive syphilis. Weight loss and night sweats are not diagnostic for SLE.

18-51   Answer B

One of the most commonly used staging systems to label the extent of a cancer is the TNM staging system. The T is for primary tumor, N is for regional lymph nodes, and M is for distant metastasis. In an example of colorectal cancer, a person classified as T1N1M0 would have a tumor that invaded the submucosa, metastasis in one to three pericolic or perirectal lymph nodes, but no distant metastasis.

18-52   Answer D

There are no generally accepted guidelines for the prevention or early detection of bladder cancer. The first problem is usually gross hematuria, followed by dysuria, frequency or urgency, and symptoms of urethral obstruction. Bladder cancer comprises approximately 4%–5% of all cancers in the United States. It is three times more common in men than women and two times more common in whites than blacks. Smoking should be discouraged and exposure to certain chemicals used in the textile and rubber industries eliminated. There is no bladder tumor marker, and annual cystoscopies are not recommended.

18-53   Answer B

A chondrosarcoma arises from cartilage and is usually located in the pelvis, femur, proximal humerus, or ribs. It is the second most common bone malignancy, seen most frequently in men between ages 30 and 60. An osteosarcoma is the most common primary bone-forming tumor, usually affecting children and young adults. It arises from osteoblast cells that multiply rapidly during periods of skeletal growth. More common in men, osteosarcomas are usually located around the knee joint, with the proximal humerus also being a common site. Ewing's sarcoma is a marrow-originating tumor consisting of small round cells. It is seen primarily in male children and adolescents. It arises most commonly in the diaphysis of long bones and in flat bones. A fibrosarcoma is a rare type of bone tumor that consists of interlacing bundles of collagen cells. It is more common in men from ages 20–60 and is commonly found in the femur and tibia.

18-54   Answer A

Alpha-fetoprotein levels may be elevated with embryonal cell tumors of the ovary or testis, hepatocellular carcinoma, and choriocarcinoma. Carcinoembryonic antigen detects colon, rectal, pancreatic, stomach, lung, breast, and ovarian tumors. Human chorionic gonadotropin detects choriocarcinoma, germ cell carcinoma, testicular teratoma, and hydatidiform moles. CA 125 is the tumor marker for epithelial ovarian neoplasms and breast and colorectal malignancies.

18-55   Answer B

The erythrocyte sedimentation rate (ESR) is a very nonspecific indicator of inflammation and is often elevated in inflammatory musculoskeletal conditions; it is not, however, diagnostic for rheumatoid arthritis. Additionally, anemia can cause an increased ESR. As people age, their "normal" sedimentation rate increases.

18-56   Answer C

Stage IV in the Rai classification system for chronic lymphatic leukemia (CLL) is the stage of thrombocytopenia where the life expectancy may be only 2 years. CLL is the only leukemia in which a staging system is commonly used because CLL has prognostic implications. A client with only an absolute lymphocytosis (Rai stage 0) may live 7–10 years or more. In the Rai classification system, stage 0 indicates a lymphocyte count greater than 10,000 mm^3, stage I indicates enlarged lymph nodes, stage II indicates an enlarged liver and/or spleen, stage III indicates anemia, and stage IV indicates thrombocytopenia.

18-57   Answer C

Before initiating cancer therapy, the first crucial step is to confirm the diagnosis using tissue biopsy. This sounds simplistic, but some practitioners "diagnose" unconfirmed cancer that cannot then be

effectively treated. The next step is to stage the disease using appropriate diagnostic means. The stage or the extent of the disease determines the prognosis and treatment. The third step is to define the goals of therapy—whether it is curative, adjuvant, or palliative—because that will influence the extent and aggressiveness of treatment. The last step before initiating therapy is to choose a treatment plan from the many therapeutic options, depending on many different client characteristics such as age, goals, wishes of the client and family, and extent of the cancer.

18-58   Answer D

Cancers with macroscopic disease that can be cured with chemotherapy include testicular and ovarian cancer and Hodgkin's disease. Bladder and breast cancers are cancers with microscopic disease that can be cured with adjuvant chemotherapy. A malignant melanoma has a low response rate or can be unresponsive to chemotherapy.

18-59   Answer A

Generalized lymphadenopathy is usually indicative of disseminated malignancy, usually hematological in nature (such as lymphoma or leukemia), collagen vascular disease, or an infectious process such as mononucleosis, syphilis, cytomegalovirus, tuberculosis, AIDS, toxoplasmosis, to name some examples.

18-60   Answer B

Pain that is poorly controlled with opioids and NSAIDs is often neuropathic in nature, meaning that it is a result of direct nerve injury, such as nerve compression. This pain may be controlled with anticonvulsants, tricyclic antidepressants, and corticosteroids. Corticosteroids may also be effective for severe bone pain. SSRIs have not had the proven results with neuropathic pain that tricyclics have, although they may prove effective in clients with cancer in general. Benzodiazepines are not usually recommended because of their sedativelike effects. The goal with cancer clients who experience chronic pain is to provide adequate pain control while keeping the client awake and able to interact with those around them and maintain as normal a life as possible.

18-61   Answer C

Clients with hepatitis A should have separate eating and drinking utensils or use disposable ones.

Most clients can be cared for at home without undue risk; strict isolation is not necessary. There is no specific medicine to treat hepatitis A.

18-62   Answer B

Smoking decreases vitamin C absorption, which is necessary for folic acid absorption. Smoking increases vitamin requirements. Clients with a folic acid deficiency should be encouraged to eat foods that are high in folic acid (asparagus spears, beef liver, broccoli, mushrooms, oatmeal, peanut butter, and red beans) daily because the liver can store folic acid for a limited time only.

18-63   Answer B

Pernicious anemia is caused by an inadequate absorption of vitamin B_{12}. The symptoms of pernicious anemia develop slowly and subtly and may not be recognized right away. In contrast, hemolytic anemias caused by the premature destruction of red blood cells (hemolysis) occur when the bone marrow cannot produce red blood cells fast enough to compensate for those being destroyed. These anemias can be acquired or congenital. Inherited conditions include hereditary spherocytosis, glucose-6-phosphate dehydrogenase deficiency, sickle cell anemia, and thalassemia.

18-64   Answer A

Smoking is not one of the risk factors for iron-deficiency anemia. The risk for iron-deficiency anemia increases in persons older than age 60; those who live in poverty; and those with a recent illness, such as an ulcer, diverticulitis, colitis, hemorrhoids, or gastrointestinal tumors. Iron supplements should be taken.

18-65   Answer B

The hemoglobin S gene is carried by approximately 8% of American blacks, and 1 birth in 400 in American blacks will produce a child with sickle cell. Prenatal diagnosis is now available for couples at risk of producing a child with sickle cell. DNA from fetal cells can be examined, and the presence of the sickle cell mutation can be accurately and definitively diagnosed. Genetic counseling should be made available to such couples.

18-66   Answer C

A serum measurement of ferritin, the body's iron-storing protein, can tell exactly how much iron is on hand in the body. It is the best way to spot an iron deficiency early before it progresses to full-blown anemia. If the ferritin level is borderline, a dietary and supplemental regimen of iron will rebuild the iron stores. Hemoglobin is the iron-containing pigment of the red blood cells that carries oxygen from the lungs to the tissues. Hematocrit is the volume of erythrocytes packed in a given volume of blood. The hemoglobin and hematocrit values give the values only at a given time, without regard for the body's stores. Reticulocytes are the last immature stage of red blood cells.

18-67   Answer C

Antibody testing may be ordered to determine whether a client has developed antibodies in response to an infection, such as hepatitis, or immunization. Antibody titers evaluate antibody-mediated responses. Serum protein is a measurement of the total protein in the blood. Albumin is a protein primarily responsible for the osmotic pressure of the blood. Globulins account for the majority of remaining serum protein. Globulins include all of the immunoglobulins and the antibodies they contain. Decreased globulin levels are noted with immunological deficiencies. Protein electrophoresis further breaks down globulin into its specific components. Analysis of specific levels of each provides cues about the immune status of the client.

18-68   Answer D

The reticulocyte count indicates the percentage of newly maturing red blood cells released into the circulating blood from the bone marrow. As the red blood cell (RBC) matures, it loses its endothelial reticulum. The reticulocyte count is elevated in cases of blood loss, as the body tries to replace the loss; it might also be elevated during treatment of anemias (e.g., iron, folic acid, Vitamin B_{12}), and bone marrow disorders, when immature RBCs are displaced by other proliferating cells. It is decreased in aplastic anemia because the bone marrow has shut down all production of cells; it is also decreased in poisonings and disorders of red blood cell maturation such as iron-deficiency anemias.

18-69   Answer C

The primary reason for newborn screening for sickle cell disease is to allow the prevention of septicemia with prophylactic medication (penicillin) and prompt clinical intervention for infection and future crises. Early detection will not prevent future crises.

Although providing information to the parents will allow them to make future decisions and have the benefit of possible genetic testing, as well as testing siblings, this is not the primary reason for early screening.

18-70   Answer B

One "pack" of platelets should raise the count by 5000–8000 mm³. One pack equals about 50 mL. A "6-pack" refers to a pool of platelets from six units of blood. Platelets may be given for decreased production of or destruction of platelets, such as occurs in aplastic anemia, acute leukemia, or after chemotherapy.

18-71   Answer A

An isograft is a transplant in which the donor and recipient are identical twins. An autograft is a transplant of the client's own tissue; it is the most successful type of tissue transplant. An allograft is a graft between members of the same species, but who have different genotypes and, in the case of humans, human leukocyte antigens. A xenograft is a transplant from an animal species to a human, such as pigskin used as a temporary covering after a massive burn.

18-72   Answer A

Sjögren's syndrome is a multisystem autoimmune disease characterized by dysfunction of the exocrine glands, specifically notable for dry eyes and dry mouth. Thus, treatment is aimed at increasing comfort and lubrication. Artificial tears can be self-administered as needed; preservative-free products are usually better tolerated. For dry mouth, increasing hydration and chewing sugarless gum may be helpful. Rinsing frequently with mouthwash, which contains alcohol, can prove more drying. Oral pilocarpine (Salagen), 5 mg qid, and cevimelene (Evoxac), 30 mg tid, have been shown to increase saliva production. Drinking milk is not recommended. Frequent removal of earwax is irrelevant to this problem.

18-73   Answer C

The first choice of therapy for a client who is HIV positive and has oral candidiasis would be clotrimazole troches (10 mg) five times daily or nystatin (Mycostatin) suspension 500,000–1,000,000 units three to five times daily. Because of the common recurrence of oral candidiasis and increased rates of

drug resistance, systemic fungicides, such as fluconazole, ketoconazole, and griseofulvin, should be reserved for severe cases, such as esophageal candidiasis and clients with dysphagia. Clotrimazole troches and nystatin suspension are the only nonsystemic medications listed.

18-74   Answer A

A fever of unknown origin (FUO) in clients with HIV is defined as temperature >101 on multiple occasions over 4 weeks' duration in an outpatient and 3 weeks' duration in an inpatient, with an uncertain diagnosis after three appropriate investigations of cultures and the like. Common causes of FUO of clients with HIV include drug fever, tuberculosis, sinusitis, cryptococcosis, lymphoma, histoplasmosis, PCP, disseminated cytomegalovirus, esophageal candidiasis, and disseminated *Mycobacterium avium*–intracellular complex. Upper respiratory infection will either resolve and/or become something more severe; likewise, a urinary tract infection has more specific, identifiable, and treatable symptoms. Although the cause of FUO may in some cases never be identified, it is not merely a systemic manifestation of disease but more likely has a specific cause.

18-75   Answer B

The most common signs and symptoms of primary HIV infection and their frequency are fever (95%), fatigue (90%), and pharyngitis (70%).

18-76   Answer C

The classic signs and symptoms of cytomegalovirus infection include cotton-wool spots ("cottage cheese and ketchup" appearance), hemorrhage, and exudates on funduscopic examination. Decreased peripheral vision, blurriness, and partial blindness are other clinical manifestations. Referral to an ophthalmologist is imperative. Cryptococcosis is a systemic fungus infection that may involve any organ of the body, including the lungs or skin, but it has a marked predilection for the brain and its meninges. In the cerebral type, headache, dizziness, vertigo, and stiffness of the neck muscles are present. Toxoplasmosis produces symptoms that may be so mild as to be barely noticeable or may be more severe and include lymphadenopathy, malaise, muscle pain, or little, if any, fever. It may result in brain deterioration. Herpes simplex is characterized by thin-walled vesicles that tend to recur in the same area, usually at a site where the mucous membrane joins the skin; however, they may be limited to the gingiva, oropharynx, or conjunctiva.

18-77   Answer C

The "gold standard" for definitive diagnosis of sickle cell anemia is a hemoglobin electrophoresis, a test that determines the presence of hemoglobin S. The client with sickle cell anemia has a decreased hematocrit level, as well as sickled cells on the smear. The baseline reticulocyte count is markedly elevated in sickle cell anemia but that is not specific to that condition. The sickle cell test is a screening test. A peripheral blood smear is used for red cell morphology. Additional testing is always required to define the hemoglobin phenotype.

18-78   Answer C

At 6 months of age, Jimmy should be immunized with diphtheria, tetanus, and pertussis (DTP); *Haemophilus influenzae* type b (HIB); hepatitis B (HBV); and poliomyelitis vaccines. Children with sickle cell disease should receive all the standard well-baby care, but in addition to the standard immunizations, they should receive the pneumococcal vaccine at age 2 years. There is no cure for this disease. Children should be treated like other children and their activities should not be limited unless they are experiencing a painful sickle cell crisis.

18-79   Answer D

Clients with sickle cell anemia should be given folic acid 1 mg PO daily. Genetic counseling, not early sterilization, is recommended for all clients with sickle cell disease; there is no routine risk in the use of oral contraceptives by women with the disease.

18-80   Answer C

Certain precautions must be taken for infants with sickle cell disease to prevent vaso-occlusive crisis. Any activity or situation that would cause dehydration should be avoided. An example is sitting in a stroller in the heat for any length of time. Children with the disease should always have access to fluids. Exposure to cold temperatures slows the circulation and can cause sickling, as can any activity that can lead to hypoxia. Immunization for Hepatitis B should be done. The infant can be taken to visit relatives, although some care should be taken to avoid exposure to children and adults with upper respiratory infections (URIs).

18-81   Answer B

Pernicious anemia is a macrocytic anemia marked by achlohydria. The parietal cells of the stomach fail to secrete enough intrinsic factor to ensure intestinal absorption of vitamin B_{12}, the extrinsic factor. This leads to a deficiency of B_{12}. Folic acid deficiency also causes a macrocytic anemia, but the B_{12} levels are normal and there are not the associated neurological symptoms seen in pernicious anemia. Vitamin D is not essential for the absorption of vitamin B_{12}. A deficiency of iron results in iron-deficiency anemia, a microcytic hypochromic anemia.

18-82   Answer D

The Schilling test is performed by giving a small, radioactive tracer dose of cyanocobalamin (about 0.5–2 mg) by mouth and then collecting and assaying a 24-hour urine sample for radioactivity. This is diagnostic of cobalamin deficiency (vitamin B_{12} deficiency). Coombs' tests ascertain the presence or absence of immunoglobulin and complement in the coating of red blood cells. The tests (direct and indirect) can differentiate between various types of hemolytic anemias; determine minor blood types, including the Rh factor; and test for erythroblastosis fetalis. The oligonucleotide probe test is a method used to diagnose antenatal thalassemia. Spherocytes are round, rather than discoid, cells.

18-83   Answer C

Sandra's symptoms indicate anemia, which is probably caused by a poor diet. She probably has an iron and folic acid deficiency. You should order iron, folic acid, and other supplements and tell her that for better absorption, she should take the iron supplement 1 hour before eating or between meals. You should also suggest that she eat foods high in vitamin C, such as citrus fruits and fresh, raw vegetables, because vitamin C makes iron absorption more efficient. Iron also will turn bowel movements black and often cause constipation, so you may want to discuss this with Sandra.

18-84   Answer D

Steroid hormones (androgens, such as fluoxymesterone [Halotestin]; estrogens, such as ethinyl estradiol [Estinyl]; and progestins, such as megestrol acetate [Megace]), are useful in cancer chemotherapy because they alter the host environment for cell growth. Antibiotics, such as doxorubicin (Adriamycin) and bleomycin (Blenoxane), interfere with DNA or RNA synthesis depending on the drug. Alkylating agents, such as chlorambucil (Leukeran) and melphalan (Alkeran), interfere with DNA replication by attacking DNA synthesis throughout the cell cycle. Other agents, such as asparaginase (Elspar) and cisplatin (Platinol), inhibit protein synthesis.

18-85   Answer C

Growth complications depend on the direct damage to the endocrine tissue. Children with acute lymphocytic leukemia, brain tumors, nasopharyngeal cancers, and orbital tumors who have received radiation therapy are at the highest risk. Approximately 50%–90% of these children will have some evidence of growth hormone deficiency. They may benefit from growth hormone therapy. Spinal radiation inhibits the vertebral body growth. Chemotherapy may result in a decrease in linear growth, but usually the child catches up when the chemotherapy is discontinued. Assuring the mother that "everything will be OK" is always a poor choice, as is negating her concern by saying "Let's worry about the cancer first, then see what happens."

18-86   Answer B

A platelet count less than 150,000/mm3 may indicate hypersplenism, as well as possible bone marrow failure or accelerated consumption of platelets. A count greater than 350,000/mm3 may indicate possible hemorrhage, polycythemia vera, or malignancy.

18-87   Answer D

A folic acid and/or vitamin B_{12} deficiency causes macrocytic normochromic anemias in which the cell size is large and irregular. Acute blood loss and most hemolytic processes cause normocytic normochromic anemias in which the cell size is normal. Infections or tumor may cause an anemia of chronic disease that produces a normocytic red blood cell. Iron-deficiency anemias are hypochromic microcytic and may result from dietary insufficiencies, as well as acute blood loss.

18-88   Answer C

Thalassemia is caused by a decreased synthesis of hemoglobin and malformation of red blood cells (RBCs) that increases their hemolysis (increased destruction of RBCs). It is an inherited disorder that

occurs primarily in Asians or persons of Mediterranean ancestry. Aplastic anemia is a depression or cessation of all blood-forming elements. An acquired hemolytic disorder is most often drug induced or autoimmune; in such cases antibodies that cause premature destruction of RBCs are produced.

18-89   Answer C

Chronic lymphocytic leukemia (CLL) has an insidious onset with weakness, fatigue, massive lymphadenopathy, pruritic vesicular skin lesions, anemia, and thrombocytopenia. Acute lymphocytic leukemia (ALL) produces fever, respiratory infections, anemia, bleeding mucous membranes, lymphadenopathy, fatigue and weakness, and a tendency to infection. Acute myelogenous leukemia has the same symptoms as ALL but less lymphadenopathy. Chronic myelogenous leukemia produces weakness, fatigue, anorexia, weight loss, splenomegaly, anemia, thrombocytopenia, and fever and can have a fulminant stage.

18-90   Answer A

Older adults have a change in their immunoglobulin (Ig) balance and a marked increase in IgA and IgG antibodies. Other physiological changes in the immune systems of older adults include a low rate of T-lymphocyte proliferation in response to a stimulus, a decrease in the number of cytotoxic (killer) T cells, and a decrease in the relative production of CD4 (T4 or helper T cells) and CD8, affecting regulation of the immune system.

18-91   Answer D

Alcohol acts as a promoter by modifying the metabolism of carcinogens in the esophagus and liver, thereby increasing the effectiveness of the carcinogens in some tissues. Because Shelley smoked cigarettes and drank alcohol, she has an increased risk for oral, esophageal, and laryngeal cancers.

18-92   Answer C

Persons who are obese have an increased risk of hormone-dependent cancers because of their excessive body fat. Because sex hormones are synthesized from fat, these people have excessive amounts of the hormones that feed hormone-dependent malignancies such as cancer of the breast, bowel, ovary, endometrium, and prostate.

18-93   Answer B

Although anyone can get skin cancer, older adults have an increased risk because of decreased pigment in their skin. People of northern European ancestry with very fair skin, blue or green eyes, and light-colored hair seem to be the most vulnerable to skin cancer, but it is a problem for all people.

18-94   Answer A

A leiomyoma is a benign neoplasm of the smooth muscle. An osteosarcoma is a malignant neoplasm of the bone tissue, a glioma is a malignant neoplasm of the neuroglia cells, and a seminoma is a malignant tumor of the germ cells of the ectoderm and endoderm.

18-95   Answer C

Carcinoembryonic antigen is a tumor marker for adenocarcinomas of the colon, lung, breast, ovary, stomach, and pancreas. Prostate-specific antigen (PSA) is the tumor marker for adenocarcinoma of the prostate; calcitonin is the tumor marker for a medullary cancer of the thyroid; and an immunoglobulin test will detect a multiple myeloma.

18-96   Answer C

Radiation therapy consists of delivering ionizing radiations of gamma and x-rays in one of two ways. In brachytherapy radioactive material is placed directly into a tumor site and delivers a high dose to the tumor and a lower dose to the normal surrounding tissues. It is also referred to as internal, interstitial, or intracavitary radiation. Teletherapy is external radiation that involves placing the source of radiation at a distance from the client and delivering a relatively uniform dosage. Radiotherapy is another name for radiation therapy. Ionization involves the passage of radioactive particles.

18-97   Answer B

In the American Cancer Society's CAUTION model to help individuals be alert to many cancers, the N is for a nagging cough or hoarseness. The C is for change in bowel or bladder habits, the A for a sore that does not heal, the U for unusual bleeding or discharge, the T for thickening or lump in the breast or elsewhere, the I for indigestion or difficulty in swallowing, the O for obvious change in wart or mole, and the N for nagging cough or hoarseness.

18-98   Answer D

With the loss of a body part, there is an initial stage of shock and denial. It is a protective mechanism and should be neither challenged nor promoted. The best response to Nancy, who refuses to look at her mastectomy scar, would be to say: "You have to accept this eventually; just glance at it today." Then every day she could spend a little more time looking at it until she is able to care for the wound herself. Saying, "You'll look at it when you're ready" may mean that she'll never be ready. She should not be forced, but you should take a matter-of-fact approach with an empathetic attitude that will assist in her eventual acceptance of the change in body image. Practitioners should always avoid saying "Everything's going to be OK" because sometimes it is not.

18-99   Answer D

Identified risk factors for hepatitis C (HCV) are intravenous drug use and, to some extent, unsafe sexual behaviors. Previously associated with transfusions before 1990 and with dialysis, the proportion of the population with these risk factors is now less common. High-risk sexual behaviors, particularly sex with someone infected with HCV, and the use of illegal drugs such as cocaine or marijuana have also been associated with increased risk. Lactose intolerance, a history of mononucleosis, and a history of sore throats and frequent upper respiratory infections are not documented risk factors for HCV.

18-100   Answer C

The most significant reason why alcohol use is discouraged in persons with HIV infections or AIDS is that alcohol decreases the ability of persons to adhere to a prescribed medical regimen. Current treatment regimens involve complex pharmacological schedules with accurate dosing, strict compliance, and regular checkups that are crucial to the success of the treatment and prevention of complications. Alcohol calories are empty and also fill up the person so that he or she may not eat important, essential food. If the client does have liver disease (which may have been caused by alcohol), it may be aggravated by the potentially hepatotoxic effects of various drugs that are commonly used.

18-101   Answer C

Routine ordering of a complete blood count (CBC) is not indicated in asymptomatic adults; it should be ordered only when a specific condition is suspected, such as an infection or a hematological disorder. Hemoglobin or hematocrit determination is recommended in pregnant women and high-risk infants, but not necessarily a CBC. There are no current recommendations for healthy adults to have a CBC as part of a routine preadmission or preoperative physical examination if little or no blood loss is anticipated, as is the case in most dental procedures.

18-102   Answer D

MCV indicates the average size of individual RBCs. Normal range, also referred to as normocytic, is 76–96 femtoliters. The MCV is increased (macrocytic) in megaloblastic anemias (vitamin B_{12} deficiency, folate deficiency), liver disease (alcohol abuse), and some drugs (e.g., zidvudine). The MCV is decreased (microcytic) in iron-deficiency anemia, defects in porphyrin synthesis (lead poisoning), and hemolytic anemias.

18-103   Answer D

A decreased MCV and MCHC is indicative of a microcytic, hypochromic anemia. To make a more final diagnosis, you need to order both a serum iron and total iron binding capacity (TIBC) level and a serum ferritin level. You would order a folate level if you had an elevated MCV and a normal MCHC, indicative of macrocytic anemia.

18-104   Answer A

Infectious mononucleosis is a lymphocytic leukocytosis that may be confused with leukemia and other disorders. The presence of heterophile antibodies (monospot test) in the context of appropriate clinical and hematological findings is diagnostic; false-positive reactions are rare. Atypical lymphocytes usually account for more than 10% of the leukocytes in the peripheral blood smear. Detection of viral capsid antigen antibody IgM (elevated) is the most accurate test confirming acute infection. White blood count may be high, normal, or low; a relative and absolute neutropenia is present in many clients. Thrombocytopenia is common, and an elevated transaminase in most clients is related to hepatic involvement.

18-105   Answer C

A decrease in lymphocytes would be most consistent with immunodeficiency disorders, long-term corticosteroid therapy, or debilitating diseases such as Hodgkin's lymphoma or lupus erythematosus. Lymphocytes are increased primarily in viral infections (hepatitis, infectious mononucleosis, CMV, herpes zoster) and only occasionally in bacterial infections (pertussis, brucellosis). Eosinophils are elevated in parasitic infections such as malaria, trichinosis, and ascariasis.

18-106   Answer D

Increased platelet count is seen in myeloproliferative leukemias, polycythemia vera, and status postsplenectomy. Platelets are decreased in coagulation disorders such as disseminated intravascular coagulation (DIC), septicemia, and eclampsia; increased destruction of platelets is seen in idiopathic thrombocytopenic purpura, systemic lupus erythematosus (SLE), and infectious mononucleosis; and decreased production of platelets is seen in aplastic anemia, most leukemias, and secondary to radiation and chemotherapy.

18-107   Answer C

Risk factors for the development of acquired thrombophilias in pregnancy include immobilization, an underlying malignancy, trauma, high estrogen levels, nephrotic syndrome, CHF and atrial fibrillation, postoperative states, and pregnancy and postpartum periods. Factor V Leiden, homocystine, protein C, and protein S are all examples of inherited thrombophilias.

Bibliography

Cheng, A, and Zaas, A: *The Osler Medical Handbook.* Mosby, Philadelphia, 2003.

Dambro, MR: *Griffith's 5-Minute Consult.* Lippincott Williams & Wilkins, Philadelphia, 2008.

Dunphy, LM, et al: *Primary Care: The Art and Science of Advanced Practice Nursing,* ed 2. FA Davis, Philadelphia, 2007.

Gates, RA, and Fink, RM: *Oncology Nursing Secrets.* Hanley & Belfus, Philadelphia, 2002.

Goolsby, MJ: *Nurse Practitioner Secrets.* Hanley & Belfus, Philadelphia, 2002.

Goolsby MJ, and Grubbs, L: *Advanced Assessment: Interpreting Findings and Formulating Differential Diagnoses.* FA Davis, Philadelphia, 2006.

Hay, WW, et al: *Current Pediatric Diagnosis and Treatment.* Appleton & Lange, Stamford, CT, 2008.

Lin, TL, and Rypkema, SW: *The Washington Manual of Ambulatory Therapeutics*. Lippincott Williams & Wilkins, Philadelphia, 2008.

Mangione, S: *Physical Diagnosis Secrets*. Hanley & Belfus, Philadelphia, 2000.

Samir, SP, and Isa-Pratt, S: *Clinician's Guide to Laboratory Medicine: A Practical Approach*. Lexi-Comp, Hudson, OH, 2000.

Speicher, CE: *The Right Test: A Physician's Guide to Laboratory Medicine*, ed 4. WB Saunders, Philadelphia, 2007.

Swartz, MH: *Textbook of Physical Diagnoses: History and Examination*, ed 6. Saunders/Elsevier, Philadelphia, 2006.

Swartz, MN: Use of antimicrobial agents and drug resistance. *New England Journal of Medicine* 337:7, 1997.

Tallia, AF, et al: *Swanson's Family Practice Review*, ed 4. Mosby, St. Louis, 2001.

Taylor, RB: *Manual of Family Practice*, ed 2. Little, Brown, Boston, 2002.

Tierney, LM, McPhee, SJ, and Papadakis, MA (eds): *2008 eCurrent Medical Diagnosis and Treatment (CMDT)*, ed 47. Lange Medical Books/ McGraw Hill, New York, 2008.

Varricchio, C (ed): *A Cancer Source Book for Nurses*. American Cancer Society/Jones and Bartlett, Sudbury, MA, 2003.

Weber, J, and Kelley, J: ed 3. Lippincott Williams & Wilkins, Philadelphia, 2007.

How well did you do?

85% and above, congratulations! This score shows application of test-taking principles and adequate content knowledge.

75%–85%, keep working! Review test-taking principles and try again.

65%–75%, hang in there! Spend some time reviewing concepts and test-taking principles and try the test again.

ISSUES IN PRIMARY CARE

Chapter 19: *Issues in Primary Care*

LYNNE M. DUNPHY
JILL E. WINLAND-BROWN

Questions

19-1 *Strategies for developing cultural competence include which of the following?*

A. Disregarding folk beliefs because they are not scientific

B. Learning basic words and sentences in the client's language

C. Explaining the pathophysiology of the disease process to the client so that he or she understands what is happening to him or her

D. Explaining your cultural beliefs to the client

19-2 *Which of the following is the best method for evaluating the efficacy of a new clinical intervention?*

A. A case report

B. A descriptive study

C. A randomized, controlled clinical trial

D. A correlational study

19-3 *Mr. Jones, age 44, is admitted to the emergency room (ER) complaining of chest pain. Which of the following actions would be the best way to establish a therapeutic relationship with Mr. Jones?*

A. Ask several quick and specific questions in rapid succession to establish the exact nature of this emergent clinical situation.

B. Ask open-ended questions to elicit pertinent clinical data.

C. Reassure the client that he is in good hands in a well-equipped ER and that all will be OK.

D. Ask the client about his anxiety level.

19-4 *According to the health belief model, motivation, or readiness to act, is determined by which of the following components?*

A. Perceived threat, efficacy, benefits of action, and perceived barriers to action

B. Education and positive reinforcement

C. Predisposing factors, reinforcing factors, and enabling factors

D. Self-efficacy theory and perceived ability to act

19-5 *Which of the following statements is accurate regarding primary care?*

A. The purpose of primary care is to provide and coordinate referrals.

B. Primary care provides integrated and accessible health-care services.

C. Primary care uses a focus group methodology to assess community needs and plan care.

D. Primary care is only for those who cannot afford specialty care.

19-6 *There are a number of barriers to full implementation of an autonomous role for advanced-practice registered nurses (APRNs) in primary care. Major barriers are*

A. the need for medical specialists because of rapidly changing technologies.

B. the increasingly complex health problems of vulnerable populations.

C. prescriptive authority, scope of practice, and reimbursement.

D. managed care organizations' views of APRNs.

19-7 *Health behaviors can be difficult to change. Which of the following is most important in influencing behavioral change?*

A. Motivation

B. Health beliefs

C. Cognitive knowledge

D. Social supports

19-8 *The marketing process is guided by a number of factors. These include*

A. the prospective pool of clients.

B. your advertising budget and what you have to offer.

C. cost, benefit, and barriers.

D. product, price, place, and promotion.

19-9 *Your Native American client is convinced that her illness has been caused by the ill will of a fellow tribeswoman. Her description of her illness is an example of her*

A. explanatory reasoning.

B. lack of understanding of scientific medicine.

C. delusional ideation.

D. cultural bias.

19-10 *Which of the following statements related to statistical techniques and their usage in research is true?*

A. Statistical significance and clinical significance are the same.

B. If a journal article you are writing is required to be limited in length, you should delete the descriptive statistics and keep the inferential statistics.

C. Correlational coefficients infer causality.

D. To determine the appropriate statistical test to use, consider sample size, level of measurement, and data type.

19-11 *To reinforce client teaching, a useful strategy is to*

A. be a role model.

B. have repeated discussions of the need for behavioral change.

C. provide additional written materials.

D. quiz the client periodically while monitoring the client's progress.

19-12 *Concrete strategies used to keep your client's attention as you institute client education include*

A. providing the education session immediately after lunch.

B. going over the materials more than once.

C. translating theoretical information into practical terms.

D. using repetition.

19-13 *The levels of evaluation and management (E/M) services are based on which types of histories?*

A. Medical-surgical

B. Psychosocial

C. Expanded problem focused

D. Preoperative

19-14 *A comprehensive history includes which of the following elements?*

A. Chief complaint; review of systems; history of present illness; and past, family, and social history

B. Chief complaint, psychosocial assessment, and risk factor analysis

C. History of present illness, immunizations, and exposure to chemicals

D. Coping mechanisms, social support, and review of systems

19-15 *The primary nursing responsibility during a crisis situation is to*

A. provide for psychotherapeutic intervention.

B. refer.

C. establish a therapeutic relationship.

D. encourage hospitalization.

19-16 *The stages of grief include*

A. shock, reality, and recovery.

B. awareness and resolution.

C. numbness, loss, and reawakening.

D. pain and loss.

19-17 *Some sources suggest that you create a marketing portfolio with documents that support what you have to offer as an APRN or nurse practitioner. These documents include*

A. your personal mission statement.

B. your scores on the certification examination or your college transcript.

C. the state nurse practice act and regulations, prescriptive authority legislation, third-party reimbursement rules and regulations, and practice protocols.

D. letters of reference.

19-18 *According to standards of care and legal prescribing, which of the following questions must you ask each client before prescribing any medication?*

A. Are you breastfeeding? Are you allergic to any medications? Are you pregnant? Have you taken this medication before? Do you have kidney or liver problems? What other medications are you taking? What medical problems do you have?

B. Are you allergic to any medications?

C. What other medications are you on?

D. Have you taken this medication before?

19-19 *Schedule IV drugs include which of the following?*

A. Morphine, codeine, fentanyl, and hydromorphone

B. Depressants such as alprazolam, clonazepam, diazepam, and flurazepam

C. Amphetamines and pentobarbital

D. Methaqualone

19-20 *Which of the following are ways one may run the risk of breaching client confidentiality?*

A. Leaving a client's record within view

B. Discussing the client with the consulting surgeon

C. Shredding duplicate records

D. Confirming the client's diagnosis over the telephone with a pharmacist

19-21 *The primary purpose of professional licensure is to*

A. protect the public by ensuring a minimum standard for competency.

B. ensure high nursing care standards.

C. standardize nursing programs.

D. grant prescriptive privileges.

19-22 *The primary purpose of certification is to*

A. document excellence and specialization.

B. regulate advanced-practice nursing.

C. enable the practitioner to obtain third-party reimbursement.

D. assure the public that an individual has a special set of skills.

19-23 *Legal authority for advanced-practice nursing rests with*

A. the Health Care Financing Administration.

B. federal statutes.

C. state laws and regulations.

D. certifying bodies.

19-24 *Credentialing means that*

A. an individual is permitted to practice advanced-practice nursing.

B. the practitioner has met certain criteria through licensure, certification, and education.

C. an individual has completed a program of study.

D. an individual has prescriptive authority.

19-25 *What factors primarily determine the ability of an APRN to obtain clinical privileges in an institution?*

A. The desires of the collaborating physician

B. Education, certification, and continuing education credits

C. Institutional policy, medical staff bylaws, state law, and Joint Commission on Accreditation of Healthcare Organizations (JCAHO) accreditation standards

D. Reimbursement and prescriptive privileges

19-26 *Goals and objectives for* Healthy People 2010 *include*

A. improving access to health care for all Americans, increasing the life span for all Americans, and mandatory emergency care.

B. instituting a nationalized health insurance plan.

C. reducing disparities in health care, increasing healthy life span, and increasing access to health care for all Americans.

D. preserving choice of provider and health-care plans for all Americans.

19-27 *"Indemnity insurer" refers to an insurer*

A. in a health maintenance organization.

B. in a preferred provider organization.

C. that pays for the medical care of the insured but does not provide that care.

D. that pays using a fee-for-service plan.

19-28 *"Usual and customary" refers to*

A. an insurance term for how a charge compares with charges made to other persons receiving similar services and supplies.

B. how an insurer evaluates the need for an ordered diagnostic test.

C. a comparison of interventions across populations.

D. how much an insurer will charge to provide coverage.

19-29 *Most health maintenance organizations (HMOs) use a reimbursement mechanism called "capitation." This means that the*

A. HMO reimburses the provider on a fee-for-service basis.

B. HMO reimburses the provider a set fee per client, per month, based on the client's age and sex.

C. fee paid to the provider fluctuates with the treatment.

D. provider is reimbursed by each individual client or family.

19-30 *When caring for a client who speaks a language different from yours, the ideal strategy is to*

A. use gestures to convey the meaning of words and use a foreign-language dictionary of medical terms.

B. rely on family members to interpret.

C. review the case first with an interpreter before beginning the clinical visit.

D. use a pad and pencil to pass information back and forth with an interpreter.

19-31 *Advance directives, such as health-care proxies and durable powers of attorney, are important for all clients to consider. In particular, persons who are unable to marry legally and those who are single by choice or circumstances may preserve their health-care wishes by*

A. executing a durable power of attorney for health care.

B. drafting a letter stating that their next of kin is not the surrogate decision maker.

C. signing an institutional document stating that the health-care provider is allowed to make all health-care decisions for the client.

D. having one partner declared legally incompetent.

19-32 *Relapse is a common phenomenon seen during behavioral change. Useful strategies for the health-care provider to institute to aid the client in a relapse situation include*

A. using fear to reinforce the need to change.

B. telling the client that the relapse is a learning opportunity in preparation for the next action stage.

C. stressing the need to stay on "the straight and narrow."

D. involving the family in stressing the need to stay "straight."

19-33 *When applying for a new position, a nurse practitioner is counseled to assess the work environment. What does this include?*

A. Call time; support staff and what they will do; supervising relationships; will you be building your own panel of clients and/or seeing those overbooked?

B. Administrative support and call time

C. Research opportunities and the nature of the supervising relationship

D. Time off and whether you will be building your own panel of clients and/or attending to the overbooked

19-34 *"Do not resuscitate" orders are decided by the*

A. physician.

B. health-care facility.

C. physician in consultation with the client, family, or surrogate decision maker.

D. interdisciplinary health-care team.

19-35 *The majority of Medicaid enrollees are*

A. young women and children.

B. unemployed, homeless clients.

C. older adults.

D. clients with a disability.

19-36 *The purpose of a block grant is to*

A. provide more comprehensive services for Medicaid recipients.

B. encourage individuals to obtain their own health insurance so that they will not need government assistance.

C. allow states to have greater flexibility in providing services to the poor.

D. decrease the proportion of state taxes that are allocated to paying for Medicare.

19-37 *Ethical responsibilities of the nurse practitioner as employee include*

A. protecting the employer's "trade secrets," such as client mailing lists, and remaining unimpaired by drugs or alcohol.

B. advertising the practice using one's own funds.

C. never indulging in any criticism of the practice regardless of the circumstances.

D. attempting to promote the role of the nurse practitioner above all else.

19-38 *Zero-base budgeting refers to a budgeting system that*

A. accounts for unexpected budget variances.

B. accounts for expected budget variances only.

C. justifies each budget on its own merits, not on the basis of the previous period's budget.

D. justifies each budget based on the previous period's budget.

19-39 *It is important to prepare for your interview as a nurse practitioner. You should be prepared to answer which of the following?*

A. How old you are and how many children you have because your child care responsibilities might affect how you are able to do your job

B. Whether you are prepared to advertise the practice from your own funds, as well as other things that you can bring to the practice

C. What you can bring to the practice and if you will be able to see clients in a 10–15 minute block of time to make yourself revenue producing

D. Why you should be hired, how many clients per day you will see, what you can bring to the practice, your willingness to work evenings and/or weekends, as well as taking calls, how independent you are in your practice

19-40 *The research function of the APRN may be operationalized as both a consumer of research findings and a researcher. Being a consumer of research findings involves a number of activities, including*

A. reading the literature, analyzing its clinical applicability, and using new interventions.

B. organizing and conducting a research study.

C. collecting data.

D. ensuring protection of human subjects.

19-41 *A good way to use an interpreter is to*

A. try to use an interpreter who is of the same sex as and older than the client.

B. have the interpreter translate word for word so that you do not receive any misinformation.

C. use more than one interpreter if necessary.

D. attempt no communication with the client other than through the interpreter.

19-42 *The Agency for Healthcare Research and Quality (AHRQ) was established to*

A. mandate treatment protocols.

B. dictate health-care policy based on voluminous research.

C. promote evidence-based practice.

D. develop cost-effective interventions.

19-43 *Which of the following statements is true regarding the consultative aspects of the APRN role?*

A. The APRN provides an ongoing supportive and educational relationship to a more junior clinician.

B. The problem is identified by someone who then may decide to call in a consultant, a recognized expert, and a nonhierarchical relationship ensues or is established.

C. The APRN consultant assumes responsibility for the client once he or she is called into a clinical situation.

D. The person who has contracted with the consultant must take the recommendations of the APRN consultant.

19-44 *According to the Joint Commission on Accreditation of Healthcare Organizations, decisions regarding policy and client care should be made based on*

A. experience.

B. clinical expertise.

C. consultation and collaboration.

D. research findings.

19-45 *Certain characteristics differentiate research from quality improvement. Which of the following is an example of research?*

A. Client satisfaction is evaluated relative to existing practice.

B. An intervention, well supported in the literature, is implemented and evaluated.

C. A standard assessment tool (e.g., risk assessment for falls) is implemented and evaluated.

D. A new intervention is implemented and compared with current practice to determine which is better.

19-46 *The primary purpose of an institutional review board is to*

A. protect human subjects.

B. evaluate the scientific merit of proposed research.

C. oversee and coordinate the research efforts of an institution.

D. oversee and coordinate the research efforts of an individual.

19-47 *Reviewing the literature refers to the ability to research existing literature about a specific problem, whether clinical or policy. The most important skill necessary to performing a thorough review of the literature is*

A. talking with colleagues about the sources.

B. attending a research conference.

C. critiquing the findings and synthesizing the results.

D. reviewing clinical journals.

19-48 *Which of the following statements is true about case management?*

A. Case management oversees the client throughout acute care hospitalization.

B. Case management is organized around a system of interdisciplinary resources and services.

C. Case management depends on physician-driven leadership to oversee the illness episode.

D. Case management is applicable to the rehabilitative portion of the episode of the illness.

19-49 *Collaboration is best defined as*

A. interdisciplinary teamwork.

B. a protocol arrangement with a physician.

C. case management.

D. cooperation with another to achieve mutual goals while not losing sight of one's own interests.

19-50 *The components that must be present to establish malpractice include all of the following except*

A. harm (damage) to the client.

B. a duty to the client.

C. deviation (breach) from the standard of care.

D. negligence.

19-51 *Which of the following are third-party payers?*

A. Indemnity insurance companies and businesses that contract for certain services

B. Free clinics

C. The Commission on Mental Retardation

D. Social organizations

19-52 *Who oversees the APRN's prescribing of controlled substances?*

A. The federal government

B. The pharmaceutical board of the state

C. The practice protocols of the hospital

D. Practice agreements

19-53 *A good resume can be crucial to your success in obtaining a job. It should include*

A. religious activities.

B. community service.

C. demographic data, including marital status and age.

D. number of children.

19-54 *Sandy, age 16, is seen by you at the women's clinic. She asks you for information on birth control. Your course of action is to*

A. provide her with birth control because most states allow you to provide contraception to a 16-year-old without a parent being present.

B. not provide Sandy with any form of birth control because she is under legal age.

C. refer Sandy to the physician in control of the clinic.

D. determine if Sandy lives away from home and manages her own affairs. If she is an emancipated minor, you can supply her with birth control.

19-55 *Mr. Griffin, age 85, has been given a diagnosis of bowel cancer, and surgery is indicated. He is mentally alert; however, he is refusing to give consent for the procedure. You respond by*

A. ordering a psychiatric consultation.

B. having your collaborating physician talk with the client.

C. respecting his wishes.

D. talking with his family.

19-56 *Mrs. Smith, age 85, lost her husband 6 months ago. Since that time, she has been overwhelmed and has* had difficulty coping. Today, she is in your office, tearful, weak, and discouraged. Her mobility is also becoming increasingly limited because of her need for a hip replacement. She is indecisive, expresses fear about the surgery, and tells you that she does not want the surgery. Your action is to

A. treat the client's psychological problems and provide support.

B. respect the client's wishes.

C. consider placing the client in an assisted-living facility.

D. explain to the client that she is depressed and will feel better after the surgery.

19-57 *A situation in which medical information may be passed on without client consent is when*

A. the client has a gunshot wound.

B. a potential employer asks for it.

C. certifying absence from work.

D. talking to another health-care provider.

19-58 *In the outpatient office setting, the most common reason for a malpractice suit is failure to*

A. properly refer.

B. diagnose correctly in a timely fashion.

C. obtain informed consent.

D. manage fractures and trauma correctly.

19-59 *As measured by the federal Health Care Financing Administration, national health expenditures are grouped into which two categories?*

A. Medicare A and B

B. Medicare and Medicaid

C. Research and medical facilities construction and payments for health services and supplies

D. Long-term care and medications

19-60 *APRNs are affected by laws and rules, although these vary from state to state. The following is an example of something affected by state law and regulation*

A. delegation of authority by physicians.

B. how many clients you must see every hour.

C. universal health-care law.

D. making no more than five referrals for one client.

19-61 *What must you do as an APRN before billing for visits?*

A. You must establish a collaborative agreement with a physician.

B. You must obtain a provider number and familiarize yourself with the rules and policies of the third-party payer.

C. You must provide evidence of continuing medical education.

D. You must have a Drug Enforcement Agency (DEA) number.

19-62 *What conditions must be met for you to bill "incident to" the physician, receiving 100% reimbursement from Medicare?*

A. You must initiate the plan of care for the client.

B. The physician must be on-site and engaged in client care.

C. You must be employed as an independent contractor.

D. You must be the main health-care provider who sees the client.

19-63 *What is important to do before negotiating a contract?*

A. Do your homework.

B. Hire a lawyer.

C. Plan a signing-of-contract dinner.

D. Stand your ground.

19-64 *If conflict arises during a job negotiation, you should consider*

A. separating the issue from the person.

B. always standing your ground.

C. getting a legal opinion.

D. basing your actions on the contract a friend of yours has secured in a local practice.

19-65 *What is the difference between a referral and a consultation?*

A. A consultation is officially telephoned in by your office and implies continued treatment.

B. A referral is a request that another provider accept ongoing treatment responsibility.

C. A consultation may occur informally.

D. In a consultation, the client is sent to another health-care provider for a more in-depth evaluation.

19-66 *What is the responsibility of the primary care provider?*

A. The primary care provider is the coordinator of the client's health care.

B. Once the client is referred to another provider for ongoing treatment, the responsibility of the primary health-care provider is relieved.

C. The primary care provider should dictate all aspects of the client's plan of care.

D. The primary care provider turns over care of the client to the specialist.

19-67 *There are advantages to owning your own practice. However, there are also barriers to the ability to do this. These barriers include which of the following?*

A. Getting and keeping a collaborative physician if required by law; getting on managed care panels; and getting privileges at hospitals

B. Getting privileges in hospitals; getting referrals from hospital emergency rooms; and lack of knowledge

C. Inability to find a collaborating physician; inability to find clients; and lack of empathy

D. Lack of legal authority to admit clients to nursing homes, to order home care, and to direct hospice services; lack of ability to manage client care without clear medical oversight and supervision

19-68 *Denial of provider status is something that seriously impedes a nurse practitioner's ability to practice. If that occurs, some steps one can take include*

A. requesting that your clients lobby on your behalf; going to the newspapers; and reapplying.

B. requesting that your physician colleagues intervene on your behalf and writing critical letters to the organization in question.

C. "bashing" the organization to others, reapplying, and contacting an attorney.

D. writing letters to the organization's president and CEO, activating others to lobby on your behalf, and reapplying after a 6-month period.

19-69 *Medicare is a federal program administered nationally by the Center for Medicare and Medicaid Services (CMS) and administered locally by Medicare carrier agencies. The CMS has developed "Guidelines for Evaluation and Management Coding," which all Medicare providers, including nurse practitioners, are expected to follow in coding client visits for reimbursement*

purposes. *Which of the following is an important consideration regarding billing practices?*

A. It is important to "undercode" so that one does not get charged with Medicare fraud.

B. The practice of "overcoding" is essential in this age of decreasing reimbursements; just provide the appropriate documentation.

C. Failing to bill for billable services will lead to unnecessarily low revenues.

D. Time spent with the client is a very important determinant of billing.

19-70 *"Advanced-practice nurse" is an umbrella term used by some states and some nursing associations to cover, collectively, which of the following?*

A. Nurse practitioners, physician assistants, and nurse anesthetists, on the basis of CMS reimbursement practices

B. Nurse practitioners, nurse anesthetists, clinical nurse specialists, and nurse midwives

C. Only nurse practitioners

D. Clinical nurse specialists, nurse midwives, and nurse anesthetists

19-71 *You have seen a client who has tested positive for syphilis. You have treated the client, tested the client for other potential sexually transmitted diseases including HIV infection, counseled the client about safe sexual practices, and scheduled the client to return at 3 and 6 months for repeat serological testing. The tests at those times demonstrated that no further syphilis was present. Should you have taken any other action?*

A. No, you have treated the client appropriately.

B. Yes, you must report the case to the local health authorities.

C. Yes, you need to notify all sexual contacts.

D. Yes, you must follow up on the client's HIV status.

19-72 *Sally, a nurse practitioner, sees Mr. Bell, who is suffering from congestive heart failure. She increases his diuretic but makes no note of his potassium and orders no replacement potassium. Mr. Bell returns a week later for routine laboratory testing. His potassium level is found to be low; however, Mr. Bell has no complaints. Sally orders a potassium supplement to begin immediately and a follow-up potassium level measurement. Is Sally guilty of malpractice?*

A. Yes, because she breached the standard of care.

B. No, because no harm came to the client.

C. No, because she took remedial action.

D. Yes, because she was negligent.

19-73 *Which of the following nonverbal communication techniques is important to the establishment of rapport with the client?*

A. Taking notes only while the client is talking

B. Making direct eye contact with the client with periodic breaks to check or take notes

C. Having a desk between you and the client

D. Wearing jeans in the clinical setting to ensure your comfort

19-74 *Which of the following verbal communication techniques is helpful in establishing rapport with the client?*

A. Not calling the client by name because you do not want to appear intrusive

B. Speaking directly to the client, introducing yourself by name, and establishing the purpose of the interaction

C. Communicating slowly and quietly so as not to upset the client

D. Very thoroughly discussing every detail of the client's history with the client

19-75 *When caring for clients from a different culture, which of the following is an important piece of assessment data?*

A. Determining the ultimate decision maker

B. Making decisions based on your general knowledge about the cultural background of the client

C. Determining the family's perception of the client's problem

D. Understanding that clients from other cultures expect their health-care provider to be an authority figure

19-76 *You are attempting to elicit a history from Mr. Barnes during his first visit to your office. He is becoming increasingly angry and belligerent. He says, "Can't you hurry up? Dr. Smith never takes this long! Why are all these questions necessary?" You respond,*

A. "I'm sorry, Mr. Barnes, but I need these questions answered."

B. "I want to provide the best possible care for you, Mr. Barnes."

C. "Perhaps your wife can assist with some of these questions."

D. "You seem very upset, Mr. Barnes. Could you share with me what is bothering you?"

19-77 *Medicare is divided into Part A and Part B. What is the difference between these two parts?*

A. Medicare Part A provides coverage for hospital care and skilled nursing facility and home care; Part B pays for outpatient fees at 80% of what Medicare determines to be reasonable.

B. Medicare Part A covers health-care expenses for individuals younger than age 65; Part B pays for individuals older than age 65.

C. Medicare Part A covers disabled individuals younger than age 65, but they are not eligible for Part B.

D. Medicare A pays for outpatient fees including home care; Part B provides coverage for hospital care only.

19-78 *Which of the following statements is true about Medicaid?*

A. Medicaid is a federal plan to provide care for all indigent persons.

B. Medicaid pays for family planning services, dental care, and eyeglasses.

C. Eligibility requirements for Medicaid are mandated by the Health Care Financing Administration.

D. Medicaid is a program for the indigent financed jointly by the federal and the state governments.

19-79 *You are working in an emergency room as an APRN. An adolescent boy is brought in, unconscious, with a head injury after being struck by a car. He has no identification and there is no parent or adult with him. What should you do?*

A. Provide the appropriate medical treatment even if it involves surgery.

B. Do everything except order a blood transfusion, although it is indicated, because you do not know the client's religious preferences.

C. Call the hospital attorney before instituting any care.

D. Contact all local police stations in an attempt to identify the client and find his parents before instituting treatment.

19-80 *The requirements for reportable communicable disease vary from state to state. Which of the following lists includes diseases that must be reported in every state?*

A. Syphilis, tuberculosis, and hepatitis

B. HIV infection, *chlamydia* infection, and syphilis

C. Gonorrhea, syphilis, and *chlamydia* infection

D. Hepatitis, syphilis, and HIV

19-81 *The gerontological population is designated a vulnerable one when it comes to obtaining informed consent to serving as a research subject because of the potential for exploitation of older adults. Safeguards you should adhere to when conducting research on a geriatric population include which of the following?*

A. Assess the competence of the individual before obtaining consent.

B. Obtain permission from the family or staff.

C. Stress how important the research is and why their participation and perspective, as an older adult, are important.

D. Determine if the research is exempt, in which case you do not need to obtain consent to participate.

19-82 *Elder abuse and neglect are increasing concerns, and it is estimated that 4%–10% of older Americans are abused or neglected. What is the legal responsibility of the health-care provider in reporting elder abuse and neglect?*

A. The health-care provider should discuss the suspected abuse or neglect with the client.

B. The health-care provider should discuss the suspected abuse or neglect with the client's family.

C. The health-care provider must report the suspected abuse or neglect to the appropriate state protective agency.

D. The health-care provider must confirm the suspected abuse or neglect before reporting it to the appropriate state protective agency.

19-83 *Mrs. Hernandez, age 79, is insisting on discharge from the skilled nursing facility where she is receiving rehabilitation after a left hip replacement. She lives alone and has very little support. You do not think she is ready for discharge. Mrs. Hernandez's insistence on discharge is an example of your client exercising her right to*

A. self-determination.

B. beneficence.

C. justice.

D. utilitarianism.

19-84 *The type of health-care delivery system that allows the client the greatest freedom of choice is a*

A. health maintenance organization.

B. preferred provider organization.

C. managed care plan.

D. fee-for-service plan.

19-85 *One way in which you, as an individual APRN, can make a difference is by*

A. reading about issues in the newspaper.

B. writing letters to the editor supporting APRNs.

C. thinking positively about the work you do.

D. supporting a Democratic candidate.

19-86 *Prescriptive authority for APRNs*

A. is permitted only under protocol.

B. is mandated by law in more than 40 states.

C. varies from state to state.

D. includes the ability to prescribe controlled substances.

19-87 *Human research subjects are entitled to all of the following except*

A. the right to informed consent.

B. the right to compensation for their participation.

C. the right to withdraw from the research without being penalized.

D. the right to alternative treatments other than the experimental treatment.

19-88 *Negotiating a salary in a practice is important. A factor to consider is*

A. the practice philosophy of the physician-owner.

B. what payment method will be used—straight salary, percentage of net receipts, base salary plus percentage, or hourly rate.

C. the socioeconomic status of the surrounding community.

D. hourly salary only.

19-89 *When negotiating a contract for employment as a nurse practitioner, there are a number of important factors to consider. What are some important questions to ask?*

A. What is the most frequently billed Current Procedural Terminology (CPT) code for this practice and what amount does the practice bill and receive, on average, for that CPT code?

B. What is the cultural mix of clients seen in this practice?

C. What is the age and sex of my supervising physician?

D. What are the arrangements for child care in this practice?

19-90 *What are some important negotiating points for the nurse practitioner seeking a job?*

A. Practice philosophy of the physician-owner

B. Salary and benefits

C. Salary

D. Salary, benefits, and work environment

19-91 *Multiple regression and analysis of variance and covariance are tests of*

A. prediction.

B. statistical significance.

C. association.

D. correlation.

19-92 *Techniques used to enhance a client's adherence to a treatment plan include*

A. stressing the dangers of missing medications.

B. giving clear written instructions and simplifying the drug regimen.

C. allowing plenty of time between follow-up visits so that the client has time to adjust to the regimen.

D. explaining the importance of the regimen to the family.

19-93 *What is the best way to monitor compliance?*

A. Obtain drug levels.

B. Use clinical judgment.

C. Ask the client.

D. Monitor the responses to treatment.

19-94 *What is a strategy that can help to foster client compliance?*

A. In-depth client education

B. Frequency of medication dosing

C. Providing positive feedback and reinforcement

D. Performing serum drug levels to assess therapeutic range

19-95 *An emancipated minor is a client who is younger than age 18 but who is considered a competent adult with the authority to accept or refuse medical treatment. How do you determine if the 16-year-old you are seeing is an "emancipated minor"?*

A. No one age 16 would be defined as an emancipated minor.

B. Although definitions vary from state to state, the term usually implies that the minor has entered into a valid marriage, is a member of the military, or has been granted this status by a court.

C. The client claims that he is free from all parental control.

D. The client is accompanied by an older friend who states that he/she will accept legal responsibility and is the client's "guardian."

19-96 *Documentation guidelines for evaluation and management of services include which type of examination?*

A. Mental, physical, and psychosocial

B. Complete and thorough

C. Single system

D. Expanded problem focused

19-97 *An effective method used to assess a client's retention and understanding of educational materials is*

A. asking the client to restate what you have reviewed.

B. providing a pathophysiology book for your client to take home and read.

C. repeating your explanations of disease pathology.

D. objective testing.

19-98 *When teaching your client about medication that you are prescribing, the most important point(s) to discuss initially is (are)*

A. the action of the drug and its adverse effects.

B. whether to take the drug on a full or empty stomach.

C. what it is for, how much to take, and when to take it.

D. what to do if the client experiences any adverse effects.

19-99 *What is the maximum number of points you should attempt to make in one teaching session?*

A. One

B. Two

C. Three to four

D. As many as you need; there is no limit

19-100 *Mr. Brill, age 50, is a house painter who has smoked two to three packs of cigarettes per day since he was 20 years old. He comes into the clinic complaining of a chronic cough. When you discuss his smoking behavior, he states, "I know I need to stop smoking, but I'm under too much stress right now." Mr. Brill is at which stage of learning?*

A. The precontemplative stage

B. The contemplative stage

C. The action stage

D. The maintenance stage

Answers

19-1   Answer B

Strategies for developing cultural competence include learning basic words and sentences in the client's language, attending special cultural events and celebrations, and relating a client's belief to your own even if it is different. It is important to recognize that clients who have English as a second language may regress back to their first language under the stress of an illness. Learning a few key phrases in the client's native language and knowing how to address the client properly can go a long way in establishing rapport and trust. Disregarding folk beliefs because they are not scientific is not a strategy to develop cultural competence. Folk beliefs must be taken into consideration because they can profoundly affect the course of the client's illness. If the client believes his or her illness is the result of a "curse," you may need to strategize ways to "undo" the curse. Explaining the pathophysiology of a disease process is not necessarily effective in countering the client's deeply held cultural beliefs.

19-2   Answer C

The best method for evaluating the efficacy of a new clinical intervention is a randomized, controlled clinical trial. Case reports, descriptive studies, and correlational studies are methodological approaches that are less reliable in establishing causal relationships, and thus the attribution of an effect to the new clinical intervention would be less clear. The effect might be attributable to other confounding variables.

19-3   Answer B

Asking open-ended questions is essential to establishing a therapeutic relationship, even in an emergency situation, and it is a good interviewing technique. Asking several questions in rapid succession may help establish the nature of the clinical situation, but it will not facilitate a therapeutic relationship or communication. To reassure the client may be unrealistic. False reassurance is considered a block to therapeutic communication. Asking the client about his anxiety level will probably only increase the client's anxiety. It is also an irrelevant question because the client would most certainly be anxious.

19-4   Answer A

An underlying assumption of the health belief model (HBM) is that behavior is determined more by a person's perceived reality than by environmental factors. Components include perceived threat, efficacy, benefits of action, and perceived barriers to action. People take actions to change their lifestyle to prevent a disease only to the extent that the disease exists in their perception. They must also perceive the benefits of action, as well as feel the confidence (often referred to as efficacy) to act. These benefits must outweigh the barriers to action. Benefits and barriers are people's beliefs rather than objective facts about the effectiveness of action. Education and positive reinforcement are not concepts associated with the HBM. Predisposing factors, reinforcing factors, and enabling factors are concepts from the precede-proceed model, which is used for comprehensive planning in health education and health promotion with individuals and communities. Self-efficacy theory and the perceived ability to act are one and the same and form only part of the HBM.

19-5   Answer B

According to the 1996 revised Institute of Medicine report, primary care addresses a large majority of personal health-care needs, provides integrated and accessible health-care services, sustains a partnership with clients, and is practiced in the context of the family and community. It is far more than the provision and coordination of referrals. Public health care commonly uses focus-group methodology to assess community needs and design a plan of care for a community. It is not meant solely to provide a source of referrals, nor is it only for those who cannot afford specialty care.

19-6   Answer C

The limitation on prescriptive authority and the scope of practice and reimbursement issues are major barriers to full implementation for an autonomous role for APRNs in primary care. The complex health problems of vulnerable populations are frequently rooted in lifestyle issues such as poverty, violence, and poor housing. These social problems are often more amenable to traditional nursing-based approaches. Managed care organizations' views are currently shifting and variable. Managed care organizations' support for advanced nursing practice continues to be variable. In some settings it is one barrier; in other settings it is something else.

19-7   Answer A

Motivation is the most important factor influencing behavioral change. Health beliefs and self-efficacy may underlie motivation for change, but it is motivation that is most strongly correlated with actual behavioral change. Cognitive knowledge and social supports have some relationships to the concept of self-efficacy, but not directly to motivation.

19-8   Answer D

The marketing process is guided by a number of factors, including product, price, place, and promotion. Referred to as the "4 P's of the marketing process," "product" stands for the service you offer; "price" is identification of the right cost for the service; "place" refers to where the services are delivered or the demands of the market where the service will be offered; and "promotion" is your ability to increase your market's awareness of what you have to offer. The prospective pool of clients, your advertising budget, and what you have to offer are only portions of a marketing plan. Cost, benefit, and barriers do not describe the marketing process in a meaningful or coherent way.

19-9   Answer A

Explanatory reasoning—reasoning that explains, in the client's view, the cause of the client's illness—has been attributed to antropologist Arthur Kleinam as the "expalanatory model." The client may have a cognitive understanding of scientific medicine, but reject it. The client's view, in this situation, is not necessarily delusional or a cultural bias.

19-10   Answer D

To determine the appropriate statistical test to use, consider sample size, level of measurement, and data type, as well as other factors. Statistical significance and clinical significance are not the same. If a journal article you are writing is limited in length, you should not delete the descriptive statistics and keep the inferential statistics. You must describe your sample and possibly a number of other things before explaining your inferences. Correlational coefficients measure the strength of the relationship between variables; correlation does not infer causality, nor can you make firm predictions based on these data.

19-11   Answer A

To reinforce client teaching, a useful strategy is to model the healthy behaviors. Role modeling is a very successful reinforcement strategy. Many people learn best by imitating the behavior of others. For example, if you are teaching exercises to your client, demonstrate them and then have the client practice them. Videos or pictures of others performing the exercises can also be helpful. Repeated discussions of the need for behavioral change are not often effective. Although providing some written materials is helpful, providing them without behavioral support may not add to the client's motivation. Likewise, although quizzing the client may provide information about his or her knowledge base, it does not positively reinforce behavior or lead to positive behavioral change.

19-12   Answer C

Concrete strategies used to keep your client's attention as you institute client education include making your point clear from the start; varying your tone of voice (speaking in a monotone may communicate a lack of interest); using various teaching methods (visual aids work best); and translating theoretical information into practical terms.

Repetition is usually not an effective strategy for keeping your client's attention. Providing an educational session immediately after eating lunch is also not necessarily conducive to learning.

19-13   Answer C

The levels of evaluation and management (E/M) services are based on four types of histories: (1) problem focused, (2) expanded problem focused, (3) detailed, and (4) comprehensive.

19-14   Answer A

A comprehensive history includes a chief complaint (CC); history of present illness (HPI); review of systems (ROS); and past, family, and/or social history. Although aspects of other data mentioned in the other answer options may be present, they do not include *all* the elements necessary for a comprehensive history.

19-15   Answer C

The primary nursing responsibility during a crisis situation is to establish a therapeutic relationship. Other nursing responsibilities include providing education regarding the recovery process, stress management and reduction, and integration of the crisis experience. The establishment of support mechanisms and the development of coping mechanisms frequently enable the client to mobilize effectively and move beyond the crisis stage. Occasionally hospitalization may be necessary during an acute crisis, and psychotherapy may be a useful intervention.

19-16   Answer A

The stages of grief include shock, reality, and recovery. The shock stage is characterized as numbness, the reality stage as deep pain, and the recovery stage as beginning to live again. Numbness, pain, loss, and resolution are all components of the process of grief. A grieving person shares many behavioral similarities with a depressed individual; however, grieving is a natural, not a pathological, process and is usually time limited.

19-17   Answer C

A marketing portfolio that will support what you have to offer as an APRN or nurse practitioner should include the state nurse practice act and regulations, prescriptive authority legislation, third-party reimbursement rules and regulations, and practice protocols. This type of information provides concrete data to potential employers and reimbursers concerning the range of services you can offer. Your personal mission statement should be used to help you personally focus your job search and options. Your scores on the certification examination and the specifics of your transcript are usually not relevant. Letters of reference should be provided only when requested.

19-18   Answer A

Answers to all questions listed in Answer A must be ascertained before prescribing medication for a client.

19-19   Answer B

Schedule IV drugs are all those listed in Answer B, plus some stimulants such as phentermine. Schedule IV drugs include depressants such as alprazolam, clonazepam, diazepam, and flurazepam; stimulants such as phentermine; and other substances such as pentazocine. Schedule I drugs include substances with little or no approved medical usage that have a high abuse potential, such as LSD and marijuana. Schedule II drugs are those with a high abuse potential with severe psychic or physical dependency but with clinical utility, such as meperidine, morphine, and methadone, to name just a few. Stimulants such as amphetamines are also included in Schedule II. Schedule III drugs have a potential for abuse, but the potential is lower than for Schedule II drugs. These drugs often contain a combination of controlled and noncontrolled substances such as Tylenol with codeine #3.

19-20   Answer A

Leaving a client's record within view, talking about a client within earshot of others, discarding unshredded duplicate records, discussing a client's condition with family members, releasing a client's medical information without written permission, and leaving a telephone message on a client's answering machine are all ways one may risk breaching client confidentiality.

19-21   Answer A

The primary purpose of professional licensure is to protect the public from unsafe practitioners by ensuring a minimum standard for competency. Licensure is a legal status granted by a regulating authority (in the case of nursing, by individual state boards of nursing). In nursing, this is accomplished by mandating passage of the National Council Licensure Exam (NCLEX-RN) by an individual before state licensure. Licensure does not ensure high nursing standards; passage of the NCLEX is designed to assess minimum competency to practice safely. The curriculum of a nursing program, although providing a foundation of nursing knowledge that will graduate a safe and competent practitioner, is not specifically geared to the NCLEX exam. Nursing programs retain autonomy over their own curricula. Although the licensing statutes may spell out prescriptive privileges for APRNs, they do not necessarily do that, nor is that the primary purpose of professional licensure.

19-22   Answer A

The primary purpose of certification is to document excellence and specialization. Certification is a voluntary process by which a nongovernmental agency or association certifies that an individual has met certain predetermined standards for competency and specialization in a particular area. Although some states mandate that an APRN pass a national certification examination before granting licensure to practice at an advanced level, this is not the case in all states. National certification may be necessary to obtain third-party reimbursement; however, that is not the primary purpose of certification, either. Although certification at the national level does provide the public with information about the skills of the practitioner, that is the realm of licensure, not the primary purpose of certification.

19-23   Answer C

Legal authority for all nursing practice, including advanced-practice nursing, rests with the individual state boards of nursing that administer the legal statutes that define nursing practice in that state. The Health Care Financing Administration oversees the administration of federal Medicare and Medicaid funds. Legal authority for professional practice was delegated to the states and territories by the Constitution and is not regulated by federal statutes. Certification by certifying bodies is a voluntary process with no legal significance.

19-24   Answer B

Credentialing means that the practitioner has met certain criteria through licensure, education, and certification. The criteria for credentialing vary depending upon the credentialing body. Hospitals, for example, may use credentialing to grant hospital privileges. An individual is permitted to practice basic or advanced-practice nursing by licensure. An academic degree is awarded when one has completed a program of study. Prescriptive authority is mandated by state statutes.

19-25   Answer C

Although the desires of the collaborating physician; education, certification, and continuing education credits; and reimbursement and prescriptive privileges may influence institutional policy and medical staff bylaws, the factors that primarily determine the ability of an APRN to obtain clinical privileges in an institution are institutional policy, medical staff bylaws, state law, and the Joint Commission on Accreditation of Healthcare Organizations accreditation standards.

19-26   Answer C

The goals and objectives contained in *Healthy People 2010* include reducing disparities in health care, increasing healthy life span, and increasing accessibility to health care for all Americans. They do not include mandatory provision of emergency care. *Healthy People 2010* does not advocate instituting a nationalized health insurance plan. Preserving choice of provider for all Americans is not one of the goals and objectives of *Healthy People 2010*.

19-27   Answer C

Indemnity insurer refers to an insurer that pays for the medical care of the insured but does not provide that care. A health maintenance organization provides the medical care, as well as the insurance of the insurer. A preferred provider organization is a network of health-care providers linked together through similar reimbursement mechanisms. A fee-for-service plan refers to reimbursement for health-care services under a fee schedule.

19-28   Answer A

The term *usual and customary* refers to comparing charges with other like charges for services and supplies received in the immediate vicinity, as well as in a broader geographic area. It does not refer to the "usual and customary" charge to obtain insurance, but rather to how much the insurer will reimburse for a service. Whether to order a diagnostic test is up to the provider's discretion, although the payer may hold the provider to the standard of care. *Usual and customary* is not a term used to compare interventions across populations.

19-29 Answer B

The reimbursement mechanism called "capitation" that some health maintenance organizations (HMOs) use is one in which the HMO reimburses the provider a set fee per client, per month, based on the client's age and sex. HMOs are prepaid, comprehensive systems of health benefits that combine both financing and delivery of services to subscribers. They may pay providers on a capitated or fee-for-service basis. Capitation is a set fee that does not fluctuate. The provider is reimbursed by the HMO and not the client. Most plans require clients to make a copayment at the time of the visit. Capitated fees for primary care range from $5 to $35 per month depending on the client's age and sex and, thus, relative risk. Fee for service refers to reimbursement for health-care services under a fee schedule that is based on a complex variety of factors. These include the number and type of services provided, the current procedural terminology, International Classification of Disease (ICD-9) codes, the geographic area (the "usual and customary" fee), and certain office and training expenses of the provider.

19-30 Answer C

Reviewing the case with an interpreter before seeing the client is the *ideal* strategy to enhance cross-cultural communication if you are in a setting where an interpreter is available. Information about the reason for the visit and the purpose of the health-care encounter can be exchanged beforehand, potentially enhancing communications. It may be necessary to rely on family members to translate, but it is not the best strategy. For example, it is often the school-age child who has the best grasp of English; however, relying on the child to interpret reverses parent-child roles and places unnecessary and sometimes inappropriate burdens on the child. It also lessens the client's sense of authority and privacy. Gesturing and relying on a dictionary may be necessary but distracts from the general flow of communication and slows the speed and comprehension of the communication.

19-31 Answer A

A durable power of attorney for health care (DPAHC) authorizes another person or agent to make medical decisions on behalf of an individual if and when that client becomes unable or unwilling to make those decisions. It is a version of the power of attorney used in commercial transactions. In the absence of such a document, in most cases, the client's next of kin (typically a spouse, parent, or child, depending on individual circumstances) is legally mandated to assume that role. Unlike the "living will," which is used for end-of-life decisions, a DPAHC is used to make decisions when the client is incapacitated.

19-32 Answer B

Useful strategies for the health-care provider to institute to aid the client in a relapse situation include telling the client that the relapse is a learning opportunity in preparation for the next action stage (positive reframing). Involving the family is not usually appropriate and stressing the need to stay "straight" may be punitive and not helpful. Using fear to reinforce the need to change usually does not work for behavioral issues.

19-33 Answer A

Although research opportunities and administrative support may be important components of the work environment for an individual nurse practitioner, the most general and inclusive answer is A. The number and role of support staff, on-call time, nature of supervision, reporting relationships, and clarification regarding which clients will be seen during the course of a day are all important parameters of the work environment.

19-34 Answer C

"Do not resuscitate" (DNR) orders are decided by the physician in consultation with the client, family, or surrogate decision maker. Advance directives may help clarify end-of-life decisions, but the lack of a documented DNR order in the chart presumes that the client desires full intervention and holds health-care providers legally responsible to initiate life-sustaining treatment. A DNR order, written by the physician, relieves the health-care providers of that responsibility. The individual decision is never made by the health-care facility, although the facility may draft generic guidelines to assist procedurally in end-of-life situations.

19-35 Answer A

The majority of Medicaid enrollees are young women and children. The majority of Medicaid funds, however, go to long-term care services for older adults and clients with disabilities.

19-36   Answer C

The purpose of a block grant is to allow states to have greater flexibility in providing services to the poor. Accelerating costs of the Medicaid program have prompted state-based initiatives for reform of the program. The federal government has considered converting Medicaid funds to block grants to allow states greater flexibility in providing Medicaid services.

19-37   Answer A

It is the ethical responsibility of the nurse practitioner to add to the goodwill that the employer has developed within the community; protect the employer's "trade secrets" such as client mailing lists; remain unimpaired by drugs and/or alcohol; provide one's best customer services at all times; maintain one's credentials and adherence to the "standard of care"; and maintain client confidentiality. The APRN has an ethical and legal responsibility to follow the standard of care. There is no ethical responsibility to advertise the practice from one's own funds; nor should the nurse practitioner promote that role above all others. The nature of the practice should be collaborative.

19-38   Answer C

Zero-based budgeting refers to a budgeting system that justifies each budget on its own merits, not on the basis of the previous period's budget. It is a process in which the budgets for succeeding budget periods are unrelated to those of earlier budget periods, but rather are justified on their own merits, as if no previous budgets had ever been prepared.

19-39   Answer D

You must be prepared to answer what you will bring to the practice, although it does not have to be put in writing. You must be prepared to answer whether you will be on-call on the weekends or evenings. You may not be willing to do this, but you must have an answer for this question. You must be able to share how many clients you may be able to see in one day, as well as how independently you are willing to practice. You do not have to share your age or the number of dependents you have and/or any arrangements in caring for them, and you are not expected to advertise the practice out of your own

revenues. You must, however, be willing to positively promote the practice in the community.

19-40   Answer A

A consumer of research findings engages in a number of activities that include reading the literature, analyzing clinical applicability, and using new interventions. Organizing and conducting a research study, as well as ensuring the protection of human subjects, are tasks of the researcher. Collecting data may be done by anyone trained to do it and does not necessarily require advanced knowledge of the research process. Research utilization, on the other hand, involves reading the current literature; critically evaluating the study, including its methods and conclusions, to evaluate applicability to practice; introducing relevant findings into clinical practice; evaluating the results of the new treatments on clients; and disseminating those results in clinical practice.

19-41   Answer A

The role of an interpreter in a health-care setting is often one of cultural broker, to act as a translator not just of words but also of cultural concepts and beliefs. Cultural values may make it more difficult for the client to discuss certain issues in the presence of an interpreter. It is helpful for the practitioner to face the interpreter and client together, maintaining eye contact with both if possible. It also facilitates observation of nonverbal cues. Using a trained same-sex interpreter, preferably one older than the client, has been found to work best. The client also needs to be reassured about the confidentiality of the information shared. For this reason, it is best to use only one interpreter and for the provider to establish rapport with the client in any way possible.

19-42   Answer C

The Agency for Healthcare Research and Quality (AHRQ) was established to promote evidence-based practice and develop databases for research and clinical guidelines. The AHRQ routinely publishes reviews of studies on clinical problems with summaries of treatment protocols and effectiveness. It does not mandate these in practice, although the provider may be held to these as a standard of care. It also does not dictate health-care policy or develop cost-effective interventions, although it does do cost-benefit analysis of the interventions.

19-43   Answer B

Principles of consultation include the identification of a problem by a professional, for example an APRN, who calls in a consultant with documented expertise in a given area; the consultant making recommendations based on his or her assessment of the situation; and the APRN remaining free to accept or reject these recommendations and retaining responsibility for the outcome of care. Classically, there is a nonhierarchical relationship between the consultant and consultee. The issue of responsibility for the outcome of care is what separates collaboration from consultation. A situation in which a senior clinician provides a supportive and educative relationship with a junior clinician is defined as "clinical supervision" and implies that responsibility for the outcome of care remains in the hands of the senior clinician.

19-44   Answer D

According to the Joint Commission on Accreditation of Healthcare Organizations (JCAHO), decisions regarding policy and client care should be based on research findings. The JCAHO mandates that decisions be based on research and rooted in and supported by scientific literature. Experience, clinical expertise, and consultation and collaboration are no longer acceptable as the rationale for policy and client-care decisions. This supports evidence-based practice.

19-45   Answer D

One characteristic that differentiates research from quality improvement is that research compares a new intervention with current practice to determine which is better. Research asks new questions that generate new knowledge when answered with a degree of generalizability. Additionally, there may be a risk implied to a human subject. Clients receiving the new and untested interventions may be at risk. Quality improvement evaluates things such as client satisfaction, for example, or the implementation and evaluation of new interventions already well-supported in the literature. It is not new knowledge but evaluation of existing knowledge. Similarly, with the implementation and evaluation of a standardized assessment tool, new knowledge is not gained.

19-46   Answer A

The purpose of an institutional review board (IRB) is to protect human subjects. The primary purpose of the IRB is ethical; it does not evaluate the scientific merit of proposed research, nor does it oversee and coordinate the research efforts of an institution or an individual. These functions are usually performed by the institution's research committee. It is your obligation as a researcher to obtain some form of IRB approval any time you are conducting research on human subjects. If you are planning a research project in a private practice setting, approval should be obtained from the IRB of some affiliating institution such as a hospital where you are credentialed and permitted to admit clients.

19-47   Answer C

Although talking with colleagues, attending a research conference, and reviewing your own clinical journals may all help identify relevant databases, the most important skill necessary to performing a thorough review of the literature is critiquing the findings and synthesizing the results.

19-48   Answer B

Case management is organized around a system of interdisciplinary resources and services; the clinical and financial aspects of care are overseen by a case manager who has a financial incentive to manage risk and maximize the quality of care. It is not physician driven. Case management is applicable to the entire episode of the illness, not just the client's acute care, hospitalization, or rehabilitative care.

19-49   Answer D

Collaboration is best defined as cooperation with another to achieve mutual goals while not losing sight of one's own interests. True collaboration combines the activities of cooperation or concern for another's interests with assertiveness. The interest considered most important in nurse-physician collaboration is the professionals' concern for the care of the client rather than the provider's personal agenda. Collaboration is essential in interdisciplinary teamwork but is not the definition of collaboration. Collaboration may include a protocol arrangement with a physician, but it is not solely defined that way. Case management is defined as managing an entire episode of illness from the standpoint of coordination of resources and services. This will involve collaboration but is a different concept.

19-50   Answer D

The components that must all be present to establish malpractice are a duty to the client, a deviation (breach) from the standard of care, and harm (damage) to the client that occurs because of the breach of duty and the deviation from the standard of care (causation).

19-51   Answer A

Medicare, Medicaid, indemnity insurance companies, managed care organizations, and businesses that contract for certain services (e.g., colleges that provide health-care services) are the major categories of third-party payers. Clients who pay their own bills are not, strictly speaking, third-party payers but still are a source of reimbursement.

19-52   Answer A

The federal government, specifically the Drug Enforcement Agency (DEA), oversees the APRN's prescribing of controlled substances. State laws vary, as do physician oversight and scope of practice from state to state. Federal registration is based on the applicant's complying with state and local laws. If a state requires a separate controlled-substance license, the APRN must obtain that license and submit a copy with an application for a DEA number. If state law does not authorize the APRN to prescribe controlled substances, the DEA will not issue a DEA number.

19-53   Answer B

A good resume should include name, address, telephone and fax numbers, e-mail address, educational background and degrees, professional employment, community service, research interests, grants written, publications, speaking engagements, consulting activities, honors and awards, professional memberships, and military history. Religious and demographic data, including number of children, should not be included to prevent candidates from being ruled out by any of these noncontributing factors.

19-54   Answer A

State laws vary on issues related to minors and you should be knowledgeable about the laws in your state. Most states consider a teenager capable of receiving birth control information and devices without the presence or consent of a parent. In the case of a teenager seeking abortion, this is not as clear. You are freer not to seek parental approval or

consent when a teenager is living on his or her own and managing his or her own affairs because the emancipated minor concept is recognized in most jurisdictions. You should not need to refer Sandy to the clinic physician.

19-55   Answer C

Respecting the client's wishes is the most correct response to this situation. You may want to consider a psychological overlay, such as depression, and be sure this is not a driving component of the client's behavior. If the client appears to be of sound mind, his wishes should be respected. Ordering a psychiatric consult or having your collaborating physician talk with the client is not necessary. Talking to his family interferes with the client's autonomy, a primary value of care.

19-56   Answer A

Your action is to treat the client's psychological problems and provide support. With Mrs. Smith, there are enough symptoms to warrant evaluation and possible intervention for psychological problems, most likely depression. Then it would be appropriate to support the client's decision. There are not enough data to evaluate the need for placement in an assisted living facility at this point. To try to convince the client that she is in need of surgery would be coercive and would violate the client's autonomy.

19-57   Answer A

One situation in which medical information may be passed on without client consent is when the client has a gunshot wound. Other situations include when the client has a sexually transmitted or communicable disease. All other situations require the client's consent for release of medical records and information.

19-58   Answer B

In the outpatient office setting, the most common reason for a malpractice suit is failure to diagnose correctly. Approximately one-third of malpractice cases brought against general practitioners involve cases of failure to diagnose in a timely manner. These cases usually involve cancer, particularly cancer of the breast (failure to diagnose promptly accounts for the highest number of liability cases), lung, colon, or testes. Failure to refer and failure to manage fractures and trauma are among the top seven allegations in malpractice cases. Failure to obtain informed consent accounts for approximately 10% of the cases.

19-59 Answer C

As measured by the federal Health Care Financing Administration, national health expenditures are grouped into two categories: research and medical facilities construction and payments for health services and supplies. Medicare and Medicaid account for more than 76% of personal health-care services. Long-term care and medications are subsumed under the other categories. Public spending for research and facilities construction totals approximately $17 billion, only a small fraction of the approximately $900 billion spent on all health care in recent years. Of that, more than 75% was dedicated to research paid for at the federal level.

19-60 Answer A

APRNs must abide by laws and rules, such as those related to scope of practice, reimbursement for health-care services, delegation of authority by physicians, quality of care, and requirements for collaboration. However, the number of clients seen per hour, universal health-care law, and number of referrals are not regulated by law.

19-61 Answer B

To bill your clients for services, you must obtain a provider or panel membership as needed and familiarize yourself with the rules and policies of each payer. Some, but not all, states require a collaborative agreement with a physician for you to practice; some states require national certification to practice, but not all do. In some states you are able to provide controlled substances, and this will require that you have a DEA number; other states do not allow you to prescribe controlled substances. Currently, there is not a requirement that you have a specific number of continuing medical education credits to bill for services provided.

19-62 Answer B

The term *incident to* implies that your services as an APRN are performed in connection with a physician. The reimbursement rate for Medicare billing "incident to" a physician is 100%. The physician must be on-site when the care is provided and must be providing medical services rather than performing administrative work. The physician must have

previously seen the client and initiated the plan of care, and the physician must see the client frequently enough to provide ongoing input into the care of the client.

19-63 Answer A

You need to do your homework. This means being prepared to present the facts clearly and succinctly. Talk with your colleagues by networking with other nurse practitioners in your area. Write down an optimal salary and benefits, as well as your required bottom-line salary and benefits to help establish a reasonable range. You do not necessarily need to hire a lawyer; you can handle most or all of this process yourself with proper preparation. It is premature and is not your best use of time to plan a signing dinner. Standing your ground is important but not if it means being unreasonable. Negotiate for agreement, not for winning or losing.

19-64 Answer A

Seeking a legal opinion might be prudent but is usually not necessary and can set up additional roadblocks in some situations. You should not base your actions or decisions on a similar situation that someone you know may have experienced. Although the experiences of others may be useful sources of comparisons, your decisions should be based on your analysis of your own situation. Standing your ground is important but not if it means being unreasonable. During the process of negotiation, an honest difference of opinion can arise. Resolving the issue is wise and prudent behavior. Always separate the issue from the person. It is about achieving a mutually satisfying outcome—a win-win situation. Clarifying misconceptions and focusing on what has been achieved thus far can be an effective strategy. You want to leave the process with positive feelings even if a work agreement is not achieved.

19-65 Answer B

A consultation implies a more informal arrangement and may occur formally or informally. It is a request from another provider for direction or guidance on diagnosis or treatment. A referral, on the other hand, is a request for another provider to accept the ongoing treatment of a client, at least in regard to one specific health problem. A consultation does not imply the continued treatment that is part and parcel of a referral.

19-66 Answer A

The primary care provider is the coordinator of all care that the client receives. The primary care provider does not necessarily dictate all aspects of the client's care—for example, the cardiologist may decide on the antihypertensive regimen, and the primary care provider may continue to monitor the client's response. But neither does the primary care provider turn over all aspects of the care to the specialist.

19-67 Answer A

Barriers to independent practice include getting on managed care panels; getting and keeping a collaborating physician if mandated in the state where one is practicing; getting referrals from hospital emergency rooms and getting privileges in hospitals; lacking legal authority in the state of practice to admit to nursing homes, offer home care services, and/or to direct hospice services. Lack of knowledge and lack of empathy should not be barriers to practice. A nurse practitioner should be able to manage client care without direct and specific physician oversight, although collaboration in some situations is essential to nurse practitioner practice just as it is when physicians call for a referral.

19-68 Answer D

There are many steps a nurse practitioner can take if denied provider status by a third-party reimburser. Going to an attorney, or contacting the newspapers, may be strategies to resort to over time, but there are many more immediate and constructive strategies to try first. "Bashing" an organization is never smart; first one should ascertain the reasons for this stance and determine whether it is the same across the board regarding nurse practitioners. If it is a consistent policy, attempt to find out why and begin marshalling evidence to overturn this stance in a constructive way. This may include having both clients and physician colleagues "lobby" on your behalf. Find out who the decision maker in the organization is and attempt to communicate directly with that person. Ascertain if there is a law in the state mandating this policy. Be prepared to testify at hearings and speak out at community meetings about this issue. Request language changes that specify "ask your doctor" and lobby to have these changes adopted. Reapplication in 6 months is reasonable. Repeated applications without attempt to change policy will not be effective.

19-69 Answer C

It is important to bill for the appropriate services and support that with appropriate documentation. Time spent with the client is not always the determining factor because it may have been time spent inappropriately. Billing is based on history taking, examination, and medical decision making. Each of these activities has specific measures and parameters to be documented. When selecting the appropriate code for ambulatory care, only face-to-face time is considered.

19-70 Answer B

The term *advanced-practice nurses* refers to nurse practitioners, clinical nurse specialists, nurse anesthetists, and nurse midwives.

19-71 Answer B

The practitioner is also responsible for reporting the case of syphilis to the local health authorities. All sexual partners of the client should be contacted; however, it is the health department that has trained staff who will perform the investigation of contacts and follow-up. Syphilis is easily treated and controllable if its presence is reported. It is not necessary to retest the client's HIV status unless there is a new clinical reason on subsequent visits.

19-72 Answer B

Sally is not guilty of malpractice because no harm came to Mr. Bell as a result of her actions. For malpractice to occur, the provider must have a duty to the client (which Sally had), a standard of care must have been breached (which Sally did when she did not check his potassium level when she increased the dosage of diuretic), and harm or damage must occur as a result of the duty and the breach of the standard of care (which did not occur). Because all of the components were not met, malpractice has not been established.

19-73 Answer B

Nonverbal communication techniques important to the establishment of rapport with the client include making direct eye contact with the client, with periodic breaks to check or take notes; avoiding having a desk between you and the client; and having personal grooming appropriate to the setting. Taking notes only while the client is talking does not help establish rapport with the client because making direct eye contact with the client aids in establishing trust. A break in eye contact, however, is important because some cultures view staring as disrespectful. Other nonverbal communication techniques that help establish rapport include sitting while interviewing the client rather than standing; standing or sitting near the client but not invading the client's personal comfort zone; and maintaining a friendly, helpful expression.

19-74   Answer B

Verbal communication techniques helpful in establishing rapport with the client include verifying the name of the client and using it throughout the conversation; speaking directly to the client, introducing yourself by name, and establishing the purpose of the interaction; and communicating in a tone of voice, speed, and choice of words that are similar to the client's. Very thoroughly discussing every detail of the client's history with the client, unless absolutely necessary, can be disturbing to the client. It is important to take cues from the client. Some areas of the history will be much more important than others. You must be astute and attuned to the client without missing important information.

19-75   Answer A

When caring for clients from a different culture, important pieces of assessment data include determining the ultimate decision maker (it may be someone other than the client; for example, it may be the male patriarch of the family); determining the client's perception of the cause of his or her problem (e.g., some clients may view it as fate or a curse); and ascertaining the client's, not the family's, expectations of the provider. It is not appropriate to make decisions based on your general knowledge about the cultural background of the client. Assuming that the client expects an authoritarian health-care provider is cultural stereotyping. The practitioner should not fall into this common trap. Each clinical visit needs to be evaluated in light of the general cultural background of the client, as well as the specific reasons for the visit.

19-76   Answer D

The most important aspect of communicating with clients is acknowledging their feelings. By responding, "You seem very upset, Mr. Barnes. Could you share with me what is bothering you?" you acknowledge Mr. Barnes' discomfort by reflecting back his feelings, and you offer to assist him. If you respond by saying,

"I'm sorry, Mr. Barnes, but I need these questions answered" or "I want to provide the best possible care for you, Mr. Barnes," you have not acknowledged Mr. Barnes' feelings. If you respond by saying, "Perhaps your wife can assist with some of these questions," you violate Mr. Barnes' autonomy and right to self-determination.

19-77   Answer A

Medicare Part A provides coverage for inpatient care, including hospital care, skilled nursing facility care, and home health care; Part B pays for outpatient fees at 80% of what Medicare determines to be reasonable. Disabled individuals younger than age 65 are eligible for Medicare A and B.

19-78   Answer D

Financed jointly by the federal and state governments, Medicaid is a program to pay for health-care services for the indigent. Each state defines income eligibility and the benefit structure. Minimally, Medicaid must provide inpatient, skilled nursing facility, and home care; physician services; outpatient care; family planning services; and periodic screening, detection, and treatment care of children under age 12. As for services such as dental care, eyeglasses, and prescription drugs, each state makes its own decisions concerning payment.

19-79   Answer A

The emergency treatment exception allows you to treat minors in emergency or life-threatening situations when a parent or guardian cannot be reached to give consent for treatment. This includes transfusions when necessary. The legal definition of an emergency medical condition is any condition that threatens the loss, impairment, or serious dysfunction of life or limb or causes severe pain.

19-80   Answer A

Of the lists presented, the communicable diseases that must be reported in every state include syphilis, tuberculosis, and hepatitis. The diseases that are notifiable by law vary by state and over time. Criteria for determining notifiable diseases have generally been based on the potential for control or prevention of additional cases of the disease. Practitioners should be familiar with what diseases need to be reported in their state; for example, invasive *Haemophilus influenzae* infection, meningitis, encephalitis, giardiasis, measles, and

Reye's syndrome are reportable in more than 40 states.

19-81   Answer A

Safeguards to follow when conducting research on a geriatric population include assessing the competence of the individual before obtaining consent, making sure the consent form is in understandable language, and obtaining verbal consent (in some situations, verbal consent is all that is required). Permission must be obtained from the client. Obtaining permission from the family or staff is usually not acceptable because it may interfere with client autonomy. Additionally, stressing the importance of the research to encourage participation is coercive. Even research deemed exempt requires consent from participants.

19-82   Answer C

If a health-care provider suspects elder or dependent-adult abuse or neglect, the provider, in most states, must report it to the appropriate state protective agency. The goals of intervention are to protect the client and prevent further injury. Although data regarding the abuse may have come from the client, depending on the situation, it is not always advisable to confront the client or the family directly. Most state laws mandate reporting of suspected abuse or neglect, not just confirmed abuse or neglect. Trained investigators can then be called in to make a more detailed assessment. Health-care providers should be involved in educating the public about the problems of elder abuse and neglect and should be aware of community resources and supports that might help clients and their families.

19-83   Answer A

Mrs. Hernandez's insistence on discharge is an example of her exercising her right to self-determination or autonomy. The principle of beneficence implies doing the greatest good for the client and preventing harm; justice implies treating individuals fairly; and utilitarianism implies doing the greatest good for the greatest number of individuals.

19-84   Answer D

The type of health-care delivery system that allows the client the greatest freedom of choice is a fee-for-service plan. A health maintenance organization,

a preferred provider organization, and a managed care plan all have greater restrictions.

19-85   Answer B

As an individual APRN, you can make a difference in advancing the role of all APRNs by writing letters to the editor on health-care issues that outline the positive impact of APRNs. Although reading newspapers keeps you well informed, it is not enough to affect others unless you also speak out in a knowledgeable fashion. Likewise, thinking positive thoughts about your role may help you communicate a positive attitude, but the communication element is essential if you are to affect others. Supporting a Democratic candidate may or may not help advance the cause of advanced-practice nursing. The stances of candidates of both parties need to be researched to ascertain each one's personal stance on this issue. There is no one "party line" on this issue.

19-86   Answer C

Prescriptive authority for APRN varies from state to state. Some states mandate the filing of a protocol that documents physician oversight, but other states do not. It is not mandated by law in more than 40 states. The ability to prescribe controlled substances varies from state to state.

19-87   Answer B

Human research subjects are entitled to the right to informed consent, the right to withdraw from the research without being penalized, and the right to treatments other than the experimental treatment. Subjects are not guaranteed any compensation for participation, although some research studies do provide compensation.

19-88   Answer B

The practice philosophy of the owner-physician is important, but it is essential that the nurse practitioner ascertain the payment methods as listed in Answer B.

19-89   Answer A

There are many important questions that a nurse practitioner seeking employment in a practice needs to ask; however, the cultural background of clients, the age and sex of the supervising physician, and specific arrangements for child care are not always appropriate questions. Things to consider are many, such as how many clients do I see per hour, day, month, and year, and how much physician consultation time is necessary will provide evidence about the speed needed in this practice setting; also important is basic information as to how the practice gets its revenues. This is why the information on frequently billed CPT codes is important and relevant. Additionally, an important question would be what percentage of practice income goes to support practice expenses, as well as the collection rate for the practice (90% is considered good). Additionally, self-assessment as to what terms of employment are essential and which can be given up helps position the nurse practitioner to be in the best negotiating position. Vacation time, sick time, health insurance, consideration of malpractice insurance, support for continuing professional education, and on-call time, as well as hospital privileges and responsibilities, are also important considerations.

19-90   Answer D

The physician may not be the owner of the practice, and although the philosophy of the "owner" is important, there are other important, concrete considerations—salary, benefits, and work environment. The neglect of one of these areas over the others may lead to discontent.

19-91   Answer A

Multiple regression and analysis of variance and covariance are tests of prediction. They are statistical techniques of inferences and imply causality, not just correlation. Statistical significance is a level set by the researcher to establish when results are sufficient to make inferences. A test of association does not exist.

19-92   Answer B

Techniques used to enhance a client's adherence to the treatment plan include giving clear written instructions, simplifying the drug regimen (such as once-a-day dosing), and having the client be an active participant (the factor most highly correlated to adherence). Negative statements that generate fear, such as stressing the dangers of missing medications, have not been found to be conducive to adherence. Positive reinforcement is best. Frequent and convenient appointments have also been correlated with higher levels of adherence. You must deal directly with the client to increase adherence, not the family.

19-93   Answer C

Although obtaining drug levels, using clinical judgment, and monitoring the responses to treatment will all assist you in assessing the degree of the client's compliance, the best way to monitor compliance is to ask the client. Most clients will be truthful.

19-94   Answer C

Strategies that help to prevent client noncompliance include providing positive feedback and reinforcement and performing careful follow-up on canceled and missed appointments. In-depth client education does not help prevent client noncompliance. Instead, client education that is short, uses multiple ways of learning, and is meaningful to the client's situation is usually more effective. Likewise, a high frequency of medication does not foster compliance but rather leads to a greater likelihood that the client will miss a dose. Monitoring blood levels to assess therapeutic efficacy does not involve the client as a partner in their health care.

19-95   Answer B

To treat this client as an emancipated minor, you need some proof of marriage, active military status, or papers from a court attesting to the minor's status as emancipated. To petition a court for emancipation, a minor must be a certain age (from 14–16, depending on the state law), not live with his/her parents or guardian, be capable of managing financial affairs, and have the ability to provide for his/her well-being. Accepting the word of someone accompanying the client, or the client himself, is not enough data for you to make the appropriate decision.

19-96   Answer D

Documentation guidelines for evaluation and management (E/M) services are based on three key components—history, examination, and medical decision making—that appear in the descriptors for office, outpatient, and hospital services, including consultations. Levels of E/M services are based on four types of examination: (1) problem focused, (2) expanded problem focused, (3) detailed, and (4) comprehensive. Although the examination may be complete and thorough, that is not the correct terminology. A single-system examination may be problem focused, expanded problem focused, or detailed.

19-97   Answer A

Methods used to assess your client's retention and understanding of educational materials include asking your client to restate or do a return demonstration of what you have reviewed, having your client keep a diary or record of his or her behaviors, and reviewing written materials with your client. Providing a pathophysiology book to your client does not help assess your client's retention and understanding of educational material. Repeated explanations of pathophysiology of disease will most likely not increase your client's retention, nor will objective testing.

19-98   Answer C

It can be difficult to find time to do client teaching; therefore, apply the rule of three S's: short, specific, and simple. The most important points you need to teach your client initially about a new drug are what the medication is for, how much to take, and when to take it. The specifics of taking the medication and what to do if there are adverse effects are also important but should be explained after the other information. Discussing the action and adverse effects of the drug might distract the client from what he or she really needs to know initially.

19-99   Answer C

The maximum number of points you should attempt to make in one teaching session is three to four. The average adult can remember only five to seven points at a time. Therefore, to enhance your client's recall, limit your instructions to three to four major points in any one teaching session. Teaching more points may overwhelm even the most advanced learner. Additionally, health-care situations are often charged with anxiety, which can further interfere with learning. Be specific about what you want the client to know, and use simple, everyday language.

19-100   Answer B

To assess Mr. Brill's readiness to learn, ask, "What do you think you should do about your smoking?" If Mr. Brill had said, "I have no problem," he would be in the precontemplative stage of learning. You would focus your teaching on increasing his awareness of his condition. Mr. Brill's response indicates that he is in the contemplative stage of learning. He is considering change but has not taken any

action. You would focus your teaching on reinforcing his understanding of the need to change, teaching him the skills needed to make the change, pointing out the positive aspects of making the change, and stressing his ability to do so. If the client had already begun to change his behavior, he would be in the action stage. You would focus your teaching on reinforcing his behavior with modeling and reward. This is a crucial stage because you do not want the client to stop the behavioral change. You must support his actions in every way possible. A client in the maintenance stage is practicing the behavior regularly. Your intervention is to continue to reinforce the new behavior and the need to maintain the change.

Bibliography

American Association of Colleges of Nursing: *The Essentials of Master's Education for Advance Practice Nursing*. American Association of Colleges of Nursing, Washington, DC, 2006.

American Nurses Association: *Nursing Social Policy Statement*. American Nurses Association, Washington, DC, 2006.

Buppert, CK: Justifying nurse practitioner existence: Hard facts to hard figures. *The Nurse Practitioner* 20:43, 1995.

Buppert, CE: *Nurse Practitioner's Business Practice and Legal Guide*, ed 3. Aspen, Gaithersburg, MD, 2008.

Burke, CE, and Bair, JP: Marketing the role. In Sheehy, CM, and McCarthy, M. *Advanced Practice Nursing: Emphasizing Common Roles*. FA Davis, Philadelphia, 1998.

Cronenweit, L: Molding the future of advance practice nursing. *Nursing Outlook* 43:13, 1995.

Dunphy, LM, et al: *Primary Care: The Art and Science of Advanced Practice Nursing*, ed 2. FA Davis, Philadelphia, 2007.

Goolsby, MJ: *Nurse Practitioner Secrets*. Hanley & Belfus, Philadelphia, 2002.

Harrington, C, and Estes, CL (eds): *Health Policy and Nursing*. Jones and Bartlett, Boston, 2002.

Hickey, JV, et al (eds): *Advance Practice Nursing*, ed 3. Lippincott-Raven, Philadelphia, 2007.

Katz, JR: Back to basics: Providing effective patient teaching. *The American Journal of Nursing* 97:5, 1997.

King, CS: Second licensure. *Advanced Practice Nursing Quarterly* 1:1, 1995.

Kovner, A (ed): *Health Care Delivery in the United States*, ed 6. Springer, New York, 2007.

Larrabee, JH, et al: Patient satisfaction with nurse practitioner care in primary care. *Journal of Nursing Care Quality* 11:5, 1997.

Mahoney, DF: Employer resistance to state authorized prescriptive authority for nurse practitioners. *The Nurse Practitioner* 20:58, 1995.

Medicare Benefit Policy Manual. CMS Services, Washington, DC, 2007.

National Organization of Nurse Practitioner Faculties: *Curriculum Guidelines and Program Standards for Nurse Practitioner Education*. National Organization of Nurse Practitioner Faculties, Washington, DC, 1995.

Parr, MBE: The changing role of advance practice nursing in a managed care environment. *AACN Clinical Issues* 7:300, 1996.

Pearson, LJ: Annual update of how each state stands on legislative issues affecting advance nursing practice. *The Nurse Practitioner* 28:1, 2008.

Pew Health Professions Commission: *Interdisciplinary Collaborative Teams in Primary Care: A Model Curriculum and Resource Guide*. The University of California, San Francisco Center for the Health Professions, San Francisco, 1995.

Pew Health Professions Commission: Nurse practitioners: Doubling graduates by the year 2000. In *Commission Policy Papers*. Pew Health Professions Commission, San Francisco, 1994.

Rustia, J, and Bartek, JK. Managed care credentialing of APNs. *The Nurse Practitioner* 22:9, 1997.

Schaffner, J, et al: Utilization of advance practice nurses in health care systems and multispecialty group practice. *Journal of Nursing Administration* 25:12, 1995.

Snyder, M, and Mirr, MP: *Advanced Practice Nursing: A Guide to Professional Development*. Springer, New York, 2000.

How well did you do?

85% and above, congratulations! This score shows application of test-taking principles and adequate content knowledge.

75%–85%, keep working! Review test-taking principles and try again.

65%–75%, hang in there! Spend some time reviewing concepts and test-taking principles and try the test again.

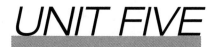
PRACTICE
EXAMINATIONS